THE BIGGEST LOSER™

BOOT CAMP

THE BIGGEST LOSER™

BOOT CAMP

the 8-week get-real, get-results weight-loss program

BY THE EXPERTS AND TRAINERS OF
THE BIGGEST LOSER

3 1336 09783 4122

NOTE TO THE READER

This book is intended as a reference volume only, not as medical advice. The information provided here is meant to help you make informed decisions about creating a healthy lifestyle. It is not intended as a substitute for any medical treatments or advice prescribed by your doctor or health professional. If you suspect that you have a medical issue, we strongly encourage you to seek the help or advice of a medical professional.

Before beginning this or any weight-loss program, consult your physician.

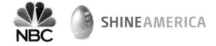

ISBN-13: 978-0-8487-4554-7
ISBN-10: 0-8487-4554-X
Library of Congress Control Number: 2014949464

contents

acknowledgments

We would like to thank the many people who have contributed their time, talents, expertise, and enthusiasm to the book:

Dolvett Quince, Jessie Pavelka, and Jennifer Widerstrom, the talented TV trainers from Season 16 of *The Biggest Loser*. Special thanks to Dolvett Quince, trainer on *The Biggest Loser* since Season 12, who created *The Biggest Loser Bootcamp* workouts and continues to inspire online Bootcampers.

Greg Hottinger and Michael Scholtz, the Nutritionist and Exercise Physiologist/Wellness Coach for The Biggest Loser Club and Bootcamp, and the experts behind Chapter 2's mental strategies.

Derek Johnson, Executive Nutrition Director at The Biggest Loser Resorts, and Chef Mark Camalleri, of The Biggest Loser Resorts Niagara, for their contributions to *The Biggest Loser Bootcamp* meal plan. Thanks also to Lesley Carey from The Biggest Loser Resorts.

Former contestants Fernanda Abarca, Lisa Rambo, and Bobby Saleem, and members of The Biggest Loser Bootcamp

Julia Smallwood, Nicole Rodgers, and many others, for sharing their experiences and tips for success.

The team at Digital Wellness, including Susy Sedano, Erin Moyer, and Tami Booth Corwin for their work in shaping and preparing the manuscript. Special thanks to Susy Sedano for her many contributions.

Stepfanie Romine for her writing and editing skills and especially for her enthusiasm and grace.

To SP Health Co. Pty, Ltd. for their contribution of recipes.

Photographers Joshua Monesson of Monesson Photography, for the workout photos, and Kerri Richardson, for the after photos of the Bootcamp success stories.

The Universal Partnerships and Licensing Team.

The Shine Team.

The team at Time Inc. for making such a great book, including Jeff Blatt, Margot Schupf, Carol Pittard, Allyson Angle, and Stephanie Braga.

Stonesong and Vertigo Design NYC.

credits

The following recipes were used by permission and are © SP Health Co. Pty, Ltd.: Turkey Wrap, p. 68; Easy Honey Mustard Chicken, p. 69; Tuna Salad Sandwich, p. 69; Quick Tandoori Salmon, p. 71; Egg Fried Rice, p. 101; Parsley & Lemon Fish, p. 102; Sesame Salmon with Rice Noodles, p. 102; Baked Apple, p. 103; Banana Yogurt Smoothie, p. 134; Quick Breakfast Couscous, p. 134; Chicken, Lemon & Orzo Soup, p. 135; Hummus & Veggie Sandwich, p. 135; Chicken & Almond Stir-Fry, p. 136; Japanese Shrimp Salad, p. 136; Warm Chicken & Quinoa Salad, p. 138 Apple-Berry Crumble, p. 139; Honey Pistachio Dip, p. 139; Italian Omelette, p. 173; Chicken & Avocado Wrap, p. 174; Vegetarian Breakfast Stacks, p. 211; Loaded Beans & Rice, p. 212; Apricot Pork with Rice, p. 213; Bacon, Lentil & Tomato Soup, p. 213; Orange & Mango Ice Pops, p. 215; Pesto Fish, p. 215; Herbed Chicken & Grapefruit Salad, p. 250; Overnight Oats, p. 250; Marinated Beef with Veggies, p. 251; Prosciutto-Wrapped Fish with Smashed Peas, p. 252; Fruit Salad with Orange Honey Syrup, p. 253; Vegetable Lasagna with Ricotta, p. 253; Carrot, Raisin & Walnut Muffins, p. 288; BBQ Spiced Chicken with Parsley Salad, p. 289; Roasted Vegetable & Couscous Salad, p. 289; Beef & Vegetable Rigatoni, p. 290; Salmon Wrap, p. 324; Garlic Shrimp, p. 326; Berry Delight Ice Pops, p. 327.

Season 16 Photos | p. 14: Trainer Jessie Pavelka with contestants Vanessa Hayden and Andrea Wilamowski; p. 16: Trainer Jennifer Widerstrom with contestant Rondalee Beardsley; p. 17: Trainer Jessie Pavelka with contestant Lori Harrigan-Mack p. 18: Trainer Jessie Pavelka with contestants Damien Woody and Howard "Woody" Carter; p. 19: Contestant Zina Garrison; p. 38: Trainer Jennifer Widerstrom with contestants John "JJ" O'Malley, Matt Miller, Sonya Jones, Toma Dobrosavljevic, Rondalee Beardsley, and Howard "Woody" Carter

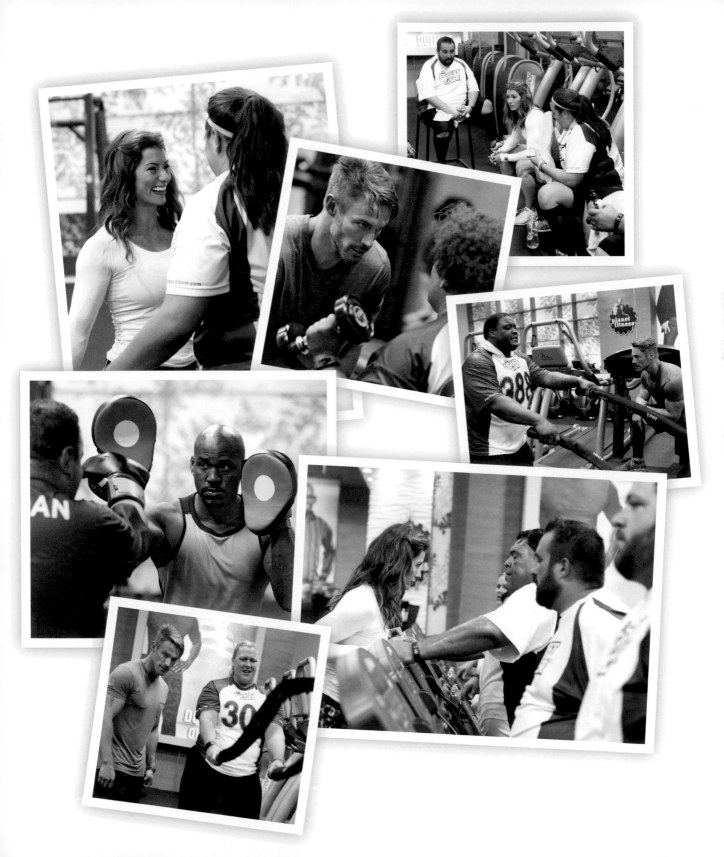

introduction

Since 2004, *The Biggest Loser* has inspired and empowered people to change their lives and believe in themselves while losing weight. Hundreds of people have lost tens of thousands of pounds on the show—and inspired millions of others watching at home to do the same. And more importantly, they've adopted healthy lifestyles that give them the energy and the motivation to live the life they always wanted.

Many contestants arrive at The Biggest Loser Ranch after years of trying to lose weight. They come with their own set of challenges, fears, and self-doubts. But they also arrive with hope that they will find the strength within themselves to turn things around.

They come with a goal in mind, and as you watch throughout the course of a season, that goal gets bigger, more focused—and then it becomes a reality. The contestants leave as totally different people. Year after year, week after week, people like you lose a big part of themselves—and end up discovering who they truly are in the process.

Whether we struggle with our weight isn't the only reason we watch the show. We all struggle at certain points in life. It's part of being human. And so we tune in because we can relate. We've been there—or we *are* there. We see ourselves in the contestants, and by cheering them on, we're cheering ourselves on as well. We start to believe

in them, and believe in ourselves as well. Through them, we are inspired to take action in our own lives.

The Biggest Loser proves that each and every one of us is special and deserves a second chance at life. It shows us that it's never too late, that you don't have to accept defeat, and that unbeatable odds were meant to be beaten. And it shows us that with the right approach—exercise, nutrition, emotional honesty, and support—it's possible for any of us to make these powerful changes in our lives!

At *The Biggest Loser*, we are always looking for ways to take the lessons from the Ranch and offer them to people who can't be on the show. So, recently we asked viewers what else they wanted in a weight-loss and fitness program. They told us that they want the same kind of program contestants get on the Ranch: the same workout style, the same nutrition, the same coaching from *The Biggest Loser* trainers, and the same emotional support to bring it all together. They wanted to be given clear, detailed daily instruction that they could trust to take the guesswork out of the process and let them focus on putting in the work and getting the results. They wanted all of this in a format that would work for them at home—and fit into their busy lives. After watching the contestants on the show, they were inspired by the hard work and perseverance they saw and were ready for a challenge—ready to set the bar higher for themselves. They were ready to take action and develop healthy, balanced lifestyles of their own, built on habits that can last. And so, we created The Biggest Loser Bootcamp, first launched as an online weight-loss and workout program and now updated and expanded in this book.

We took the life-changing training style that is used on the Ranch and condensed it into a powerful eight-week program that delivers real results. Just as Dolvett and the other trainers, including newcomers Jessie Pavelka and Jen Widerstrom, help the contestants on the show lose 40, 50, even 100 or more pounds, this plan will help you! And if you don't have 50 or 100 pounds to lose, this program can help you increase strength, build stamina, and gain energy to fuel an active life.

The Biggest Loser Bootcamp provides a comprehensive set of tools to help you lose weight and reach your goals: daily motivation from our experts, challenging workouts appropriate for all levels, plus delicious, easy-to-make meals.

And in the book, we have the opportunity to delve deeper into the emotional and mental aspects of the program, elements that are key to what works for contestants' success on the show—and are missing in most other approaches. If you're already a member of The Biggest Loser Bootcamp online, think of this book as a comprehensive companion. If you're new to the program, it's a complete stand-alone guide.

Because this is a *Biggest Loser* program, there's also a focus on accountability—no phoning it in! Though you won't have a trainer counting down your reps for you while you're working out or encouraging you through the tough times, you will have daily check-ins to keep you focused on your goals.

This program is designed for people of various health and fitness levels. Our trainers' can-do attitudes and tough-love approach can take you from couch potato to gym junkie. The Bootcamp will provide a beginner with all the tools needed to succeed and provide avid exercisers with an extra boost of daily motivation, guidance, and fresh new workouts. It's worked for the contestants on the show, and it's worked for our online Bootcamp members. Now it's your turn… let's get started!

the bootcamp philosophy

the biggest loser bootcamp program and experience is about getting real and getting results. Forget excuses. Forget shying away from something because it might be hard. You're committing to a lifestyle change, and it doesn't happen just in your kitchen or only while you're doing physical activity. These changes apply to all aspects of your life.

Each season, trainers on the Ranch guide people who have spent their entire lives giving up and making excuses as they take on big challenges and discover that they are made of tougher stuff than they ever thought. And that stuff? It's not a secret ingredient they add to their smoothies or some fancy gadget that does the work for them. It comes from inside. It's been there all along, just waiting to be uncovered. We are here to help you tap into the same stuff inside you. It's in there— and we know it's just waiting for you to rediscover it. A big part of that process is opening your mind and embracing some key imperatives:

- Get Real
- The Whole Package
- Believe in You
- Challenge Yourself

1. get real

This program is about getting real and keeping it real. That goes for the expectations you have about the process, the food in your meal plans, the hard work you'll put in during your workouts, and the accountability that will keep your eyes on the prize. Most importantly, it's about getting real from the inside out and remembering what it is that's inspiring you to do this. That's right; you're going to take a long, hard look at the person in the mirror and discover what it is that's holding you back. Together, we're going to help you be who you've always wanted to be.

If you want to get results, you've got to get real. Here's how we'll help you make that happen.

REAL FOOD: As you'll hear throughout the program, the keys to weight loss are found in the

meet your trainers

Fitness experts Jennifer Widerstrom and Jessie Pavelka joined veteran trainers, including Dolvett Quince, on *The Biggest Loser* in Season 16.

Committed to helping people live their best lives through health and fitness, Jennifer was a star of the NBC series *American Gladiators*. She strives to make her workouts challenging yet inclusive. A native of Lisle, Illinois, Jennifer is very experienced in guiding people through the dramatic changes that take place — both physically and emotionally — while losing weight.

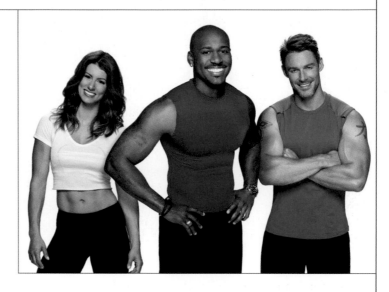

Jessie Pavelka is an internationally recognized fitness expert known for helping others develop practical solutions to lose weight and live a healthy lifestyle. A native of Corpus Christi, Texas, and a former professional bodybuilder, Pavelka's passion for fitness inspired him to become a trainer and help others embrace health and wellness.

A leader in the field of health and fitness, Dolvett Quince joined *The Biggest Loser* in Season 12. Known for his passion, regimens, and dramatic transformational results, Dolvett is one of the most in-demand fitness specialists in the country.

kitchen. No matter how much work you put in at the gym, you can't outrun a bad diet, and you can't load up on junk food, thinking you'll just burn off the calories during your workout.

"Eat clean. It's for you and no one else."
—Nia, Arlington, Massachusetts

WHAT GOES INTO YOUR BODY IS WHAT YOU GET OUT OF IT: If you want to see results and have energy for your daily workouts (not to mention the rest of your life), you've got to eat real food—that is, whole foods that are minimally processed and packed with nutrients to fuel your body and help you create this new life.

One of the reasons the contestants post such huge losses those first few weeks on the Ranch is that they're eating real, clean food—no more processed sugar and no more fast food. Without all that salt, sugar, and the bad kind of fat, the body can focus on fueling itself, growing stronger, and keeping you healthy and happy.

Though you'll be eating clean and healthy foods, we also know that indulging from time to time is part of life. Therefore, it's also part of the program. We show you how to balance special-occasion eating with your everyday clean meals and snacks. As long as you're counting your calories, measuring your portions, and making smart food choices, you can indulge sometimes. You will learn that you don't have to deprive yourself to reach your goals. This helps you develop a healthy relationship with food and can even end the cycle of emotional eating.

One essential step in achieving your goals— whether or not they involve weight loss—is getting your head around giving up on junk food, diet food, and starving yourself of calories. Those tactics don't work, and we're going to help you repair your relationship with food and eating.

REAL WORK: Changing your diet is necessary if you want to lose weight, but you'll quickly hit a weight-loss wall if you don't also include exercise. And working out is key to building a stronger, leaner body with the energy to live the full, active life you want to live. Our program includes six days of workouts a week, with one active rest day, one do-your-own-workout (DYOW) day, and five prescribed daily workouts created by Dolvett. (Of course, you should listen to your body and rest as needed, especially if you're new to exercise. We also encourage you to see your doctor or health professional before starting a workout plan.)

The workouts won't be easy, especially in the beginning, but they were designed with beginners and more advanced exercisers in mind. They'll challenge regular exercisers, yet they're suitable for those unaccustomed to breaking a sweat. You can do them at home or in a gym, and you don't need any equipment beyond a towel. We even give common modifications for those with physical limitations. The workouts use your own body weight as resistance to burn calories and build muscle, which will help you look leaner and more toned as you slim down. Building muscle will also help you burn more calories.

If it doesn't challenge you, it doesn't change you. You're going to be challenged, and if you do the work, you can change over the next eight weeks. It doesn't matter where you're starting. We all start somewhere. What matters is that you keep coming back, day after day, and strive to be a little bit better than you were yesterday. No matter what happens, just don't quit.

❝I often tell my friends that the reason *The Biggest Loser* diet worked for me is because I didn't have to cut anything out of my diet. I'm allowed to eat fruits, rice, pasta, and even an occasional candy or sweet treat. The main thing I keep in mind is that it's all about portion control and I can continue to eat almost anything I like, within reason.**❞** —Lenida, Sunnyvale, California

REAL ACCOUNTABILITY: Using a "Challenge Yourself— Don't Settle" philosophy, *The Biggest Loser Bootcamp* is designed to get results. To see those results, you have to commit to the changes—physical and mental—that are coming. This program is never just about the physical; it's about getting to the core of your issues and working through the mental roadblocks as much as the physical ones.

You're here because you're ready to change. You're ready to make time for you and become the person you know you can be. You owe it to your current and future self to be accountable. Do your workouts. Stick to the meal plan. Get stronger, fight harder, and keep reaching higher—one step at a time. Soon these changes will become habits, and these meal and exercise plans will become your lifestyle.

FIRST AND FOREMOST, YOU HAVE TO SET GOALS: An overall program goal, weekly goals, and even daily goals. Goals provide us with direction and a vision; that direction and vision can be anything from an old pair of jeans you want to fit back into, to a photograph of yourself at a healthier stage in your life, or a number on the scale that you've set your sights on. You're going to vary your weekly and daily goals, not focusing on one thing, but instead concentrating on the overall experience, or "the journey."

The contestants on the Ranch have the added pressure of losing weight while the whole country watches. You don't have all those eyes on you, but you also have to take a little more personal responsibility from day one.

> **"MOVE THE BODY; THE MIND WILL FOLLOW.** Did you wake up not feeling into the workout today? That's your mind. Get up, gear up, and go. Make it happen. A body in motion makes the decision for the mind.** —*The Biggest Loser* trainer Jessie Pavelka

No one but you will know if you sneak an extra slice of pizza in the kitchen after dinner. No one but you will know if you ate fries in your car before bringing a salad back to your desk. And no one but you will know if you skim a few reps off your workout. But that doesn't mean those things didn't happen. Every action you take, either positive or negative, will contribute to your weigh-in each week and, more importantly, your overall success in the program. We don't want anything holding you back from reaching those goals.

Mike from Season 13 struggled with emotional eating, but creating new, healthy habits helped him stay strong and focused. "A lifestyle is nothing more than doing it 'til it's just what you do, as easy as tying your shoes!" he said.

Throughout the book, you'll get the tough love you expect from *The Biggest Loser* team. That doesn't mean it's all going to be tough—there's just as much, if not more, love in this program as well.

REAL RESULTS: The Bootcamp's comprehensive program will challenge you to stop relying on quick fixes and instead learn to rely on yourself. We're here with you every step of the way as you build a new, healthy lifestyle. After years of yo-yo dieting, this approach to weight loss will feel like a tremendous relief. We help you strip away the last of your excuses and distractions, and you're left with nothing standing between you and your goals. You can finally reach your full potential—nothing's holding you back.

Embrace what's real, what you instinctively know will work—real food, hard work, and a belief in yourself—and you'll get real results that can last a lifetime.

2. the whole package

The reason the Bootcamp is so effective is that it's based on the same whole-person plan contestants use on the Ranch. We don't want you to just cut calories and move your body; we want you to integrate a combination of powerful motivational, emotional, and behavioral strategies to help you deal with the reasons you got to this place in your life. Sure, the big prizes on the show go to those who have the most weight-loss success, but they couldn't have achieved those goals without addressing other aspects of their health and well-being.

For Season 14 winner Danni, the biggest obstacle was mental. "Sure, the physical and nutritional changes were hard, but really digging deep into the 'why am I the way that I am?' was truly eye-opening," she said. She had to get uncomfortable and question herself, exposing "some demons that I wasn't willing to face in the past." The first couple of episodes, Danni was falling apart and in danger of giving up. "My weight has stolen my confidence, without a doubt," she said through

tears in Episode 2. No one would guess that she would go on to be The Biggest Loser.

Once she got real with herself, she was able to work to overcome those demons and focus on getting her whole self healthy and happy. Danni says she's more comfortable with herself, and the awareness and strength she's developed make tackling emotional issues that much easier, which directly impacts her overall health and lifestyle choices.

To achieve real, lasting weight loss, you have to connect the dots not just between diet and exercise, but also motivation and goal setting, emotional health, and behavioral modifications. These aspects of the plan are interconnected, and we'll show you how they work together to get you real results.

NUTRITIONAL: The better you eat, the better you feel. Jackson, a fan favorite from Season 14, was so busy during the day with work and volunteer activities that he wouldn't eat until just before bed. Then, he would cram in up to 4,000 calories—twice what his body needed—in an hour. His blood sugar was on a roller coaster, and all that sugar, fat, and salt made him feel awful.

Shifting to a whole-foods diet with regular, portion-controlled meals and snacks helps him balance life. He gets to enjoy foods he loves without going overboard like he used to.

We hear similar stories from our Bootcampers and our contestants on the Ranch about their poor diets, and we think many of you can relate.

Do you ever:

- skip meals, then overeat?

- eat healthy foods in public, then binge on fast food when you're alone?

- turn to sugary quick carbs for comfort, then feel too tired to get up and get moving?

- reward yourself with food, or punish yourself by withholding it?

- eat when you're bored, tired, or stressed?

- finish other people's food, so it doesn't go to waste?

- zone out while eating and consume far more food than you realize?

- lie about what you've eaten?

- drink too many sugary beverages?

- eat late at night?

You don't have to write down the answers, but be honest with yourself as you think about the questions we've just shared. If you've answered yes to any of them, that's OK. You can use the next eight weeks to start to change your eating habits and patterns. Shifting your diet is the first step toward breaking the cycle of emotional eating and achieving lasting weight loss, our Bootcampers have discovered.

the point of physical discomfort? Have you eaten sugary foods that give you an instant rush of energy and then an hour later make you want to take a nap? You're not alone. Combining your workouts with a clean-eating plan helps give you the energy you need to get moving—and keep moving.

Exercise is a high-yield, guaranteed investment, but you have to spend energy to get energy from your workouts. That is, exercise will repay you by giving you the energy you need for your daily life, but you have to work for it. The good news is it gets easier—no matter if you are currently working out or not exercising at all.

Biggest Loser website member Chris started his 102-pound weight-loss journey by following meal plans and using his food diary. Eventually he transformed himself from junk food addict to gym junkie and says his newfound stamina is also making him more productive at work. "When I start work in the morning, I am ready. Before, it would take me three or four coffees to get going, so I wasn't really ready until lunchtime," he said. "I think this new productivity is a combination of sleeping better, feeling better, and being happier in general."

Chris discovered another aspect of exercise: the emotional benefits that can help you overcome stress and anxiety—and even become a better employee, parent, and partner.

PHYSICAL: Food is fuel, and without the right fuel, exercise becomes that much more difficult. Have you ever eaten to

"After eight weeks of eating healthy and working out, I no longer feel extremely hungry between meals—smaller portions are more satisfying. I no longer crave sweet treats, and find fresh fruit satisfies my sweet tooth." —Julia, Durham, North Carolina

EMOTIONAL: The saying "you are what you eat" really does hold true. Chow down on sugary snacks or fast food all day, and in addition to feeling little to no energy, chances are you won't feel very cheerful or upbeat. Changing your diet can boost your mood and make it easier for you to identify and cope with life's triggers and stresses. Add exercise to the mix, and you'll get a double dose of feel-good energy.

The Biggest Loser takes it one step further and asks you to set goals to help you stay on track despite life's ups and downs. In this Bootcamp, we help you find your areas for improvement, provide you with strategies to cope, and then assist you in finding the strength within to not only lose weight but also become a whole new you.

Lisa Rambo did it. She came to the Ranch plagued by self-doubt and left feeling stronger than she ever had. She is now a motivational speaker who travels the country helping others find the strength and courage to lose weight and get healthy. Before joining the show in Season 14, she had weighed more than 200 pounds for her entire adult life.

"For me, the biggest obstacle came from inside," she said, crediting her trainer, Dolvett, for her mental shift. "I had to get over my self-doubt. Once I believed I could actually do it, I began to do it."

"I went on a show to lose weight, and by the end of it, it wasn't about my weight at all," she said. "There's nothing more empowering and encouraging than seeing yourself get stronger and healthier."

3. believe in you

Each season, contestants arrive at the Ranch with a goal to lose weight. As they set out on their journey, they start exercising, push through their mental roadblocks, completely change their diets, and go on to reach those weight-loss goals successfully. But more importantly, they discover a power and belief in themselves that allows them to make things happen in their lives that they never believed possible.

We know what it's like to try a diet and give up. We know how frustrating it can be to start an exercise program after years of being inactive. A key to sticking with a new healthy habit is to believe you can reach the goal, not doubting your physical or mental abilities. But you do have to know that we believe in you—and you have to learn to believe in yourself. Throughout the eight-week program, you will be given the tools to help retrain your mind to put aside unhealthy patterns. We'll walk you through this mental and emotional work each week and put it into an actionable plan—just as you see contestants do on the show.

We all have a story. Whether you used to be thinner, fitter, faster, or more active, or whether you've struggled your whole life, it doesn't matter. You're starting over today, and this is your clean slate. You can do this, and you can succeed, as long as you trust yourself and stick to your plan.

This is an important revelation—it's not just about believing in you, but believing in your investment. You decided to buy this book and put your time, your money, and your goals on the line. You're committing to this, for eight weeks. That's 56 chances to wake up, recommit to goals, and fight for your life. You decided now was the time to do this. And you decided that this Bootcamp is the way to reach your goal. You took the first steps. Now, trust us to guide you as we help you find success.

4. challenge yourself

Weight loss is not only about improved health and physical appearance; it's about that more powerful truth, the truth of untapped potential in each of us. The weight-loss journey forces everyone, as it will force you, to dig deeper than ever and discover things long hidden or lost: strength, resilience, and trust in ourselves to succeed. It's that discovery, not the act of shedding the pounds, that makes this journey life-changing.

NO EXCUSES: Here's where you need to ask yourself if you're ready. You bought the book, you've taken the time to read it (at least up to this point), and you've begun the journey. What makes this time different from any other? In this program we want you to ask yourself the hard questions and not be afraid of the answers or the emotions those questions might stir up. If you're ready, we're ready to help you.

We've all used excuses, quite often unintentionally. Excuses are a big roadblock to getting real. They come in many shapes and sizes, and you're probably familiar with most of them—no time, physical limitations, no money for healthy foods, not a good time to start, not enough willpower, and so on. Are excuses holding you back? As you get ready to dive in, think about your own excuses. Write them down and then question why you're making them. Is it fear of failing? Fear of hard work? Fear of *succeeding*? If you can bring them to the front of your mind instead of letting them chip away at you subconsciously, it will go a long way toward getting them out of your way. You can do this!

> **❝**I love this quote from Glinda in *The Wizard of Oz*, and it sums up my journey: 'You've always had the power, my dear. You just had to learn it for yourself.' Until I started this journey, I had no idea how strong I was or what I could accomplish if I set my mind to it. It has been life-changing.**❞** —Julia, Shawnee, Kansas

lisa found the potential within

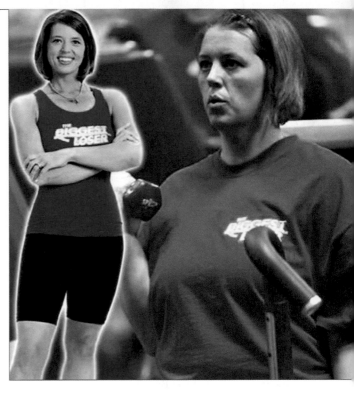

Lisa Rambo tried out for *The Biggest Loser* three times before being selected for Season 14. The 38-year-old mother of four from Wisconsin arrived on the Ranch at 246 pounds. "It feels like my dreams are coming true," she said the day she was chosen to be on the show. "I love taking care of other people, but for the first time ever, I'm on a 'me mission'... so I can be the most amazing, greatest mom to my kids that I could ever possibly be."

But deep down, Lisa wasn't sure she had it in her to change. Then, she met her trainer, Dolvett Quince. "He looked at me when I was an obese, insecure woman and saw something different," she said. "He looked at me and saw all my potential."

And did Lisa have potential! She was sent home during Week 5, but that didn't stop her.

She credits it all to the "Challenge Yourself—Don't Settle" philosophy Dolvett instilled in her on the Ranch. We'll share the same tactics she learned from him during her time on the Ranch, an essential part of the Bootcamp philosophy.

"I've been a yo-yo dieter my whole life. With Dolvett's lessons and *The Biggest Loser*, I finally quit *trying* to lose weight and decided to *do* it," Lisa said. "For the very first time I believed that I could do it. I could dream it and just believe it, then achieve it."

Lisa's at-home life is now more active than ever. And one of her biggest accomplishments is being able to be active with her family, her kids in particular. Lisa rides her bike along with her kids, and her mother, now in her 50s, picked up running. In fact, they even ran a half-marathon together.

Despite all the hard work, Lisa says this new life isn't difficult. It's just her life. Thanks to *The Biggest Loser* and the Bootcamp principles, Lisa has found a permanent solution to a lifelong struggle with obesity.

mental strategies

close your eyes for a moment and think about what it means to you to be healthy. Would you like to sleep better, deal more effectively with stress, be more productive during your day, or spend more quality time doing the things you love with the people who matter most?

Would you like to have the energy to go out and grab life by the horns? If so, *The Biggest Loser Bootcamp* can help you get there. On the next page, we will introduce you to Nicole, who not only lost weight but feels like she's truly living again. She joined the Bootcamp because she saw herself reflected in the contestants on the show, and we think you'll see much of yourself in her.

This Bootcamp is eight weeks long, but it's designed to help you maintain healthy behaviors for a *lifetime*. That's a lifetime of feeling alive, feeling empowered, and feeling in control of your health—perhaps for the first time ever. This chapter helps you prepare mentally for the Bootcamp and sets you up for a successful transition beyond these next eight weeks. You will be able to apply what you learn to the rest of your life. You're in

the driver's seat. You're in control. You can begin to write your own success story by *believing* that you'll never go back to your old habits. Ever.

We're rewriting your story, and it starts today. Many people lose focus and regain weight—that might have even been your story at one point. Your new story has a happy ending. Many people are making the connection between better health and living the life they want, and you can, too. Throughout this Bootcamp, you'll discover what truly matters to you, and you will find out first-hand how being healthier and stronger helps you get it—even if what you want has no obvious connection to your physical self. That connection becomes motivation that lives inside you. That's the "big secret" to losing weight. And what you're about to read will help you find it.

i'm alive again!

NAME: Nicole Rodgers

AGE: 40

STARTING WEIGHT: 200.5

ENDING WEIGHT: 171

CURRENT WEIGHT: 140

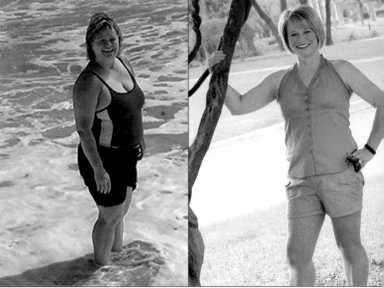

For years, I felt like a fake. I'm a physical therapist, and I work with patients to get strong and healthy and change their lives, but I was 200 and a half pounds—60 pounds overweight. When I told them that they needed to eat right and exercise, I knew they were thinking, "Well, why aren't *you* doing it?"

Since joining The Biggest Loser Bootcamp in February 2014, I feel like a new person. It's taught me how to live again—my life isn't centered on food anymore. I feel confident and more like me.

I wasn't always overweight. In high school, I was a multi-sport athlete and never had to think about my weight. I played college basketball, but an injury freshman year sidelined me. I became depressed and felt like a failure for not playing anymore, and I turned to food as comfort. I stopped being active and started eating whatever and whenever I wanted. It seemed like overnight that I was pushing the 200 mark. I was devastated and was willing to try anything and everything—and I did.

I tried pills, drinks, supplements, joining a gym, you name it. I was able to lose some weight here and there, but then anytime I had a strong emotion—sadness, joy, grief, celebration/elation, I would always turn to food.

A friend recommended I try The Biggest Loser Bootcamp. I found happiness like I haven't had in a long time. I lost 30 pounds during the first eight weeks and 60 total. I now weigh 140. I have learned so much and am loving life now. I have become a runner. I never thought I would do that. Now I wake up before my alarm, looking forward to my workout.

After Bootcamp, I rode 22 miles on my bike, which I have not been able to do in a long time. I want to do a 100-mile bike race here in the Texas heat. I can't thank Dolvett and The Biggest Loser Bootcamp enough for changing my life.

The story-changing motivation strategies you're about to learn don't stop when you move on to the next chapter. We have integrated coaching exercises into each week of the program. They include some of the best tools and exercises we use with The Biggest Loser Bootcamp online, and they will help you change the way you think. The first phase is about *getting on track* and *strengthening your thinking*. You need the structure of a plan that you can trust. The Bootcamp's eating and exercise plans will give you that structure. The program is designed to jump-start your progress and give you ideas about what works well for you and what does not. During the first five weeks of the Bootcamp, our coaching exercises will help you develop powerful mental tools including discovering the "why" behind your journey, how to stay focused on the positive, and learning to be self-compassionate—not self-critical.

The second phase is about transitioning to what comes next and learning to stay on track for good. In Week 6, while you still have the safety net of the Bootcamp underneath you, we'll ask you to begin thinking about what's next. For Nicole, completing a 22-mile ride led to the goal of planning a 100-mile odyssey on her bike. Where will your success in Bootcamp lead you? The coaching exercises in Weeks 6, 7, and 8 will begin to open up a whole new world of possibilities for you. You'll identify the areas that you're most excited about and the changes you're most confident you can continue. And you'll learn how to chart your course and stay focused in the months ahead.

Are you ready to begin your journey?

finding direction

You cannot be "talked into" doing something you do not want to do or that you are not ready to do. If you want to succeed at any goal, it has to be something *you* want to achieve. Your doctor, your best friend, and even your family might suggest that you lose weight, for example, but to have the best chance of achieving your goals, the motivation has to come from within. Your goals should be set of your own free will—not imposed by someone else. Experts call this *autonomy*. On the Ranch, we see contestants make this shift every season. They start out doing something (usually exercise) because their trainers tell them to do it or because all their teammates are doing it—and we watch them struggle. They seem miserable, and they want to quit. Once we witness their mental shift, and they start to make healthy choices on their own, they begin to experience lasting success—and they reach their goals, week after week.

Lasting change comes from focusing on what *you* truly want, and not what someone else tells you or even encourages you to do. Goals you set on your own are more exciting and empowering than doing things for somebody else, and they help you take on bigger challenges and stick to them when the going gets tough. Autonomy is the reason that, while we insist you set a goal each week, we don't tell you what that goal should be.

However, staying in touch with your wishes and your values is easier said than done—especially in today's busy, hyper-connected world. And, without a deep understanding of your true self, you risk falling into one of two types of traps: compliance and defiance.

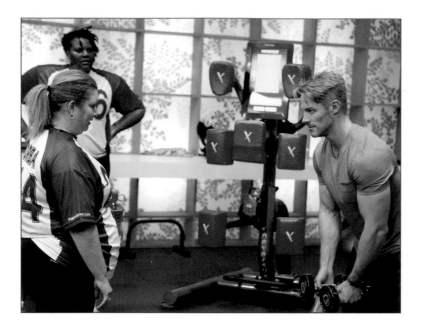

Compliance is giving in to what others expect or demand of you, be it a friend or loved one or an authority figure in your life. You might find yourself trying to please them, or you might even begin to act out the beliefs of others without even being conscious of it. You might, for example, change how you eat or begin exercising because you think you "should" or you "have to." You've internalized the expectations of the world around you to such a degree that you think you're making a choice based on what you want, when, in reality, you're acting the way the rest of the world wants you to act.

On the flip side is *defiance*—you push back against the demands of others even though you want to change. When this happens you might find yourself eating unhealthy foods or quitting your exercise program just to show someone else they can't control you. And, you'll make these choices even though you like some of those healthy foods or have found an exercise plan that you enjoy.

In both examples, your choices are based on your reaction to what others want from you or expect of you, not on your own values and what you want and need in order to remain true to those values.

When Season 15 contestant Bobby Saleem first arrived on the Ranch, he kept telling himself "you can't do this." By Episode 7, when he clocked a 9-pound weight loss, he was hearing himself say "you can do this." "I'm so proud of that mental shift in me, and I really feel confident.

"This journey pretty much represents a soul-searching expedition for me," he said on the show. "I came to *The Biggest Loser* so lost in myself. This journey has really, really helped me define who I am as a person. Bobby is a strong person, Bobby is a smart person. I know these things now, but those are things I didn't know when I first started on *The Biggest Loser*."

Sent home after nine episodes, Bobby went on to lose a total of 188 pounds, which he couldn't have done without autonomy.

Tapping into the power of autonomy like Bobby did means doing some self-discovery. You need to know your own personal and compelling reasons for making changes. Two of your exercises involve making and examining personal choices.

In Week 1 (see p. 45), you will consider what your reasons are for doing the Bootcamp right now. In Week 6 (see p. 217), you will begin thinking about what you want to focus on once the Bootcamp is completed.

you're not in this alone

Having the support of others like you is a powerful tool for getting on track and experiencing long-term weight-loss success—and one that is often overlooked. It's so helpful to have someone who knows exactly what you're facing and how significant it is to shed pounds and maintain a healthier body weight. Research shows that many overweight individuals believe that they got into their predicament alone and *should* be able to get out of it on their own. And yet, what we've seen is that having others in your corner 24/7 can make a huge difference in sustaining a change, especially when you're struggling.

For Nicole, the turning point was the support she found online. Weight-loss forums, such as those on *The Biggest Loser* website, offer a way to connect with others just beginning their journey as well as those who've had great success. And it is important to note that you can benefit greatly by *giving* support to others as well, lifting them up in tough times and celebrating their victories with them. There is evidence to show that when you identify yourself as a role model for others, such as your child, a significant other, or even another person in your exercise class or support network, your commitment to stay on your path will deepen.

You'll work on your own support team during Week 2 (see p. 73).

strength you can't see

There is no quality more important for making and sustaining changes than *resilience*, which is your ability to recover from or adjust easily to setbacks or change. The reality is that life is filled with curveballs and you will need to become stronger mentally to be ready for them. In Episode 3 of Season 15, Dolvett's Red Team got stuck with baking equipment and supplies in *The Biggest Loser* fitness auction. Instead of giving up, they used those heavy bags of sugar and flour as pieces of exercise equipment. That's resilience! "I've been in worse predicaments with less equipment," Dolvett said. "There's nothing that's going to stop us from getting our burn!" And burn they did!

Three tools that have been shown to be effective in building resilience are:

1. practicing more self-compassion

2. focusing on what is working well

3. shifting from a black/white approach to one that has more flexibility

You can begin strengthening your resilience with these tools starting today, and we'll walk you through it again in Weeks 4 and 5 (see pp. 141 and 179).

be nice to yourself

You might be surprised to hear that we are encouraging you to be kinder to yourself as a way to be more successful on your weight-loss journey. What we mean here is changing the way you talk to yourself, moving from a "cold, stiff-upper-lip" tone, which at times might be downright mean, to a compassionate voice that is soothing and comforting. Choosing kindness, when at the core of a model of self-compassion, can improve behavior and change outcomes. You might wonder if being kinder to yourself will make it easier to bail out on the hard choices you have to make to be successful on your weight-loss journey. Research has found the opposite to be true: Having more self-compassion will lead you to take more responsibility for your choices. When you don't beat yourself up for making a mistake, you are able to take *more* responsibility for your choices, even the poor ones, and not get derailed in the process.

It worked for Fernanda Abarca, who joined the show in Season 15 feeling horrible about herself and beating herself up for her food choices. "I had no confidence. I was dead. I existed but I wasn't living," she said.

"Now I'm feeling good about myself," she told viewers before the finale. "For the first time in a long time, I'm starting to love myself, and that feels really good." Fernanda has lost 97 pounds and isn't finished yet.

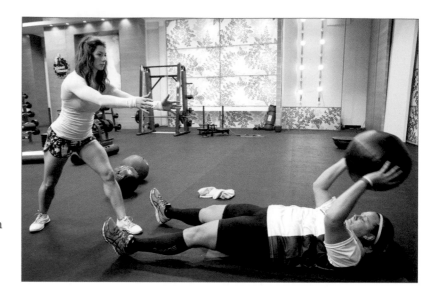

You'll work on improving your self-talk like Fernanda did in Week 3 (see p. 104).

the power of positivity

The next tool for building resilience is to shift your focus from what isn't going well to the areas that are working and taking a moment to savor these positives. Positivity is more than just putting on a "happy face" or looking at the bright side, and it is definitely not accomplished by ignoring problems and challenges. Rather, positivity is a way of approaching life, both its moments of celebration and its trials, in a positive frame.

Take, for example, Cate Laughlan from Season 14. She left the Ranch after just three weeks, but she didn't let that stop her from continuing her journey at home and finding success. She credits a mental shift—and her positivity.

"Dolvett, in this short time, has completely rearranged the furniture in my mind," she said after being told she was going home. "Being here for these three weeks has taught me that being healthy isn't a chore. It's a gift! And I don't *think* I can do this at home—I *know* that I can.

"Thanks to *The Biggest Loser*, I don't watch my dreams fade away—I go after them."

The best way to describe how positivity affects change is the "Broaden and Build" theory developed by Barbara Fredrickson, PhD. Positivity broadens our minds, making us more creative and able to see more possibilities. Ironically, by focusing on the possibilities versus the problem, we see many more ways to overcome the problem. This makes us more willing to take on a tough task with an uncertain outcome and more adept at altering our course, when necessary, to reach a goal.

creating a vision of your future

All expectations are not created equal! Sometimes your expectations of the future get you excited about what is to come. You look forward to the focus, effort, and achievement. Or you relish the coming relaxation and rejuvenation. But other times, expectations bring pressure—lots of it. You fret over what you have to do or what you have to sacrifice. You worry about the outcome. Ultimately, you get sidetracked by life or paralyzed by the very thought of doing whatever task or goal you had in mind, and you end up frustrated and disappointed.

What makes the difference between expectations that undermine your motivation and those

that fire you up? One thing is those self-directed goals we discussed earlier in the chapter. Making sure the goals you set are *yours* and yours alone is vitally important. But another important factor is the balance between what you give and what you get back: the effort and the reward.

When the effort/reward balance is off, you might see the effort as daunting and the return as bland and boring. For example, you might think you have to give up everything you like to eat or that you have to exercise every day. It seems as if you have to be "perfect" to achieve your goals. And perhaps what you imagine in return is that you will "feel better" or "tone up." Those are very dull rewards! You see them on the cover of health

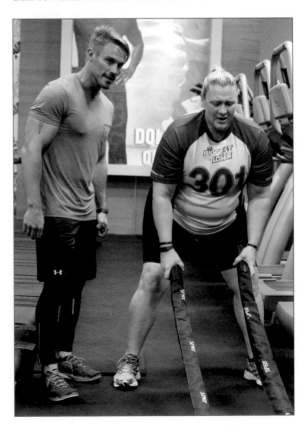

magazines and hear them promised by fitness programs everywhere. To you, they do not have any deep, personal meaning. And that means you're not truly drawn to them. To help tip the effort/reward balance back in your favor you will need to make changes to both sides of the equation.

First, it is important to shift your thinking about the effort involved. It is not necessary or possible to be "perfect." Everyone makes less-than-healthy choices from time to time. Sometimes it's on purpose, like having a slice of birthday cake. And other times you slip, the result of temptation overcoming your ability to make the healthier choice. The good news is that by making healthy choices most of the time, you can achieve your goals for living a healthier life. This is the 80/20 model of change.

The second part of the equation is all about upping the ante of the reward from bland and boring to compelling and thrilling. Ideally, what you imagine for yourself is deeply personal, aligns with your values, draws you toward it like

a magnet, and jolts you into action! This is the essence of a *wellness vision*.

Success depends on having a good enough reason—think about David Brown from Season 15. He cared for his first wife as she battled cancer for years, promising her he would be there for their girls. He came to the Ranch to lose weight and be the father he promised he would be, and that's what kept him motivated. David's vision helped him fight week after week, ultimately losing 222 pounds and becoming the runner-up.

In Week 7 (see pp. 256–257), you can create your own vision for yourself. This vision will be what gets you out of bed in the morning to do your workout and what you can be reminded of when you're trying to find the resolve to pass up dessert.

What behaviors do you need to do consistently if your vision is to come true? For example, your vision of being healthier might mean changing how you eat, doing more exercise, or getting more and better-quality sleep. These are great ideas, but they are not specific enough for you to "see" yourself doing them.

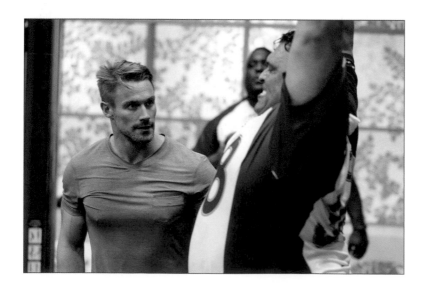

In Week 8 (see pp. 294–295), you will create three-month and weekly goals that are more specific and measurable. For instance, you will take a general goal like "change how I eat" and make it laser-specific like "eat at least three servings of vegetables each day." And, when you know exactly what you're working on each week, you'll be on your way to achieving lasting changes and, ultimately, your wellness vision.

the bootcamp diet and exercise plan

thousands of bootcampers have not only embraced this plan, they've also reported success. Energized by their daily workouts and fueled by whole foods, they told us they had never felt this great—some people even stopped dreading their morning alarms and actually started looking forward to getting a healthy start to the day.

While the overall program has many components, this chapter explains the food and the exercise you'll need to put in to reach your goals. And to help you get those results, you'll be following a daily meal plan in addition to your workouts. You've heard it before, and you'll keep hearing it throughout this book: Diet and exercise go hand in hand. Unless you have a physical limitation or a dietary restriction that prevents you from following our plans as we have developed them, we recommend committing to both the diet and exercise components. And if you do have a limitation or restriction, find ways to adapt the plan to fit your lifestyle and participate as it relates to your specific needs. Don't worry, it's doable! Once you get used to the plan, it starts to become second nature. And the results are worth it!

You will be following a meal plan crafted to help you integrate *The Biggest Loser* nutrition guidelines into your life. It's packed with a variety

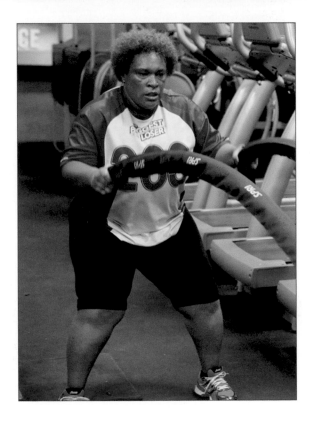

of delicious and satisfying recipes and quick meal options, such as Spicy Turkey Breakfast Quesadilla, Hearty BLT Salad, and Spaghetti Squash Chicken Alfredo. The plan provides you with all the essential nutrients your body needs on a lower-calorie diet to promote health and weight loss. It will be what fuels you through your daily workouts.

To create the Bootcamp workouts, we reached out to *The Biggest Loser* TV Trainer Dolvett Quince and asked him to help us create a program that allows people to do the workouts at home, no equipment necessary. Using the same "body confusion" training techniques Dolvett uses with his team on the Ranch, we created 30- to 45-minute workouts that include resistance moves and short cardio sequences.

There are five of Dolvett's workouts each week of Bootcamp—40 over the eight-week program.

Every workout is unique, each using a handful of movements combined in a different way. The repetition allows you to see improvements in specific movements, but they're always arranged in a fresh new way, so you won't get bored. So when you see "air jump rope" or "rear lunges" repeated, don't get frustrated if they feel challenging. Think of this as another opportunity to get better and stronger.

Now that you have a general understanding of the meal plan and the workouts, let's talk details. There's a lot of information in the coming pages, so don't get overwhelmed. Just take it one page at a time. Take as much time as you need to soak it all in, and really learn the basics. But also know that we lay it all out for you in the program section, so it will be crystal clear what to eat to stick to the plan.

the diet plan

We do the heavy lifting for you by providing you with a meal plan. It's up to you to add or subtract calories based on anything else you eat or drink during the day. We recommend you track your meals and snacks, either online or in a notebook. Taking the time to journal your food intake has several benefits. First, you'll keep yourself accountable. Keeping yourself honest might prevent you from either choosing the wrong type of food or overeating. Plus, it's a terrific way to see where your calories are coming from.

The Biggest Loser Bootcamp meal plan is based on 1,500 calories daily, an amount that will yield consistent, healthy weight loss for most people. However, if you have an active job or your starting weight is more than 250 pounds, you might need additional calories; if you are sedentary, you might need fewer calories each day. You can easily adjust your meal plan to suit your needs by consulting the charts we have provided.

If the charts show you need to eat more calories, you will supplement the meal plan with

daily calorie targets

To reach these numbers, we consider your everyday activity level and then deduct a certain portion to achieve the "negative energy balance" required for weight loss.

A negative energy balance means your energy in is less than your energy out. In other words, you're using more energy through everyday activity and exercise than you're consuming through food and drink.

	DAILY ACTIVITY LEVEL	RECOMMEND FOR 1-2 LBS PER WEEK	DAILY CALORIE TARGET AND ESTIMATED AVERAGE WEEKLY WEIGHT LOSS
WOMEN <250 LBS	Office worker or sedentary	1,500	1 lb: 1,500 calories 1.5 lbs: 1,200-1,300 calories
	Active and on the go	1,500	1 lb: 1,700-1,800 calories 2 lbs: 1,200-1,300 calories
	Physical laborer	1,750	1.5 lbs: 1,700-1,800 calories 2 lbs: 1,500 calories
WOMEN >250 LBS	Office worker or sedentary	1,500	1 lb: 1,700-1,800 calories 2 lbs: 1,200-1,300 calories
	Active and on the go	1,750	1.5 lbs: 1,700-1,800 calories 2 lbs: 1,500 calories
	Physical laborer	2,000	1.5 lbs: 2,000 calories 2 lbs: 1,700-1,800 calories
MEN <250 LBS	Office worker or sedentary	1,750	1 lb: 1,700-1,800 calories 1.5 lbs: 1,500 calories
	Active and on the go	1,750	1 lb: 2,000 calories 1.5 lbs: 1,700-1,800 calories
	Physical laborer	2,000	1.5 lbs: 2,200-2,300 calories 2 lbs: 2,000 calories
MEN >250 LBS	Office worker or sedentary	1,750	1 lb: 2,000 calories 1.5 lbs: 1,700-1,800 calories
	Active and on the go	2,000	1.5 lbs: 2,000 calories 2 lbs: 1,700-1,800 calories
	Physical laborer	2,250	2 lbs: 2,200-2,300 calories 2.5 lbs: 2,000 calories

additional healthy and approved snacks and portion-controlled servings. If the charts show you should eat fewer calories to achieve your goals, you can cut out one or more of the snacks.

Your daily calorie intake is divided like this:

BREAKFAST: 350–400 calories

LUNCH: 350–400 calories

DINNER: 400–500 calories

SNACKS: 200–300 calories total

With the types of food you will be enjoying, that breaks down into 45 to 65 percent of calories from carbohydrates, 10 to 35 percent of calories from protein, and 20 to 35 percent of calories from fat.

Each day, you will eat:

CARBOHYDRATES: 170–245 grams

PROTEIN: 40–130 grams

FAT: 30–58 grams

SATURATED FAT: less than 20 grams

SODIUM: less than 2,400 mg

FIBER: more than 20 grams

FRUITS AND VEGETABLES: 5–7 servings

LEAN PROTEIN: 3–5 servings

LOW-FAT DAIRY: 2–3 servings

WHOLE GRAINS: 3–5 servings

a few food rules & simple substitutions

The meal plan is simple: Choose whole foods. But beyond that, there are a few "rules" to follow that will keep your body burning calories while fighting off hunger.

- Eat any fruits and vegetables (except white potatoes).

- Choose whole grains instead of white rice, bread, or pasta.

- Limit added sugar to only natural sources, and use as little as necessary.

- Avoid artificial sweeteners.

- No trans fats, which are harmful to the body.

- Limit your saturated fat. Choose meats that are at least 94 percent lean.

- Drink skim milk, and opt for other dairy products that have no more than 1 percent milk fat.

To help you swap out these foods that won't do anything for your weight loss, here's a chart of simple substitutions:

INSTEAD OF...	... TRY
Mashed potatoes	Cauliflower puree
Cream in your coffee	Skim milk or almond milk
Bacon	Turkey bacon
Italian sausage in your spaghetti sauce	1 part sausage to 3 parts extra-lean ground turkey
Tortillas for your tacos and burritos	Romaine lettuce leaves or lightly steamed collard leaves (stem removed)
Chips	Thinly sliced carrots, jicama, or peppers
Sour cream	Fat-free Greek yogurt
Ice cream	Pureed frozen banana "soft serve"
White rice with your stir-fry	Minced and steamed cauliflower or brown rice
Pasta	Zucchini "noodles" or spaghetti squash
Diet soda	Green tea or carbonated water with fruit
Pizza crust	High-fiber tortilla or a chicken breast, pounded thin
Sandwich rolls or buns	Romaine lettuce leaves or high-fiber wraps

filling out your meal plan

If our charts advised you to eat more, here is an easy way to increase a meal by 200 calories and keep it balanced. Add:

- 1 oz. extra protein (e.g. fish, chicken, beef, tofu, or beans), plus

- 1 oz. extra noodles or pasta or ⅓ cup cooked rice, plus

- 1–2 cups extra vegetables or salad

As you may have noticed, some days in your menu plan will be a few calories under or over your daily calorie target. Why? It's almost impossible to design an appetizing, practical daily menu that's a perfect 1,500; 1,800; 2,200; or whatever number of calories your target might be.

Being a little over or under your meal plan each day isn't a concern for our program. What matters is that you're sticking to your suggested caloric target (within reason) and doing so by choosing the right foods.

If you are struggling to reach your recommended level of protein, we suggest incorporating some of the following foods to increase your intake and ensure you're meeting your daily need—protein is given in grams. And as we mentioned earlier, don't be afraid to experiment with preparation; try incorporating these and other foods in creative and tasty ways. Be sure to record any additions or substitutions in your food diary:

- 10 almonds (3 grams)

- ½ cup edamame, shelled (8 grams)

- 1 hard-boiled egg (6 grams)

- ½ cup quinoa (4 grams)

- 1 cup cottage cheese (13 grams)

- 1–2 scoops protein powder (prepare as a beverage with water or milk, or add to foods like oatmeal or yogurt) (up to 16 grams)

what if I'm still hungry?

Our Bootcamp meal plan is designed to sustain you through your busy day, including workouts. However, if you've been eating far more calories than you need on a regular basis, it might take a short time for your appetite to regulate itself. Usually what we mistake as hunger is one of two things: thirst or boredom, in this case known as "brain hunger." If you feel hungry even after a meal or snack, start by drinking a glass of water. It is easy to confuse the feelings of hunger and thirst. If you drink a cup of water and your "hunger" subsides, it was thirst. If it is hunger, consider whether it is true hunger coming from your stomach *needing* food—or your brain telling you it *wants* food. As you adjust to your new meal plan, you'll soon be able to tell the difference and find other things to do to occupy your mind instead of eating.

If it is true hunger and you feel you need more food than your meal plan provides, check out the list of snacks in this chapter for healthy, filling options that will not add many calories to your meal plan. You can also increase portion sizes or add mini meals.

You can swap out snacks if you want to eat something that is not on the menu, but you should still ensure you have two to three servings of low-fat or fat-free dairy and five to seven servings of fruits and vegetables each day. And be sure to track your food—it really helps for weight loss!

what about water?

Water is an important part of weight loss and can even help you diagnose true hunger, as you have learned. Aim for eight glasses a day, and don't wait until you're thirsty to drink. Sip steadily throughout the day to keep your energy levels high, fight fatigue, reduce bloating, and keep your body healthy.

Drink 16 ounces within two hours before you work out. During exercise, aim for 8 ounces every 20 to 30 minutes, then consume another 16 ounces within an hour of completing your workout. If you're a heavy sweater, you will need to drink even more.

Your urine can tell you if you're drinking enough; it should be pale yellow.

Though herbal tea and flavored water do count toward your water quota for the day, we recommend sticking with plain water as much as possible.

what else can I eat?

We know there are times when sticking to the meal plan isn't possible, such as business dinners, family gatherings, or travel. However, you can usually stick to a clean-eating, whole-foods plan without too much extra effort. Don't hesitate to ask your server at a restaurant to hold the butter or oil in a dish, ask for foods to be steamed or sautéed rather than fried, or ask for extra vegetables. It never hurts to ask, and it can make all the difference in helping you hit your daily calorie target. At family dinners or potlucks, offer to bring a healthy side dish, and stick to one plate and one trip to the buffet table. Pack healthy snacks with you when you're on the road to avoid temptation and hunger-induced overeating.

Use the portion control guidelines in this chapter and in the "Prep Week" chapter, choose whole foods even when you're not preparing your food, and fill half your plate with fruits and vegetables and one-fourth each whole grains and lean protein.

portion control

While the Bootcamp meal plan is based on whole foods to fuel your body, it pays to be mindful of portion sizes no matter what is on your plate. Even healthy foods can lead to weight gain when eaten in excess of what your body needs.

We recommend that you weigh and measure your food and drinks throughout the entire Bootcamp and for as long as possible, until you get used to correct portion sizes.

Weighing and measuring will be keys to your weight-loss success, because so many of us eat and drink supersize portions, both at home and when eating out. We consume far too many calories without even realizing it.

We recommend using a food scale and measuring cups and spoons. By weighing and measuring your food, you will begin to understand what a normal serving should look like. Once you get the hang of estimating portion size, you'll be able to look at any food and know if it's over or under. It takes a little practice, but it makes all the difference in helping you reach your goals. Here are some tips to help make planning and prep easier.

weighing foods

Place a plate, bowl, or piece of parchment paper on your electronic kitchen scale. Follow the manufacturer's directions to clear the weight of the plate or bowl. (This usually means simply pressing the Reset or On button.) Add the food you want to weigh—it may take a couple of seconds for the scale to settle and display the final reading. Add or remove food to achieve a serving.

We recommend weighing meat and fish, as well as cheese.

If you do not have a food scale, use the original packaging to help you determine the proper portion. A block of cheese, for example, is 8 ounces, but a serving is 1 ounce. Divide the block in half, then divide each half two more times. You'll end up with eight pieces that can be stored in a resealable plastic bag. This prevents "creative" cuts later on.

> **"**Convenience rules. I always have a snack on hand —it's got to be easy and handy. One of my go-to favorites is an apple with a tablespoon of peanut butter. Feel free to substitute for any natural nut butter. Convenient, quick, and filling.**"**
> —*The Biggest Loser* trainer Jessie Pavelka

estimating portion size

When you're away from home or it isn't possible to weigh and measure your portions, you can use images of familiar household items to estimate how much you're eating.

OBJECT	SERVING SIZE	USED TO MEASURE
Deck of cards	3 ounces cooked/4 ounces raw	meat or fish
Tennis ball	1 cup	pasta, grains, or ice cream
Domino	1 ounce	cheese or chocolate
Baseball	1 serving	fruit
Die	1 teaspoon	fat (oil, butter, or margarine)
Computer mouse	1 small	baked potato
Golf ball	2 tablespoons	condiments (jam, peanut butter, or salad dressing)

measuring foods

Use measuring spoons for energy-dense foods such as oil, butter, sugar, and honey. Keep the measure level by flattening off the top of the spoon with a knife, so that it's leveled instead of heaped. One heaped tablespoon of peanut butter, for example, could add an additional 50 calories.

Use measuring cups for foods such as breakfast cereal. You can also use them as measuring scoops, especially for cooked rice, pasta, and noodles.

snacks and hunger busters

Nibbling fruits, veggies, whole grains, and low-fat dairy between meals will not only help you get a grip on your hunger levels, but it can actually help boost your metabolism, too.

Choose the right snacks and you could see your fruit and vegetable intake skyrocket until you're getting all your fruit and veggie servings each day without even trying.

Regular snacking on healthy foods could even help keep a lid on stress by balancing your energy levels throughout the day.

Fill your body with the right fuel by snacking on some of these healthy options.

snacks under 50 calories

- 1 cup vegetable sticks with 1 tablespoon salsa, 29 calories

- 1 cup vegetable sticks with 1 tablespoon low-fat (1% milkfat) cottage cheese with herbs, 35 calories

- 1 small piece of fresh fruit, 44 calories

- ½ cup fruit salad, 46 calories

- 1 cup mixed berries, 48 calories

snacks under 100 calories

- 1 brown rice cake topped with 2 tablespoons low-fat cottage cheese, 56 calories

- 10 almonds, 69 calories

- 1 hard-boiled egg, 78 calories

- 2 cups mixed salad with 2 tablespoons low-fat shredded cheese and 2 teaspoons fat-free dressing, 79 calories

- 1 medium piece of fresh fruit, 89 calories

- ½ cup fat-free frozen yogurt, 96 calories

snacks under 200 calories

- 6 strawberries dipped in ½ ounce dark chocolate, 102 calories

- 1 cup fat-free milk blended with ½ cup berries and 1 teaspoon honey, 128 calories

- 1 slice raisin bread topped with 2 teaspoons reduced-fat peanut butter, 133 calories

- 1 slice whole-wheat bread topped with 2 tablespoons hummus and ½ tomato, 137 calories

- 1 whole-wheat English muffin topped with 2 teaspoons jelly, 172 calories

- 1 slice whole-wheat bread topped with ¼ avocado and 1 slice low-fat cheese, 198 calories

the workout plan

Now that you know how you'll be fueling your body to give you the energy you need to get up and get moving, let's talk more about those workouts Dolvett designed for you.

Your program kicks off with great cardio and strength interval workouts to get you started burning lots of calories. His style is "body confusion" (mixing it up to maximize fat loss), so you'll be switching between cardio and classic body-weight exercises that will prepare you for tougher moves later on. No equipment is necessary, but you can use a hand towel, hand weights, or a resistance band to create some resistance in some of the moves. Have fun with it, and don't be afraid to push yourself!

In creating the Bootcamp, we considered how to cater to all of you—those who are just starting

out and those who are already really into fitness. The solution was time and intensity.

TIME: Rather than complete a prescribed number of repetitions, you'll do the resistance exercises for a certain amount of time. The fitter you are, the more work you can complete during an interval. If you are newer to exercise, you can still work at a slower pace. For example, a beginner member might be able to complete 15 squats per minute, and an advanced member, 25 to 30.

Over time, you'll see improvements. In Week 1, you might complete 10 squats per minute, and by Week 4, you'll have doubled that amount. The key is to challenge yourself. Don't settle for the same easy option; continue to set those daily and weekly goals. You never know what you're capable of completing until you try. Remember: You are your only competition. You only have to be better than you were yesterday.

INTENSITY: The cardio intervals suggest intensity on a scale of 10, with 1 being not moving and 10 being as hard as possible. "Hard" cardio should feel like a 7 out of 10. For some of you, that might be walking in place; for others, that might be "quick feet" or jumping rope. "Easy" cardio, including your warm-ups and cooldowns, should be a level 3 or 4. You should feel like you could keep going for a long time, and you should be able to carry on a conversation.

If you have back or knee problems, or any health issue that might prevent you from doing the workouts as they are laid out in the book, you can still complete this program using modifications to suit your body. After getting clearance to exercise from your physician, do what you can. Walk in place, march while sitting in a chair, or step instead of jumping. Do what you can, and consult the chart for modifications for some of the exercises you'll encounter in the program.

We know that at first it might feel like nothing is ever going to change and that this will be "hard" forever. Soon, as if by some miracle, it will get easier. You will notice that you can do this.

You might be able to do things you hadn't done in months or even years!

We know that many of you might not have exercised in a very long time. That's OK. Many of the contestants were once in your shoes. Everyone starts somewhere. Just take it one day at a time and do what you can. Focus on what you can do, rather than what you can't do. If you're not ready to try some of the strength moves, swap in the ones you can do. If you are limited to walking or chair workouts, do those. As long as you're moving, you're doing this!

IF YOU HAVE ISSUES WITH ...	... TRY THIS
Jumping (such as skater jumps or air jump rope)	Step and land softly
Getting down on the floor (such as Russian twists)	Try the move from a chair
Kneeling down (such as with knee walks)	Stand, and do high knees
Balancing (such as in lunges)	Hold onto a chair or stick with moves that use both legs (such as squats)
Doing "compound" movements (such as rear lunges with a one-armed row)	Do each move separately
Your low back (such as in seated abs exercises)	Plank

As Dolvett says, "There's nothing that's going to stop us from getting our burn." Use these modifications along with any others you need to make the program work for your body. We just want you to move—how you move isn't as important. As you progress in the program, you might just surprise yourself at what you can do physically. Keep working, keep moving, and keep trying. We know you can do it.

It's OK to do the workouts on different days to better suit your schedule. For example, every Wednesday we've programmed a freestyle day where you can do your own workout (DYOW). That could be your favorite Zumba class, your weekly basketball game, etc. Every Sunday is a rest day, but your schedule might require you to take your rest day on a Tuesday, for example. As long as you get it done, we don't mind if you switch up the workouts!

the workouts

Each workout is made up of three parts: the warm-up, the workout, and the cooldown (usually stretching). Warming up and cooling down are just as important as the workouts themselves, so don't skimp on them—or skip them altogether.

Each day you'll do the same warm-up and cooldown, which we share on the next few pages, but your workout will never be the same. (We share the steps of the warm-up and the cooldown with you again on Day 1.)

Most of the moves we use in the daily workouts are variations on body-weight moves that will seem familiar to you, even if you haven't done a push-up since high school gym class. However, there are some that might be new or more complicated, and we're explaining some of those here.

> **Too much of one thing isn't good—you don't want one result, you want overall results.**
> —*The Biggest Loser* trainer Dolvett Quince

tip

WHAT'S COMING NEXT

Confession: We weren't being 100 percent honest when we said "it will get easier." What we should have said is it will *feel* easier as you get fitter, faster, and stronger, but the workouts themselves aren't going to get any easier. If you are someone who hates exercise, that's OK. You will learn to like it, the more you do it. And the feeling you get when you complete the workouts is amazing! Your energy and confidence increase daily!

Expect the workouts to gradually get harder and longer. Each week, we'll introduce some new moves to keep challenging you both physically and mentally. Remember: We're all in this together, and we know you can do it.

As the workouts progress, you get to choose your intensity, so you'll continue to compete only against yourself.

You'll have detailed photos of each move in the daily workouts, but you can refer to these pages if you have any questions.

You do have the option of using weights for an added challenge on certain movements, but that is absolutely not necessary. The option of adding weights is there for those of you who are already working out and want more resistance, but if you use only a towel or your body weight, you'll still get a great workout. If you choose to add hand weights, opt for a weight that's heavy enough to challenge you but light enough that you can complete all your exercises. We recommend 2- to 8-pound weights, and if you have access to multiple weights, you can change it up.

warm-up

"Dolvett said 'you need to fall in love with the gym,' and it's happening. It's happening! When he told me that, I thought 'Yeah, right. This is Hell. I'm never gonna love Hell!' But the transition is beginning, and I'm getting excited to get in there and do these workouts!"
—Cate, Season 14

1
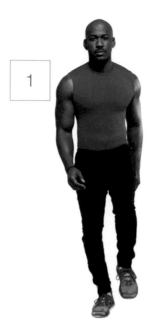

2
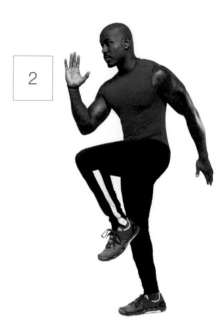

3a
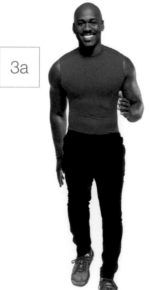

3b
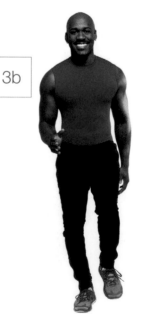

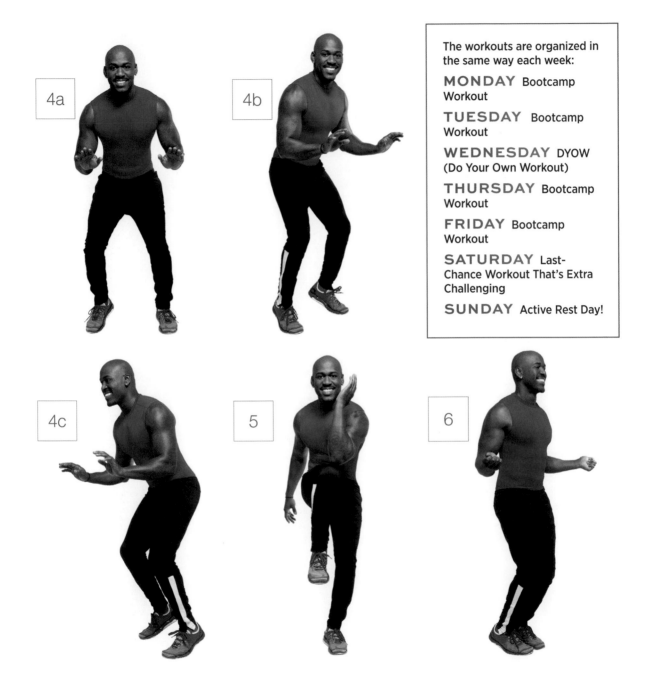

4a

4b

4c

5

6

The workouts are organized in the same way each week:

MONDAY Bootcamp Workout

TUESDAY Bootcamp Workout

WEDNESDAY DYOW (Do Your Own Workout)

THURSDAY Bootcamp Workout

FRIDAY Bootcamp Workout

SATURDAY Last-Chance Workout That's Extra Challenging

SUNDAY Active Rest Day!

cooldown

1a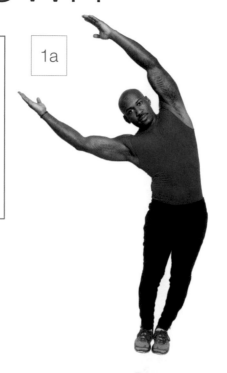

1b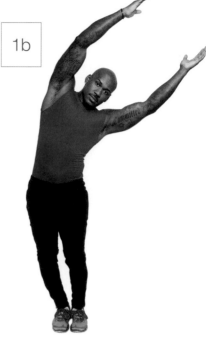

2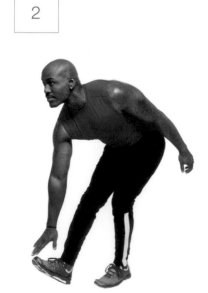

3a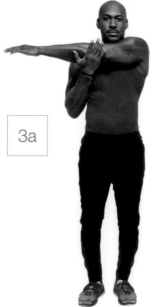

3b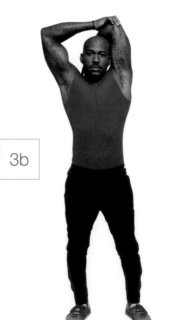

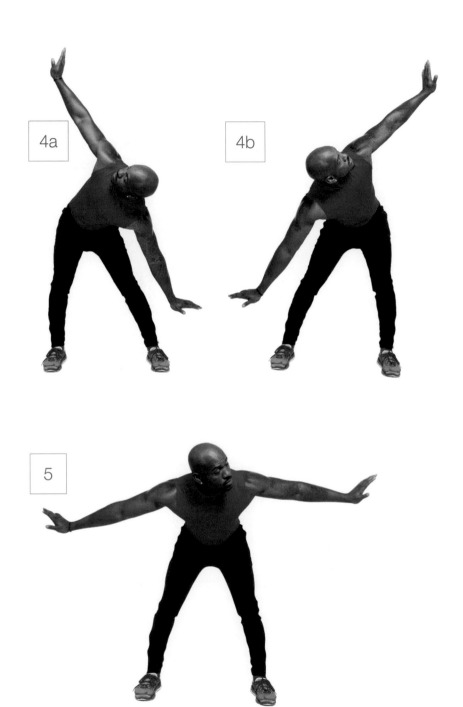

workout exercises

These are some of the excercises you'll be doing throughout Bootcamp:

BICEPS CURLS TO OVERHEAD PRESS:
Stand with feet slightly wider than your hips. Hold a towel between your fists, and pull out to create resistance. With your arms in tight against the sides of your body and your palms facing up, begin with your fists on your legs. Curl your arms all the way to your shoulders, then straighten your arms as you push the towel toward the ceiling and pull your fists apart to keep resistance.

BURPEES: Bring your hands down to the floor, shoulder-distance apart. Step or jump back into a plank. Jump or step your feet forward, and stand up. Repeat.

CHEST PRESSES: Lie down flat on your back. Extend your arms overhead, holding the towel between your hands. Use resistance by pulling your hands apart (still holding the towel) as you bring your hands toward your chest, arms out to the sides. Use resistance as you lift your arms back overhead.

FRONT PRESS HOLDS: Go down into a squat position, and bring your arms out in front of you as you hold onto a weight or a bag of rice or heavy books. Hold the squat with your arms out in front of you.

HIP BRIDGES: Lie down flat on your back, palms by your side, hands flat on your mat. Press down with your feet to raise your hips. Squeeze tightly at the top, then come back down.

LAT PULLDOWNS: Use a hand towel to add resistance. Pull that towel as hard as you can, palms across from each other. Take your arms overhead, and continue that resistance by pulling with all your might, separating your hands from each other.

LUNGE TWISTS: Step your right foot back into a lunge, then twist your torso and upper body to the left side. Twist back to center as you step your feet back together, then repeat on the other side.

MOUNTAIN CLIMBERS: Get down on all fours. Bring your knees in toward your chest one at a time, as if you were climbing. Keep your heels up high. Slow down if needed.

REAR LUNGES: Start with your feet hip-width apart. Step your right foot back, dropping your knee toward the floor as your left leg bends toward 90 degrees. Repeat on the other side. Make sure the knee of your front foot doesn't go forward beyond your toes. Take your time going down to really feel the muscles working. Focus on "exploding" and emphasizing your movement.

REAR-STEPPING LUNGES WITH ONE-ARM ROWS: Start with your feet hip-width apart and arms by your sides, holding a weight or a heavy object, such as a gallon of water, in your right hand. Step your right foot back, dropping your knee toward the floor into a lunge as your left leg bends toward 90 degrees. Once you're in the lunge, pull your arm straight up with the elbow pointing behind you. As you step forward and come out of the lunge, bring the arm back down by your side.

Repeat on the other side. Make sure the knee of your front foot doesn't go forward beyond your toes. Take your time going down to really feel the muscles working. Focus on "exploding" and emphasizing your movement.

RENEGADE ROWS: Start in a plank position, with or without weights. Lift your right arm, drawing the weight up to your shoulder, keeping your elbow pulling back. Return your right hand or weight to the floor, and repeat on the other side.

RUSSIAN TWISTS: You can use a medicine ball for this move, but it isn't necessary. Sit down and balance with your heels down and toes up. Twist your torso to one side, touch the floor, and twist to the other side. Repeat.

SEATED WOODCHOPS: Sit down on the floor with your heels down and toes up. Contract your abs. Reach down next to you on the left, then lift your arms up and overhead to the right.

SIDE LUNGES WITH SINGLE ARM LATERAL RAISES: Starting with a weight in your right hand and your feet wider than hip-width, step to the left and lunge your left leg. Once you're in the lunge, lift your right arm straight up in front of you, palm facing down. As you return to center, lower the arm. Repeat on the other side.

SKATER JUMPS: Start with your feet hip-width apart. As you push off the right foot, place it behind the left foot as you jump over to the side. Make sure you land very softly and with a bent knee.

SQUATS WITH BICEPS CURLS: This is a combination movement with both squats and biceps curls. You only need a towel. Hold the towel between your hands, and bring them shoulder-distance apart. Squat down and bend your elbows to 90 degrees, pulling your wrists away from each other. As you stand up, bring your arms back down.

SQUATS WITH REAR FLY: Begin by standing with your feet wider than your hips. Take your arms out to the sides, palms facing up. Squat down, then bring your hands together in front of your body. As you stand up, return your arms to your sides.

SQUATS WITH OVERHEAD PRESS: This is a combination movement with both squats and an overhead press. You only need a towel. Hold the towel in your hands, and pull your fists apart to add resistance. Stand with your feet hip-width apart and bring your fists in front of your shoulders.

TRAVELING SQUATS: With your feet hip-width apart, step one foot out to the side and squat down. As you come up, bring your feet back to hip's distance. Step the other foot out wide, squat down, and bring your feet closer as you come up. Repeat.

TRAVELING SQUATS WITH PIVOT: Follow the same instructions as the Traveling Squats, but as you go down into the squat, pivot the outside foot and come right back up. Switch sides halfway through.

TWO-ARM ROWS: Hold a towel between your hands, with your arms straight out in front of you. Pull your arms strongly toward you, letting your elbows come out to the sides, away from each other. Bring the towel in toward your chest, feeling your back muscles work, then press it back out in front again.

WALK-OUT PUSH-UPS: Bend over, touch your toes, then walk out to a plank, lower into a push-up, and come back to a plank. Walk your hands back in, stand up, and repeat.

WARRIOR 1: Step your feet apart, with your right toes pointing forward and your left foot in at an angle. Point your hips toward your right foot. Bring your arms overhead, palms together. Switch sides halfway through.

WARRIOR 2: Step your feet apart, with your right toes pointing forward and your left foot in at an angle. Turn your hips to the left side. Extend your arms out, and bend your right foot into a lunge, looking out over your right fingertips. Switch sides halfway through.

WOODCHOPS: Stand with your feet slightly wider than hip's distance. Hold a weight (or a bottle of water) upright in both hands, with your fingers interlaced, then swing your arms overhead and to the right. Drop your arms diagonally across the bottom to the left, being careful not to hit your hips. Allow your torso to twist, which works your obliques. Switch to the other side halfway through.

DYOW ideas

If you're new to exercise or still haven't learned to like it, it might be challenging to figure out what to do on those DYOW (Do Your Own Workout) days. Cardio exercise is any activity that helps your cardiovascular system function and strengthens your heart. It doesn't need to involve running, jumping, or even walking!

Here's a list of fun workouts that you can do with little to no equipment—no gym membership required:

- Take a walk with a friend.
- Walk laps around the field during your child's soccer practice.
- Go bowling.
- Play touch football, baseball, or basketball with your kids.
- Walk the dog.
- Take a hike.
- Clean the house.
- Ride your bike.
- Ride an exercise bike while watching a movie.
- Walk laps around the mall.
- Dance to your favorite music.
- Jump on a trampoline!

prep week

your meal plan: get your diet right

The diet you'll be following during Bootcamp is based on the energy equation, which is the foundation of every successful diet. In Chapter 3, you read the basis of the plan and decided on your personal calorie target. Just like with your goal, you're not aiming for perfection—you're going to keep to it as closely as possible.

Your meal plan is designed to help you get the most out of the program. Our meal plan is approximately 1,500 calories, which is adequate for most people who want to lose 1 to 2 pounds a week while being active most days. You can refer to Chapter 3 for more information on adjusting the meal plan.

The meal plan is an example of a very balanced diet with lots of variety and a few treats which may appear as a snack or dessert.

If you don't want to use the meal plan, you can do your own thing. Just remember to track what you're eating (honestly!), and make sure you're eating:

- lots of fresh fruit and vegetables
- lean protein (lean meat, chicken, fish, tofu, eggs)
- low-fat dairy
- whole grains

We'll have lots more on nutrition over the next eight weeks, so stay tuned.

Remember: The keys to weight loss are in the kitchen, so if you're not following the meal plan, be sure to log your food and drinks so you can keep your calories in check, using the guidelines laid out in Chapter 3.

If you want to get the best results and you respond better to structure, you have to trust the meal plan. The Bootcamp was designed for you.

As one Bootcamper from Alexandria, Virginia, said: "I thought I was active before and eating healthy, but I was really kidding myself. The menu plan makes it easier to eat healthy and enjoy it."

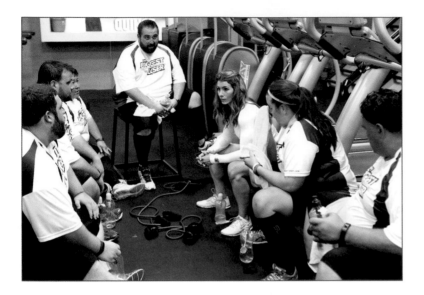

into this workout plan. (Please remember to clear this and all workouts with your physician.)

It's important to listen to your body. If it needs a break, you can take a rest day, but make sure it's your body talking and not your mind. If we all waited until our minds were ready to lose weight, we wouldn't ever achieve our goals.

There's not much you need to do to get ready for the fitness part of the plan, which was designed with first-timers in mind. The workout plan can be done with no equipment except a towel for added resistance in some exercises. You can do these workouts at home or at the gym with just a comfortable pair of sneakers and some workout clothes.

To be more comfortable during your workouts, you might also want:

- music, headphones, and something to hold your phone or player

- sunglasses and sunscreen if you exercise outside

- headband or hat to keep sweat out of your eyes

- compression shorts (Some people find that wearing compression shorts under workout clothes reduces friction and chafing.)

Lenida said she couldn't have dropped four dress sizes without the meal plan. "If I'd had to come up with a menu on my own, I don't think I would have done as well."

And not to worry: You'll be able to swap in additional meals or snacks if there's something on the plan you don't like or can't eat.

move it to lose it

Exercise is a huge part of the Bootcamp. The plan is set up with six workouts a week, and one rest day. Whether you do every workout or take an additional rest day is up to you. As you hear Dolvett say to contestants, "If you're not moving, you're not losing." But we also know some of you are just starting out and will need to ease

❝Don't wait, don't settle, and don't quit!❞ —Lisa Rambo, Season 14

PLANNING FOR TOMORROW
When Bootcamp starts, the most important thing is to read each day the night before, so you can get the benefit of the morning motivation and plan for the day ahead. This might mean that you need to adjust your evening schedule slightly. We think that reading about tomorrow each night will help you stay on track at one of the most tempting times of day—after dinner, when many of us tend to snack!

make time for you

This Bootcamp was designed for real life—we know you're not quitting your job or sending your friends and family away for the next eight weeks. You still gotta live your life. But to stick with this, you need to plan ahead and make time for *you*. No excuses! You have to get your life in order. This week, grab your calendar and start looking at what you *have* to do versus what you *want* to do over the next two months. When will you do your workouts? Don't just guess. You need to make time for them six days a week. Schedule them—then honor those commitments just as you would a doctor's appointment or work meeting. You also get to pick your rest day, so schedule that as well.

You've got to keep your eyes on the prize and make time for your meals and exercise. Tell your mind to get out of your body's way.

It's not going to be easy. The first few days will be the hardest. But the more you move, the more you'll be *able* to move. The more often you pick healthy foods over unhealthy ones, the easier the decision to stick with it will become.

Keep telling yourself that you've got to keep pushing through. When you are tempted to give up on yourself, remember all the hard work you put in during the week. No matter how much weight you lose, soon you'll be telling yourself: "I'm not the person I was when I started this program."

Just two episodes into Season 15, the eventual winner, Rachel, noticed a huge attitude adjustment. "I can see the work I'm putting in, and I can feel how proud I am becoming of myself, and it's just a wonderful feeling," she said during an interview on the show. Rachel was just starting her journey. As the season progressed, she grew stronger inside and out. The former state swimming champion conquered a fear and did laps for Dolvett after years away from the pool. She lost weight and gained confidence. No longer was she the young woman who hid in her home and turned to food for comfort. She was smiling, laughing, and truly living her life.

The reason you're reading this book is to get your body healthy and fit so that you can finally live the life you always wanted. That won't happen without a commitment to make this about you. You can't get sent home, but you can certainly get off track. We're here to make sure that doesn't happen.

In addition to workouts, you need to:

- Set your goals each week.

- Weigh in on Sundays.

- Grocery shop and prep healthy snacks.

- Prepare your meals: Cook dinner, pack lunch, and prep breakfast and snacks.

Whether you use an online or paper calendar is up to you, but we recommend printing out your meal plan, fitness schedule, and even your goals and placing them where you'll see them several times a day: on the bathroom mirror, at your desk, and on the fridge, for example.

you're not alone

Since you're not doing this on the Ranch, you get to do this with the support of your loved ones! This week, sit down as a family and explain the changes that will happen during the Bootcamp. Divide up the meal prep, shopping, and cleanup duties, and get them involved with your Prep Week planning.

Remind your family that they're your "team," and if they resist, explain to them that you're doing this for yourself but also for them. This is your second chance at life. You'll be a better partner, a better parent, and a better friend because of this.

And if you live alone, you're not going it alone. Reach out to your friends, your family, and your co-workers for support. This book will walk you through everything you need to know, day by day and step by step.

get your mind in the game

Here comes the hard part. It's time to get real and look at yourself in the mirror. Why are you doing this? This week, we want you to spend some time thinking—really thinking—about why you're doing this. There are no right or wrong reasons. There are only *your* reasons. So what are they? Why aren't you continuing with the status quo of life?

Every season, contestants come to the Ranch for a variety of reasons:

- I don't want to die young, like my father did.
- I had to have a follow-up mammogram because I was so big.
- I can't start a family because of my size.
- I want to ride horses with my sons.
- I want to lose the weight I gained while I cared for my dying wife.

We heard similar stories from our Bootcamp Success Stories:

- I was at my wit's end. I was so tired of having no energy. I was angry and bitter.
- I was tired of feeling a failure in the battle of the bulge.

tip

BE HERE OFTEN One of the most important things you can do on this program is carry this book with you as much as possible and read through each day ahead of time. You'll get a daily boost of inspiration and you'll get to build healthy habits that will make this journey easier and more rewarding.

- I had tried every diet out there.

- I swore I'd never see 300 pounds on the scale; I joined the Bootcamp when I weighed 299.6 pounds.

- My sister and I did it together to cope with the death of our brother.

- I watched Season 15 and recognized myself in the contestants.

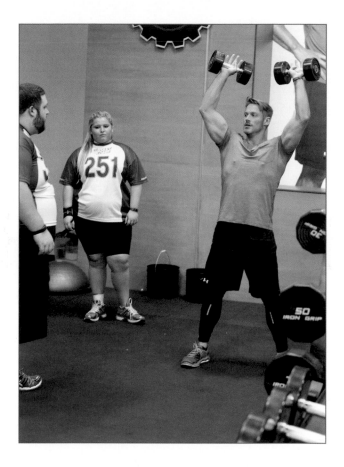

These people come from all over the country, a variety of ages, professions, and lifestyles. And yet they have one thing in common: They wanted to change their lives—and they did.

So why do *you* want to do this?

This week, consider what you could accomplish in seven days. You've watched the show, and you've seen contestants achieve incredible results in just one episode and throughout the entire season—and not just on the scale. That can be you! So what can *you* do?

Write a list of what you want to get from this. Where will you be in a week, two weeks, four weeks, eight weeks? And even though the Bootcamp ends after eight weeks, your journey will continue. So where will you go from there?

In addition to weighing yourself this week, we also want you to take measurements, then record it all in a notebook or online. These numbers will help you track your progress.

We also want you to take a Bootcamp "before" selfie. Share it, if you want, on Instagram and tag @biggestlosernbc so we can cheer you on. Or find us on Facebook: https://www.facebook.com/the-biggestloserclub. Over the next eight weeks, we want you to look back at that photo to see where you started—and how far you've come!

❝ Just be better than yesterday! ❞ *—The Biggest Loser* trainer Dolvett Quince

weekly goals help build healthy habits

One of the most difficult challenges that contestants faced in Season 15 was the "Diner Challenge." The White Team—down to just three people—had to work all week on their feet in a diner, *then* head back to the Ranch for their workouts. Jay, Marie, and Tumi all reached or exceeded their goals, losing 6, 6, and 9 pounds, respectively. They knew that the additional work would make it harder to keep their motivation levels high, so they focused on their goal: to stick with their workouts even during such a challenging week.

"We really wanted to prove to America that people can work *and* they can lose weight, because it's something I'm going to face when I go home," said Marie.

"It's been constant change. It's been unrelenting," said Tumi, who, despite losing 75 pounds over nine episodes, was still doubting herself. That 9-pound weight loss was her turning point. It took just one week—her hardest week yet on the Ranch—to prove to herself that she could do this. "I can do it. I can do it," she said through happy tears. "That 9 (pound loss) was everything to me!" She eventually lost 175 pounds. Tumi's confidence in herself, which gave her the strength to keep working after she was sent home, all started with that one weekly goal.

We believe in goals—grandiose, long-term ones as well as small, achievable goals. Those small, achievable goals are the ones you'll set (and crush) every week. Why set weekly goals?

- A week is a realistic time to plan ahead.
- It gives you a chance to celebrate success regularly.
- It helps you build the healthy habits required to achieve your bigger goals, and maintain your weight well beyond this program.

focus on progress, not perfection

You'll notice that throughout Bootcamp, we avoid "all or nothing" goals each week. Instead of setting a goal like: "Do *every* workout" we suggest: "*Do at least 3* of the Bootcamp workouts."

That's because we're not looking for perfection. We are looking for you to always be better

tip

WHEN SHOULD I WEIGH IN?
The Bootcamp runs Monday through Sunday. The day you weigh in is up to you, but we recommend weighing in on Sundays, which is scheduled as your rest day. Weighing yourself at the same time of day, on the same day of the week, and in the same place each week will ensure you get a more accurate reading. Your weight can fluctuate by several pounds throughout the day based on what you've eaten, how much water you've consumed, and whether you've gone to the bathroom, so creating a routine helps you get a better idea of your fat weight loss rather than water weight loss.

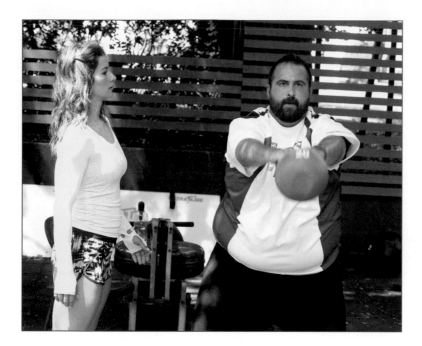

Each week when you achieve that goal, we want you to record it at the end of the chapter, then SHOUT about it to your family and friends!

We also want you to tell US! Just because you're not on the Ranch doesn't mean you're not part of *The Biggest Loser* family. Facebook, Twitter, Instagram, you name it—come on over and tell us what you've achieved.

It's so important to celebrate your goals; achieving them makes you happy, and people want to be around happy, successful people like you. But let's

than yesterday. Sure, we hope you do the workouts every day, but no one goes from zero to hero. If you've done zero exercise since... college? high school? birth? it might not be realistic to exercise every day. If you can, go for it—but if nothing else, just be better than yesterday. (You're going to hear that a lot throughout this program!)

not celebrate with food or beverages. Manicures, yes. New sneakers, yes. Candy and cocktails, no. If you don't achieve every goal, that's OK, too, as long as you keep trying and working hard. It's about the journey! Sometimes you'll set goals and realize that you can't or just don't want to reach them. As we explained in Chapter 1, it's not about the scale. This is about something much, much bigger: It's about believing in yourself, trying new things, and sticking with it even if you encounter hurdles and setbacks.

celebrating your goals

Make space in a notebook or journal to record your goals. We also encourage you to write down your weekly goals and post them in places where you'll see them frequently.

Think of all the things you've wanted to do for so long but have never had the confidence to do. Now you're going to be able to do them—and much more. You've been given a second chance to create the best version of yourself. What you do with it is up to you.

Let's get started.

week 1

today is the day!

It's Day 1 of Bootcamp. We hope you're excited to kick off this journey. Eight weeks may seem like a long time, but it isn't. We are diving right in, and you're going to start working on a new you right away.

Starting a new program is exciting (and maybe a little overwhelming, we know), but don't sweat it. You've already made the commitment to be here, and that's the first step to success. You're not doing this on your own: We've anticipated the hurdles, the setbacks, and the challenges—and we're going to be with you each and every step of the way. We'll be here to motivate and guide you, but this is not a one-way street: There are a couple of things we ask of you.

commitment

You have to keep coming back to the program, doing your workouts, and setting your goals. You will get so much more out of this Bootcamp if you pick up your book each evening to plan ahead for tomorrow and each morning read the Morning Motivations or Nutrition Bites, which contain tips and inspiration to keep you focused.

goal setting

By now you've read through the Prep Week chapter, so you know that you're going to set a goal each week of the program. Goals are critical to success, so take the time to record yours now. You can use that same notebook to keep track of how many workouts you did each week!

We all know how great it feels to complete something—and we know you'll work hard to reach your goal this week.

WEEKLY WORKOUTS

MONDAY	Ready To Rock
TUESDAY	I Heart Cardio
WEDNESDAY	Do Your Own Workout (DYOW)
THURSDAY	Do It For Dolvett
FRIDAY	Be Better Than Yesterday
SATURDAY	Last-Chance Workout—Danni
SUNDAY	Active Rest Day

coaches' corner

WHY NOW? AND WHY DOES THIS MATTER TO YOU? The Bootcamp provides you with the tools you need to eat healthier, exercise regularly, and lose weight, but of course, you are the one who will need to put it into action. It will take a concerted effort on your part, and that means you'll need some serious motivation to make it through Bootcamp.

A key strategy for building motivation is to think about the pay-offs you're expecting and exactly how these payoffs will make a difference in your life. This week, write down at least five reasons why the best time to start the Bootcamp is right now. What will you gain? What will be better in your life? What are you going to do differently or do more often as the weight begins to come off?

The next step is to elaborate on these payoffs by "digging" deeper into the changes that are really meaningful for you. Here's how it works. Look at each of the five reasons you've written down and beside each ask yourself: "... and why does this matter to me?" As you identify a specific reason, again, ask yourself why it matters. Continue the process until you can't go any further. Here is an example:

Why do Bootcamp? "To have more energy." ...and why does this matter to me? "So I can spend more time playing in the yard with my children." ...and why does this matter to me? "So I can encourage my children to do more physical activities." ...and why does this matter to me? "I want to be a role model for them growing up healthy and for them to remember me playing with them as a reason they love to be active."

WEEK 1 MEALS

MONDAY

B Breakfast Bacon & Egg Grilled Cheese

L Caprese Chicken Pita

D Quick Tandoori Salmon

TUESDAY

B Peanut Butter Toast

L Turkey Wrap

D Grilled Pork with Honey BBQ Sauce

WEDNESDAY

B Chocolate, Banana, Peanut Butter Smoothie

L Leftover Grilled Pork with Honey BBQ Sauce

D Two-Bean Chili Con Carne

THURSDAY

B Morning Oatmeal

L Two-Bean Chili Con Carne Stuffed Sweet Potato

D Philly Cheesesteak Stuffed Tomatoes

FRIDAY

B Yogurt with Granola & Fruit

L Roasted Red Pepper Hummus Wrap

D Two-Bean Chili Con Carne

SATURDAY

B Morning Oatmeal

L Hearty BLT Salad

D Easy Honey Mustard Chicken

SUNDAY

B Oatmeal Pancakes

L Tuna Salad Sandwich

D Quick Chicken Parmesan

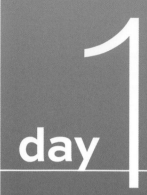

day 1

nutrition bite:

I Will Eat A Healthy Breakfast.

Eating a healthy breakfast not only fuels your body and mind to prepare you for your day ahead, eating breakfast is also linked to weight loss. In some studies, people who are dieting and skip breakfast actually end up eating more calories by the end of the day than people who eat a healthy breakfast! So go ahead and eat up to fuel up and slim down.

ready to rock

33 MINUTES

It's time for your first workout! Today we're offering this little pep talk before you get started, but as of tomorrow you'll dive right into the workout—no intro or explanation. Dolvett's style is "body confusion"—mixing it up to maximize fat loss—so you'll be alternating between cardio and classic body-weight exercises that will prepare you for tougher moves later on. Have fun with it, and don't be afraid to push yourself!

Start with this five-minute Warm-Up. We use the same warm-up and the same cooldown for each of the Bootcamp Workouts, so you'll memorize it quickly. Today is the only day we'll list the individual exercises. You can refer back to this page or Chapter 3 if you forget any of the moves in your warm-up or cooldown.

WARM-UP

1 Walking X 30 seconds
2 High Knees X 30 seconds
3 Jogging X 30 seconds
— High Knees X 30 seconds
4 Quick Feet X 30 seconds
5 High Knees with Torso Twist X 1 minute
— Walking X 30 seconds
6 Air Jump Rope X 60 seconds

For photos of this warm-up, see pp. 30–31.

THE WORKOUT

2 ROUNDS

— High Knees X 30 seconds

1 Jogging X 30 seconds

— Air Jump Rope X 30 seconds

2 Squats X 1 minute

— Jogging X 30 seconds

— Air Jump Rope X 30 seconds

3 Skater Jumps X 30 seconds

4 Push-Ups X 1 minute

5 High Knees X 30 seconds

— Jogging X 30 seconds

— Air Jump Rope X 30 seconds

6 Plank X 1 minute

— Jogging X 30 seconds

— Air Jump Rope X 30 seconds

— Skater Jumps X 30 seconds

7 Lat Pulldowns X 1 minute

Repeat for Round 2

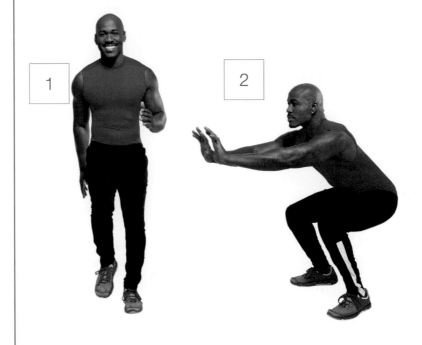

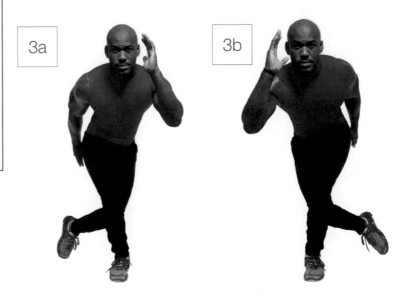

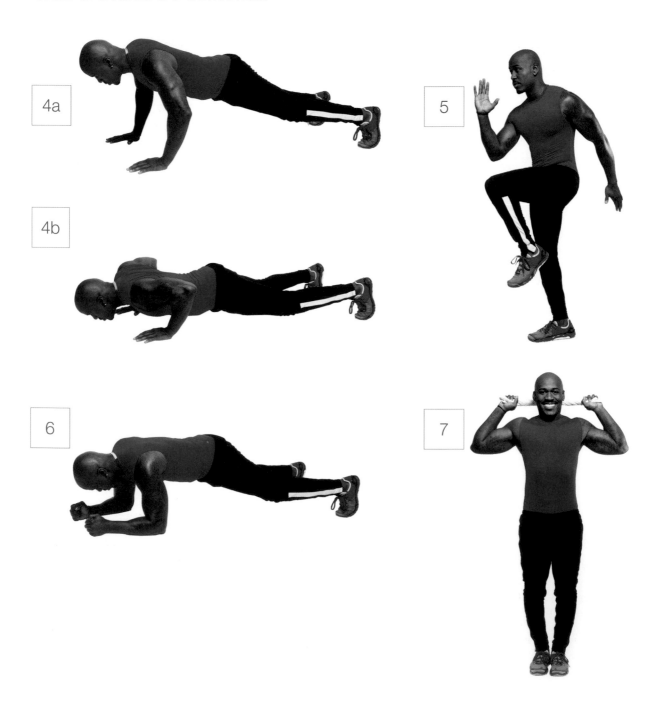

COOLDOWN

1 Side Stretch

2 Hamstrings Stretch

3 Triceps Stretch

4 Sunrise Stretch

5 Horizon Stretch

For photos of these stretches, see pp. 32–33.

tip

NUTRITION INFO Throughout the Bootcamp meal plans, the nutrition info provided is for the recipe or quick meal only—not any sides or extras. You're going to be tracking your food online or in a journal, and by sharing the nutrition info for only the main dishes, you have more freedom to choose vegetables and side dishes that suit your tastes and your calorie budget.

MEALS

BREAKFAST

breakfast bacon & egg grilled cheese

Serve with 1 orange and 1 cup skim milk.
Spread 1 tsp. margarine on 1 slice whole-wheat bread. Toast the bread on 1 side in a skillet, then top with 2 cooked egg whites, 1 slice crumbled turkey bacon, ½ cup chopped fresh spinach, and 2 Tbsp. shredded reduced-fat cheddar cheese. Continue cooking over low heat until the cheese has melted.

VEGETARIAN OPTION Sub in 1 slice tempeh bacon or omit the bacon entirely.

NUTRITION INFO: *Calories 221, Fat (g) 11, Sat fat (g) 3, Protein (g) 19, Carbs (g) 14, Fiber (g) 2, Sodium (mg) 460*

LUNCH

caprese chicken pita

Serve with ½ cup low-sodium pasta sauce for dipping, plus a medium-size banana.
Layer 3 oz. shredded cooked chicken, ¼ cup part-skim mozzarella, 1 sliced medium-size tomato, and fresh basil on half a whole-wheat pita. Toast until the cheese melts.

VEGETARIAN OPTION Sub in ½ cup mashed white beans for the chicken.

NUTRITION INFO: *Calories 309, Fat (g) 6, Sat fat (g) 3, Protein (g) 38, Carbs (g) 24, Fiber (g) 2, Sodium (mg) 480*

DINNER

quick tandoori salmon

See recipe on page 71. Add ¼ cup unsalted and shelled sunflower seeds to the salad.

SNACKS

Choose up to 300 calories of snacks to reach your calorie goal for the day. See the lists in Chapter 3 for snack ideas.

day 2

morning motivation:

Love Yourself Now.

It's so important to learn to love yourself. You are worth loving and taking care of. You might think that you should be loving or taking care of other people first, but that's backwards. Give your family the best version of yourself—by loving yourself no matter what.

WORKOUT
i heart cardio
30 MINUTES
WARM UP FOR 5 MINUTES

Today's workout is called "I Heart Cardio"! You might not love it now, but you will by the end of the Bootcamp! Today you'll experience the first of many cardio interval workouts designed to burn fat and build fitness.

THE WORKOUT

1 Jogging X 1 minute
2 Walking X 1 minute
3 High Knees with Torso Twist X 1 minute
— Walking X 1 minute
4 Quick Feet X 1 minute
— Walking X 1 minute
5 Air Jump Rope X 1 minute
6 High Knees X 1 minute
— Jumping Jacks X 1 minute
— High Knees X 1 minute
— Air Jump Rope X 1 minute
— High Knees X 1 minute
— Jumping Jacks X 1 minute
— High Knees X 1 minute
— Quick Feet X 1 minute
— Walking X 1 minute
— High Knees with Torso Twist X 1 minute
— Walking X 1 minute
— Jogging X 1 minute
— Walking X 1 minute

COOL DOWN FOR 5 MINUTES

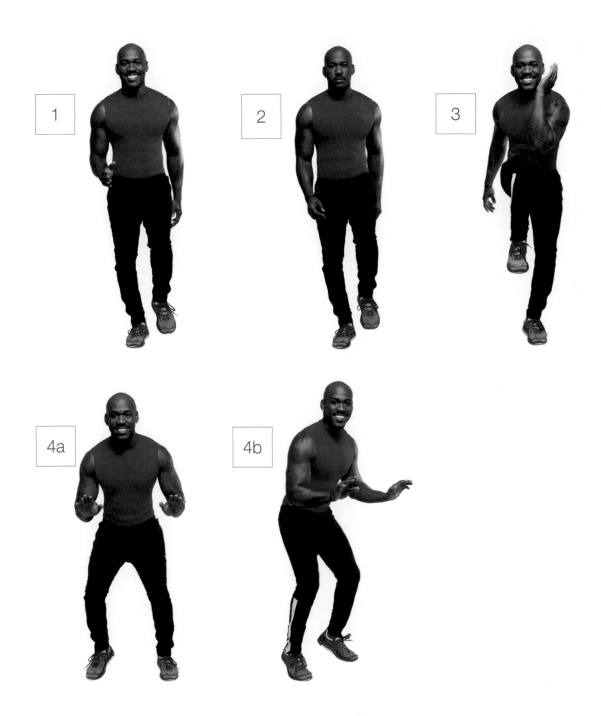

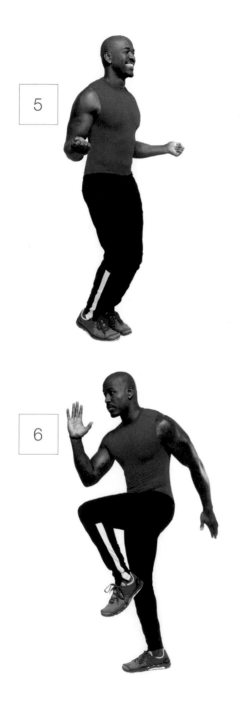

MEALS

BREAKFAST
peanut butter toast

Serve 2 slices whole-wheat bread, 1 Tbsp. peanut butter, and 1 orange with 1 cup skim milk.

NUTRITION INFO: *Calories 395, Fat (g) 10, Sat fat (g) 1, Protein (g) 20, Carbs (g) 59, Fiber (g) 7, Sodium (mg) 390*

LUNCH
turkey wrap

See recipe on page 68.

Serve with 1 stalk celery and 1 Tbsp. natural peanut butter.

DINNER
grilled pork with honey bbq sauce

See recipe on page 70.

Serve with 1 peach, 1 piece corn on the cob, and a quick slaw. To make the slaw, combine 2 cups broccoli slaw with 2 Tbsp. light vinaigrette. You'll save half the pork for tomorrow's lunch.

NOTE Broccoli slaw is shredded broccoli stems, often with cabbage and carrots added. It is only vegetables—no dressing. You can find it with the bagged lettuce at the supermarket. We like it in slaw-style salads as well as stir-fries.

day 3

it's day 3, wednesday,

which means you've almost made it through half of the week.

How are you doing? Don't hold back! If you've missed a few workouts or made some spontaneous unhealthy food choices, don't worry—you have four days left this week. You've got this!

WORKOUT

do your own workout (dyow)

Every Wednesday of Bootcamp is DYOW—Do Your Own Workout! This is an opportunity for you to squeeze in your favorite class, sweat it out with your favorite workout DVD, or go for a walk/run/ride/swim/surf/ski. You can also DYOW by gardening or shoveling snow.

If you're stuck for ideas, simply repeat or flip ahead to one of the workouts in this week, or see the list of suggested exercises in Chapter 3.

For beginners, it's OK to take this workout as an extra rest day, but only if your body needs it.

❝Just say yes. Be open to all types of food and fitness. You've made the decision to change your lifestyle. Now's the time to add new items to your docket and plate. Have fun! Who knows what will happen. I think you will surprise yourself! ❞

—*The Biggest Loser* trainer Jessie Pavelka

MEALS

BREAKFAST
chocolate, banana, peanut butter smoothie

See recipe on page 67.

LUNCH
leftover grilled pork with honey bbq sauce

Serve the second portion of pork in a whole-wheat tortilla with 1 cup broccoli slaw.

DINNER
two-bean chili con carne

See recipe on page 70.

Serve with 1 tablespoon shredded reduced-fat cheddar cheese and ½ cup cooked brown rice. You'll save one portion for tomorrow's lunch and one for Friday's dinner.

SNACKS
Choose up to 300 calories of snacks to reach your calorie goal for the day. See the lists in Chapter 3 for snack ideas.

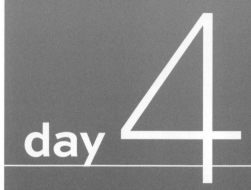

day 4

morning motivation:

Anything Is Everything.

How you do anything is how you do everything. This is a principle to live by, or to try to live by. How you prepare each meal, write a Facebook post, recite this Morning Motivation—it's how you do everything. Think about that today.

WORKOUT do it for dolvett

33 MINUTES | WARM UP FOR 5 MINUTES

THE WORKOUT

2 ROUNDS

1 High Knees X 30 seconds

2 Jogging X 30 seconds

3 Air Jump Rope X 30 seconds

4 Rear Lunges X 1 minute

— Jogging X 30 seconds

— Air Jump Rope X 30 seconds

5 Skater Jumps X 30 seconds

6 Chest Presses X 30 seconds

— High Knees X 30 seconds

— Jogging X 30 seconds

— Air Jump Rope X 30 seconds

7 Hip Bridge X 1 minute

— Jogging X 30 seconds

— Air Jump Rope X 30 seconds

— Skater Jumps X 30 seconds

8 Two-Arm Rows X 1 minute

Repeat for Round 2

COOL DOWN FOR 5 MINUTES

We called this workout "Do It For Dolvett" to remind you that whenever you feel like skipping a workout for no good reason, remember that Dolvett put a lot of sweat into these sessions, so the least you can do is do it for him.

Today's workout is a similar format to Monday's workout in that it alternates cardio with strength moves. But the moves are new, so it will feel like a very different workout.

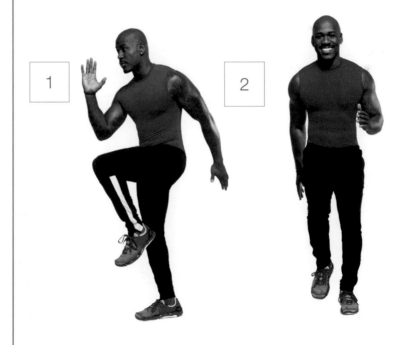

55

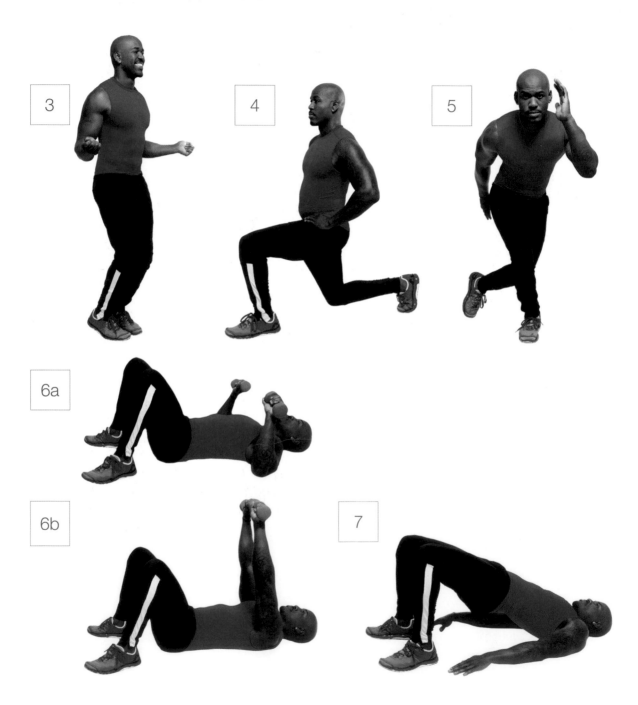

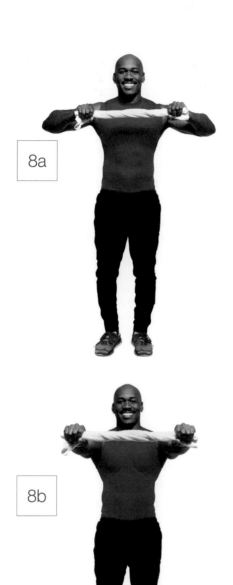

8a

8b

MEALS

BREAKFAST

morning oatmeal

Prepare ½ cup oats with ½ to ¾ cup water. Top with 1 sliced peach and 7 chopped walnuts (½ oz.). Serve with 1 cup skim milk.

NUTRITION INFO: *Calories 387, Fat (g) 12, Sat fat (g) 1, Protein (g) 17, Carbs (g) 58, Fiber (g) 7, Sodium (mg) 121*

LUNCH

two-bean chili con carne stuffed sweet potato

Stuff 1 small baked sweet potato with leftover chili from last night.

DINNER

philly cheesesteak stuffed tomatoes

Serve with ½ cup brown rice.
Core 2 small tomatoes. Top with 3 oz. lean beef, 1 cup sautéed onions and peppers, and 1 slice reduced-fat Swiss cheese. Heat until the cheese melts.

NUTRITION INFO: *Calories 294, Fat (g) 9, Sat fat (g) 3, Protein (g) 30, Carbs (g) 27, Fiber (g) 5, Sodium (mg) 88*

SNACKS

Choose up to 300 calories of snacks to reach your calorie goal for the day. See the lists in Chapter 3 for snack ideas.

day 5

nutrition bite:

What Do You Need Right Now?

That's a powerful question to ask yourself when you're feeling the pull of unhealthy foods. A follow-up question is: "Am I really hungry?" If the answer is no, think about what would help you feel better in the next 10 minutes. Take a shower. Put on your favorite music. Get some fresh air. Switching gears when you find yourself struggling will help you resist temptation.

WORKOUT
be better than yesterday

30 MINUTES | WARM UP FOR 5 MINUTES

It's all we ask of you during this program: to be better than yesterday. That's all any of us can do, and it's something to reflect on while you sweat it out in today's cardio intervals workout.

> "Take the lead and do you. Make decisions, speak your true voice and be you! Lead by example. "
> — *The Biggest Loser* trainer Jennifer Widerstrom

THE WORKOUT

1 Jogging X 1 minute

2 Walking X 1 minute

3 High Knees with Torso Twist X 1 minute

— Walking X 1 minute

4 Air Jump Rope X 1 minute

5 High Knees X 1 minute

6 Quick Feet X 1 minute

— High Knees X 1 minute

7 Jumping Jacks X 1 minute

— Walking X 1 minute

8 Skater Jumps X 1 minute

— Walking X 1 minute

— Air Jump Rope X 1 minute

— High Knees X 1 minute

— Quick Feet X 1 minute

— High Knees X 1 minute

— Jumping Jacks X 1 minute

— Walking X 1 minute

— Skater Jumps X 1 minute

— Walking X 1 minute

COOL DOWN FOR
5 MINUTES

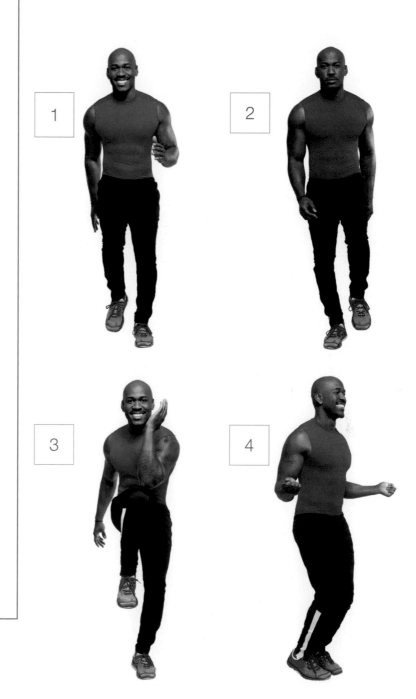

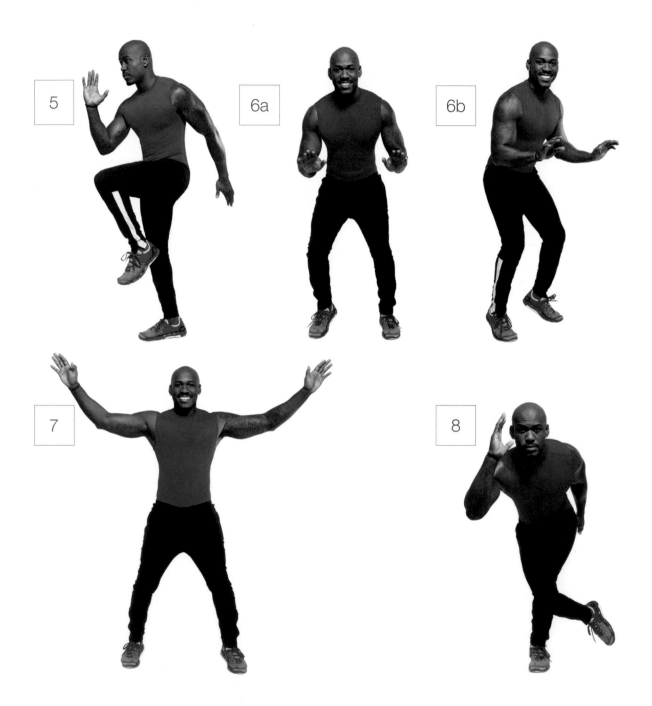

MEALS

BREAKFAST

yogurt with granola & fruit

Serve 1 (6-oz.) container plain fat-free Greek yogurt with ¼ cup low-fat granola, 7 chopped walnuts (½ oz.), and 1 cup strawberries.

NUTRITION INFO: *Calories 417, Fat (g) 12, Sat fat (g) 1, Protein (g) 31, Carbs (g) 52, Fiber (g) 9, Sodium (mg) 102*

LUNCH

roasted red pepper hummus wrap

See recipe for Roasted Red Pepper Hummus on page 68.

Serve ¼ cup hummus with 3 oz. lower-sodium deli turkey and 1 cup vegetables of your choice inside 1 whole-grain wrap or half a whole-grain pita, or between 2 slices whole-grain bread.

DINNER

two-bean chili con carne

Serve leftovers from Wednesday atop 1 small baked sweet potato with 1 Tbsp. shredded reduced-fat cheddar cheese.

DESSERT

yogurt-covered blueberries

Toss ½ cup blueberries with ¼ cup fat-free vanilla Greek yogurt. Place on a sheet of parchment and freeze for at least an hour.

NUTRITION INFO: *Calories 95, Fat (g) 0, Sat fat (g) 0, Protein (g) 7, Carbs (g) 14, Fiber (g) 2, Sodium (mg) 36*

SNACKS

Choose up to 300 calories of snacks to reach your daily goal. See the lists in Chapter 3 for snack ideas. Don't forget to include your dessert in your food journal (dessert gets included with your snack calories).

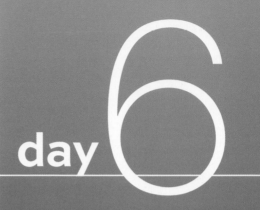

day 6

You should be proud of yourself each time you complete a workout, but these Last Chance workouts are more challenging than your other workouts through the week. Be even more proud of yourself for finishing this one! Have some fun with it—and don't be afraid to push yourself.

last-chance workout—danni

41 MINUTES

WARM UP FOR 5 MINUTES

Every Saturday during Bootcamp, you'll end the week with a "Last-Chance Workout"—that's one last chance to sweat it out, end the week on a high, and earn the rest day that's coming up tomorrow.

Expect these "last chances" to be a little tougher than the previous workouts. This particular workout uses all the moves you've learned this week as well as back-to-back exercises for the same body part. This lack of rest between strength exercises makes your body dig a little deeper.

We're dedicating today's Last-Chance Workout to Season 14 winner Danni Allen. She's proof that you can achieve amazing weight loss following *The Biggest Loser* philosophies, and keep it off. Think of Danni today when you do this workout. She did it, and so can you!

THE WORKOUT

2 ROUNDS

1   High Knees X 30 seconds

2   Jogging X 30 seconds

3   Air Jump Rope X 30 seconds

4   Squats X 1 minute

5   Rear Lunges X 1 minute

—   Jogging X 30 seconds

—   Air Jump Rope X 30 seconds

6   Skater Jumps X 30 seconds

7   Push-Ups X 1 minute

8   Chest Presses X 1 minute

—   High Knees X 30 seconds

—   Jogging X 30 seconds

—   Air Jump Rope X 30 seconds

9   Plank X 1 minute

10 Hip Bridge X 1 minute

—   Jogging X 30 seconds

—   Air Jump Rope X 30 seconds

—   Skater Jumps X 30 seconds

11 Lat Pulldowns X 1 minute

12 Two-Arm Rows X 1 minute

Repeat for Round 2

COOL DOWN FOR 5 MINUTES

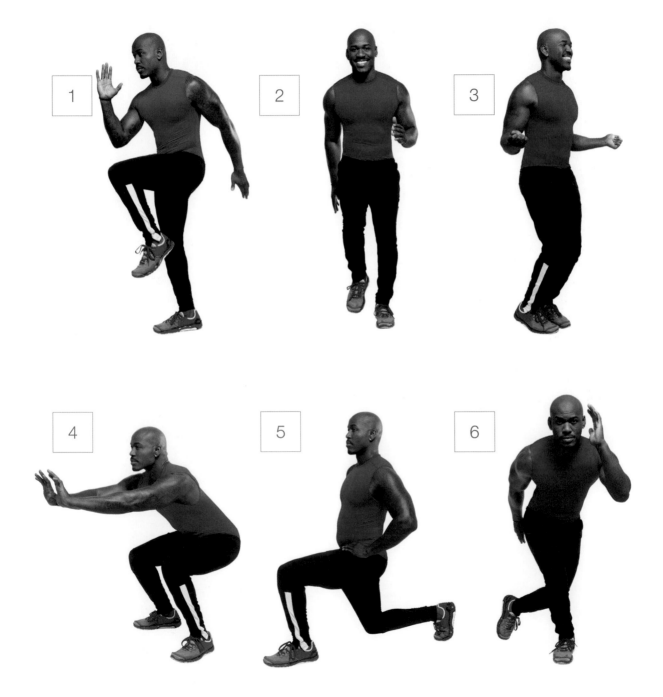

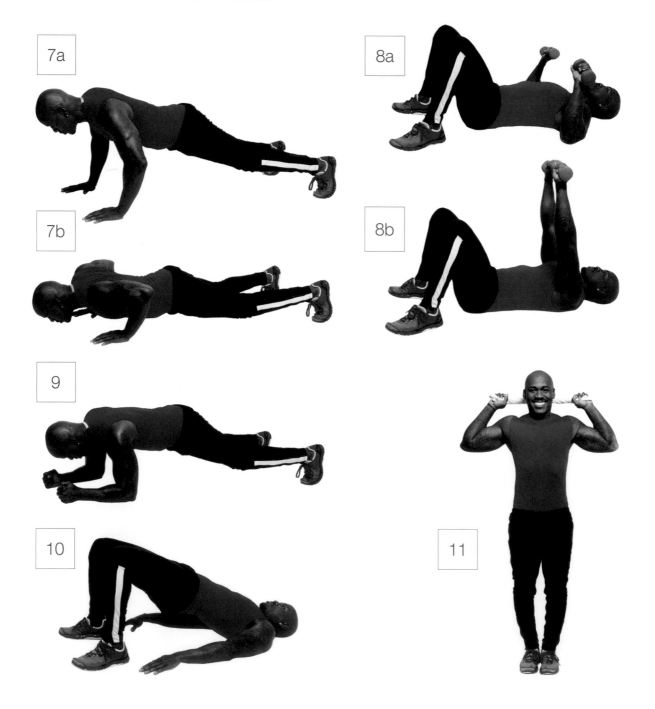

7a

7b

8a

8b

9

10

11

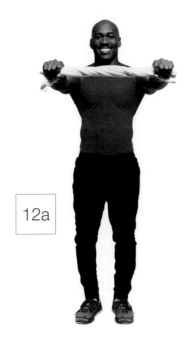

12a

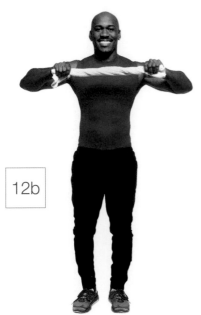

12b

MEALS

BREAKFAST

morning oatmeal

Prepare ½ cup oats with ½ to ¾ cup water. Top with 1 sliced peach and 7 chopped walnuts (½ oz.). Serve with 1 cup skim milk.

NUTRITION INFO: *Calories 387, Fat (g) 12, Sat fat (g), 1 Protein (g) 17, Carbs (g) 58, Fiber (g) 7, Sodium (mg) 121*

LUNCH

hearty blt salad

Start with 3 cups chopped romaine lettuce. Add 2 slices chopped turkey bacon, 1 cup chopped tomatoes, ½ cup (thawed) frozen corn, ½ cup chopped cucumber, 2 Tbsp. unsalted sunflower seeds, and 2 Tbsp. fat-free ranch dressing.

VEGETARIAN OPTION Skip the bacon; sprinkle on some smoked pepper or paprika.

NUTRITION INFO: *Calories 330, Fat (g) 13, Sat fat (g) 1, Protein (g) 17, Carbs (g) 39, Fiber (g) 7, Sodium (mg) 482*

DINNER

easy honey mustard chicken

See recipe for Easy Honey Mustard Chicken on page 69.

SNACKS

Choose up to 300 calories of snacks to reach your calorie goal for the day. See the lists in Chapter 3 for snack ideas.

day 7

morning motivation:

You're Not Perfect.

Nobody's perfect. We don't expect you to be perfect—that's not what this program is about. We want you to be become more aware of how your choices are affecting your life, and work on always being better than yesterday. Pause for a moment and think about yesterday. What did you do well? Did you have any moments where you wished for a re-wind or "do-over" button? If so, how will you do better today? This isn't a race, there are no winners, and there is no single "right" path. You're doing this your way, so cut yourself some slack even as you strive each day to become the person you know you can be.

active rest day

Today is a chance to kick back and let your body, and your mind, have a rest. We've called it an "Active Rest Day" because you don't have to be a coach potato. If you feel like it, include some light exercise such as a walk or a gentle yoga class.

Remember that this was your first week—you've already done a great job by getting started. Whether you did all the workouts as written, rested an extra day, or modified every move, you should be proud of yourself. It's not about being perfect; it's about progress! No matter what, honor yourself for any efforts you made and take this motivation with you into the next week.

MEALS

BREAKFAST
oatmeal pancakes

Serve with 1 cup blueberries and 1 Tbsp. maple syrup.
Blend 2 egg whites with ½ cup oats and ½ banana,
plus a pinch of cinnamon and ¼ tsp. vanilla extract.
Pour into a greased skillet and cook as you would
pancakes.

NUTRITION INFO: *Calories 342, Fat (g) 4, Sat fat (g) 0, Protein (g)
14, Carbs (g) 69, Fiber (g) 6, Sodium (mg) 113*

LUNCH
tuna salad sandwich

See recipe on page 69.

Serve with 1 cup grapes, 2 carrots, and 2 Tbsp.
hummus.

DINNER
quick chicken parmesan

Top 1 cooked chicken breast (3-oz. portion) with 2
Tbsp. part-skim shredded mozzarella, ½ cup low-sodium pasta sauce, and 1 tsp. shredded Parmesan. Bake at
350° until bubbly, about 10 minutes (or microwave).
Serve over 1 cup whole-wheat pasta with 1 cup sautéed
mushrooms.

VEGETARIAN OPTION Sub in a low-sodium veggie burger
for the chicken.

NUTRITION INFO: *Calories 405, Fat (g) 6, Sat fat (g) 1, Protein (g)
40, Carbs (g) 48, Fiber (g) 5, Sodium (mg) 433*

DESSERT
chocolate peanut butter
fudge *See recipe on page 71.*

SNACKS

Choose up to 300 calories of snacks to reach your daily
goal. See the lists in Chapter 3 for snack ideas. Don't
forget to include your dessert in your food journal (dessert gets included with your snack calories).

WEEKLY RECIPES

BREAKFASTS
chocolate, banana,
peanut butter smoothie

This decadent smoothie is served at The Biggest
Loser Resorts Niagara.

SERVES 1   PREP TIME 5 minutes

- 1 small banana
- 1 cup unsweetened almond milk
- 1 serving chocolate protein powder
- 1 Tbsp. ground flaxseed
- ¼ cup plain fat-free Greek yogurt
- 2 tsp. powdered peanut butter

Combine all ingredients in a blender. Blend until
smooth. Add ice as needed to reach desired consistency.

NUTRITION INFO: *Calories 370, Fat (g) 5, Sat fat (g) 0, Protein (g)
33, Carbs (g) 54, Fiber (g) 9, Sodium (mg) 257*

note

This and all the delicious and nutritious
recipes provided by The Biggest Loser Resorts
Niagara were shared by Chef Mark Camalleri,
a Culinary Institute of America graduate and
native of western New York, where he trained
and honed his craft at some of the region's
most exclusive restaurants and clubs.

roasted red pepper hummus

Store-bought hummus is often packed with salt. This version, from The Biggest Loser Resorts Niagara, has only five ingredients and is low in sodium. Spread it on sandwiches or use as a dip with vegetables.

SERVES 10 (serving size 2 Tbsp.)   PREP TIME 5 minutes

- 1 (14.5-oz.) can garbanzo beans, drained
- ¾ cup roasted red peppers
- 1 Tbsp. lemon juice
- 1 tsp. ground cumin
- 2 oz. extra-virgin olive oil

Combine all ingredients in a blender or food processor. Puree until smooth. Serve chilled, and refrigerate leftover hummus for up to 1 week.

NUTRITION INFO: *Calories 122, Fat (g) 7, Sat fat (g) 0, Protein (g) 4, Carbs (g) 13, Fiber (g) 3, Sodium (mg) 44*

turkey wrap

Dried cranberries add a nice twist to the usual turkey sandwich!

SERVES 1   PREP TIME 5 minutes

- 2 Tbsp. dried cranberries
- 2 Tbsp. plain fat-free Greek yogurt
- 1 (8-inch) whole-wheat tortilla
- 1 cup spinach
- 2 oz. lower-sodium deli turkey
- 1 mandarin orange

Mix the dried cranberries and the yogurt. Fill tortilla with spinach, turkey, and cranberry mixture, and roll the tortilla over the ingredients. Cut into 2 pieces.

Serve with a mandarin orange.

VEGETARIAN OPTION Swap in ½ cup mashed white beans for the turkey.

NUTRITION INFO: *Calories 282, Fat (g) 1, Sat fat (g) 0, Protein (g) 19, Carbs (g) 50, Fiber (g) 7, Sodium (mg) 484*

tuna salad sandwich

Who doesn't love a healthier version of a classic sandwich?

SERVES 1   PREP TIME 5 minutes

- 1 (2.6-oz.) pouch low-sodium tuna packed in water
- ¼ cup chopped red bell pepper
- 1 scallion, greens and whites chopped
- 1 Tbsp. light mayonnaise
- 2 slices whole-wheat bread
- 2 slices tomato
- 1 cup lettuce

Combine tuna, bell pepper, scallion, and mayonnaise in a small bowl.

Spoon tuna mixture over 1 slice of bread, and top with tomato and lettuce.

Add the other slice of bread to make a sandwich. Toast, if you prefer.

VEGETARIAN OPTION Swap in ½ cup cooked chickpeas combined with a pinch of powdered seaweed for the tuna.

NUTRITION INFO: *Calories 250, Fat (g) 5, Sat fat (g) 1, Protein (g) 17, Carbs (g) 32, Fiber (g) 5, Sodium (mg) 407*

DINNERS

easy honey mustard chicken

This delicious dinner is full of flavor, thanks to a sauce made from just two simple ingredients.

SERVES 1   PREP TIME 15 minutes   COOK TIME 45 minutes

- 1 small sweet potato
- 1 Tbsp. honey
- 2 tsp. yellow mustard
- 4 oz. chicken breast
- 2 cups broccoli florets

Preheat the oven to 375°. Pierce the sweet potato with a fork several times and place in the pre-heated oven. Bake for 45 minutes.

Combine honey and mustard, and coat the chicken evenly.

While the sweet potato is baking, steam or saute the brocccoli. Spray a nonstick skillet with cooking spray and cook chicken over medium heat for approximately 3 minutes on each side or until cooked through.

VEGETARIAN OPTION Sub in 3 oz. tofu for the chicken.

NUTRITION INFO: *Calories 346, Fat (g) 1, Sat fat (g) 0, Protein (g) 35, Carbs (g) 49, Fiber (g) 7, Sodium (mg) 294*

grilled pork with honey bbq sauce

This sweet and tangy supper is ready in 30 minutes.

SERVES 2   PREP TIME 5 minutes   COOK TIME 20 minutes

¼ cup BBQ sauce
1 Tbsp. rum
1 Tbsp. honey
8 oz. lean pork

Prepare grill.

Combine barbecue sauce, rum, and honey in a medium saucepan; bring to a boil. Cook 2 minutes or until reduced to ¼ cup. Reserve 1 Tbsp. sauce for serving. Use remaining sauce for basting.

Place pork on grill rack coated with cooking spray; grill 8 minutes. Turn and baste pork with sauce; cook 8 minutes. Turn and baste with sauce. Cook 4 minutes or until a thermometer registers 160° (slightly pink). Let stand 5 minutes; cut into thin slices.

Spoon 1 Tbsp. sauce over each serving.

Refrigerate one portion for later in the week.

NOTE If you don't want to use rum, swap in 1 Tbsp. cider vinegar instead.

VEGETARIAN OPTION Sub in 3 oz. tofu or tempeh for the pork.

NUTRITION INFO: *Calories 226, Fat (g) 5, Sat fat (g) 2, Protein (g) 23 Carbs (g) 17, Fiber (g) 0, Sodium (mg) 311*

two-bean chili con carne

Chili is usually an all-day dish, but this one just tastes like it cooked for hours!

SERVES 4   PREP TIME 13 minutes   COOK TIME 26 minutes

2 large green bell peppers, chopped
1 large onion, chopped
3 cloves garlic, chopped
8 oz. extra-lean ground beef
1 tsp. salt-free Mexican seasoning
1 (14.5-oz.) can no-salt-added diced tomatoes
1 (14.5-oz.) can dark red kidney beans, drained
1 (14.5-oz.) can black beans, drained
¼ cup salsa
1 Tbsp. plain fat-free Greek yogurt, to serve

Coat a Dutch oven with cooking spray; place over medium-high heat until hot. Add pepper, onion, and garlic; cook, stirring constantly, 3 to 5 minutes or until tender. Add ground beef, and cook until beef is browned, stirring until it crumbles. Drain well.

Stir Mexican seasoning into beef mixture; cook 1 minute. Add tomatoes and next 3 ingredients, stirring well. Bring to a boil. Cover, reduce heat, and simmer 20 minutes, stirring occasionally.

Ladle one portion of the chili into a serving bowl and top with Greek yogurt.

Refrigerate two portions for later in the week; share or freeze the remaining portion for up to 1 month.

NOTE For added convenience, substitute frozen chopped green pepper and frozen chopped onion for fresh in this recipe. Keep a bag of each in the freezer, and measure out the amount you need at any time.

VEGETARIAN OPTION Sub in 1 additional can of beans for the beef.

NUTRITION INFO: *Calories 286, Fat (g) 3, Sat fat (g) 1, Protein (g) 24, Carbs (g) 47, Fiber (g) 13, Sodium (mg) 169*

quick tandoori salmon

Yogurt and tandoori spices yield a juicy, savory salmon dinner.

SERVES 1 PREP TIME 5 minutes COOK TIME 10 minutes

- 1 tsp. tandoori paste
- 2 Tbsp. fat-free Greek yogurt
- 4 oz. salmon fillet
- 2 cups salad greens
- 2 Tbsp. plain fat-free vinaigrette
- ½ cup cooked brown rice

Combine tandoori paste with the yogurt, and coat the salmon fillet.

Spray a nonstick pan with cooking spray and heat over medium heat; cook the salmon for 3 minutes on each side or until just cooked through.

Serve with the salad and rice.

VEGETARIAN OPTION Sub in 3 oz. tofu or tempeh for the salmon.

NUTRITION INFO: *Calories 316, Fat (g) 5, Sat fat (g) 1, Protein (g) 35, Carbs (g) 29, Fiber (g) 1, Sodium (mg) 418*

DESSERTS

chocolate peanut butter fudge

This simple, decadent fudge is low in fat, thanks to the evaporated milk and powdered peanut butter. Choose high-quality chocolate for this dish, which is courtesy of The Biggest Loser Resorts Niagara.

SERVES 4 PREP TIME 5 minutes COOK TIME 5 minutes

- 2 oz. chocolate (at least 50% cacao)
- 2 Tbsp. fat-free evaporated milk
- 2 Tbsp. powdered peanut butter
- Dash of vanilla extract or other extract

Melt the chocolate, using a double boiler. Heat the evaporated milk in a small saucepan. Add the powdered peanut butter and vanilla to the warm evaporated milk, and then slowly add the melted chocolate until fully incorporated and smooth. Do not let mixture boil, or the cocoa butter will separate. Pour into a small dish lined with parchment paper. Spread the fudge fairly thin. Cool to room temperature or put it in the refrigerator. When cooled and set, cut into 2" x 2" pieces (1 oz. each). Try rolling into truffles topped with cocoa powder.

Share the other servings or freeze them.

NUTRITION INFO: *Calories 113, Fat (g) 6, Sat fat (g) 1, Protein (g) 3, Carbs (g) 12, Fiber (g) 2, Sodium (mg) 36*

week 2 congratulations

on your amazing effort in Week 1. You did it. You showed up, participated, and now here we are starting Week 2. The weeks will soon be flying by!

Starting a new program can be exciting and a little overwhelming. You've made a commitment to be here: That is the first step to success. When it gets tough, just breathe; we are here together.

When you start working out with this type of intensity, you are going to be sore. That is normal, and it is OK. Keep doing what you are doing and modify the moves if needed. Don't let the soreness keep you from working out—keep going. You can go slower or modify any moves that feel too challenging for you.

Listen to your body and rest when you need to. Remember, though, that it is normal for you to feel sore after a workout—that's your muscles telling you that they're getting stronger! Soreness is not the same as injury. It's normal to be tired or sore in the days after a workout, but you should never feel sharp, sudden, or stabbing/throbbing pain during or after a workout. Soreness won't cause swelling or be felt only in one body part. If you have any questions about whether you are sore or injured, please call your physician immediately.

set a goal—that's an order!

We said it last week and we'll say it again: We believe in setting small, achievable goals. Most importantly, we believe in setting goals every week. We want you to start this week by setting a Week 2 goal that you can conquer by this coming Sunday.

Your goal this week could be a repeat of last week's goal. Or it could be something you struggled with in Week 1 that you want to improve on.

Avoid setting too many goals for the week: Focus on something realistic that is within your control. This ensures that you "win" often and keep that good feeling going. Don't underestimate how important it is to set yourself up for success— this will be a long journey for many of you, and you're going to need small victories often to help you stay focused on your long-term goal.

WEEKLY WORKOUTS

MONDAY	Curtsy To The King
TUESDAY	Honor
WEDNESDAY	DYOW
THURSDAY	No Challenge, No Change
FRIDAY	Don't Hate Us For It
SATURDAY	Last-Chance Workout— Patrick
SUNDAY	Active Rest Day

coaches' corner

WHO'S WITH YOU? A support network and a list of local resources are both important for keeping your journey interesting and on track.

First, think about who you have in your life that you can truly count on to support you unconditionally. These are people with whom you can share your victories, your challenges, and your slips or lapses, and they will remain solidly in your corner. They don't try to "fix" you by telling you how you should be doing things. They're just good listeners and are there to help you find what you need to be successful. There is no pressure to come up with someone. Be picky. As your support group comes to mind, make a list. If you think of several, limit your list to your top five. These people are your "inner circle."

Next, do some research and locate some resources that can help you stay on track. These resources can be online, like The Biggest Loser Club, or in your community, like

your local gym, walking club, or church group. If you think of several, limit your list to your top five.

To help you recall your lists and put them to use, you might try some of the following ideas or make up your own:

- Create a fitness or healthy eating "challenge" that includes your inner circle and/or uses one of your resources.

- Take pictures of your inner circle and keep them somewhere that reminds you they're there for you.

- Create a private Facebook group where you and your inner circle can share your stories and motivate one another.

- Ask someone in your inner circle to exercise with you on a consistent basis.

- Increase your accountability by asking a close friend to agree to share daily or weekly updates.

WEEK 2 MEALS

MONDAY

B   Protein Mocha Shake
L   Confetti Quinoa
D   Egg Fried Rice

TUESDAY

B   Egg White Scramble
L   Bahn Mi Salad
D   Cheesy Quinoa & Broccoli

WEDNESDAY

B   Slim Bagel Sandwich
L   Cheesy Quinoa & Broccoli
D   Parsley & Lemon Fish

THURSDAY

B   Peanut Butter Toast
L   Open-Face Turkey & Swiss Melt
D   Mark's BBQ Sauce with Chicken

FRIDAY

B   Breakfast Quinoa Bowl
L   BBQ Chicken Pizza
D   Egg White Scramble

SATURDAY

B   Breakfast Bacon & Egg Grilled Cheese
L   Grown-Up PBJ
D   Sesame Salmon with Rice Noodles

SUNDAY

B   Spicy Turkey Breakfast Quesadilla
L   Roast Beef Lettuce Pocket with Horse-
    radish Mayonnaise
D   Tempeh Vegetable Stir-Fry

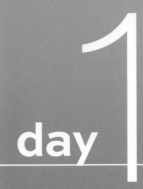

day 1

nutrition bite:

Rethink Your Splurge.

Splurges happen, and so do cravings. Oftentimes, such as with a holiday or special event, you know it's coming. Other times they come out of nowhere, but you can't think about anything else! A key to weight-loss success is to keep your indulgence to just the meal or the day and not the entire weekend. Try "bookending" your splurge by working out hard and eating extra healthy the day before and the day after and sticking to the principles of healthy eating: portion control and stopping when you're nearing fullness. What matters most after an indulgence is letting it go and getting back on track quickly. Have that cupcake, and get on with the rest of your life.

WORKOUT curtsy to the king

30 MINUTES | WARM UP FOR 5 MINUTES

THE WORKOUT

INTERVAL A

1 Jogging X 30 seconds

2 High Knees X 30 seconds

3 Traveling Squats X 30 seconds

Then do

4 Squats X 1 minute

5 Side Lunges X 1 minute

INTERVAL B

1 High Knees with Torso Twist X 30 seconds

2 Rear-Stepping Lunges with Woodchops X 30 seconds

3 Jumping Jacks X 30 seconds

Then do

4 Push-Ups X 1 minute

Repeat Interval A, then do

5 Forward Lunges X 1 minute

6 Curtsies X 1 minute

Repeat Interval B, then do

7 Lat Pulldowns X 1 minute

(CONTINUES)

In today's workout you'll curtsy to the king! We couldn't wait any longer to introduce this FAVORITE move—the curtsy. It's a great booty exercise, and we hope you love it as much as we do. Note that there are two rounds of intervals that you'll repeat throughout this workout and also intersperse new moves.

INTERVAL A

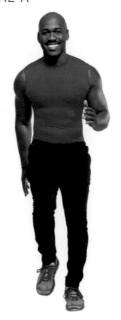

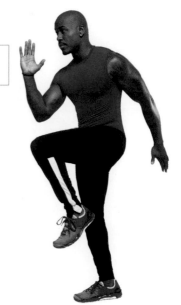

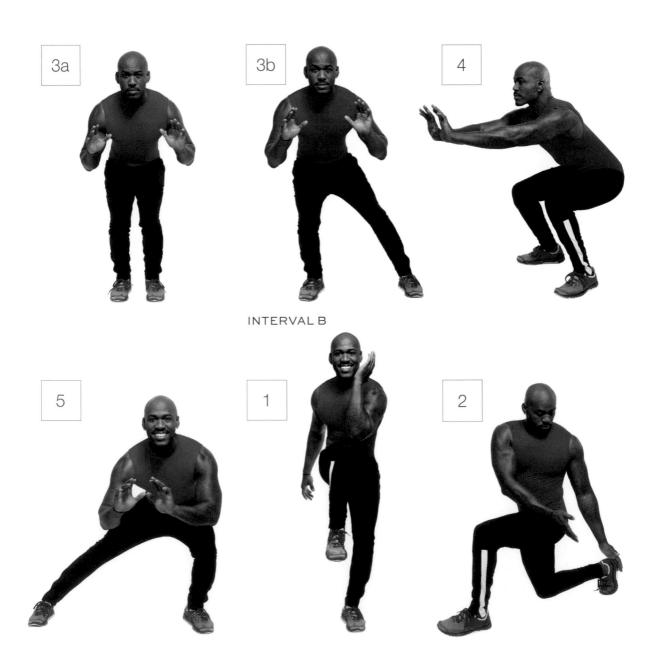

3a

3b

4

INTERVAL B

5

1

2

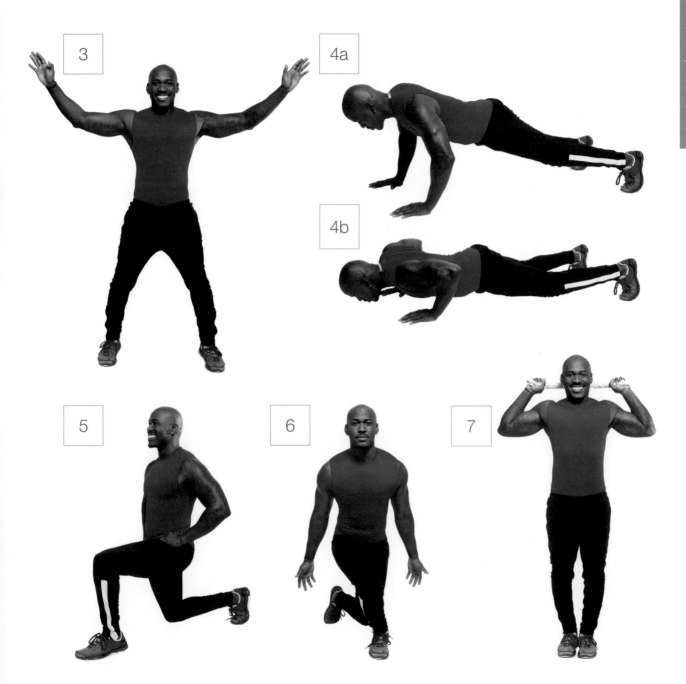

THE WORKOUT

CONTINUED

Repeat Interval A, then do

1 Side Lunges X
1 minute

2 Curtsies X 1 minute

3 Bicycle Crunches X
1 minute

COOL DOWN FOR
5 MINUTES

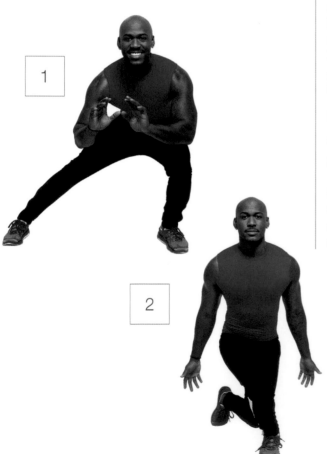

MEALS

BREAKFAST

protein mocha shake

Serve with 7 walnut halves (½ oz).
In a blender, combine 1 cup skim milk, ½ cup ice, 1
scoop chocolate protein powder, 1 banana, and 1 tsp.
instant coffee.

NUTRITION INFO: *Calories 296, Fat (g) 2, Sat fat (g) 0, Protein (g)
28, Carbs (g) 44, Fiber (g) 6, Sodium (mg) 170*

LUNCH

confetti quinoa

Toss ½ cup cooked quinoa with ½ cup shelled edamame, ½ cup shredded carrots, ½ cup chopped yellow
bell pepper, 2 Tbsp. chopped red onion, 1 Tbsp. dried
cranberries, and 1 Tbsp. reduced-fat feta cheese.
Drizzle on 1 to 2 Tbsp. fat-free balsamic vinaigrette.

NUTRITION INFO: *Calories 374, Fat (g) 9, Sat fat (g) 2, Protein (g)
21, Carbs (g) 56, Fiber (g) 10, Sodium (mg) 396*

DINNER

egg fried rice

See recipe on page 101.

SNACKS

Choose up to 300 calories of snacks to reach your
calorie goal for the day. See the lists in Chapter 3 for
snack ideas.

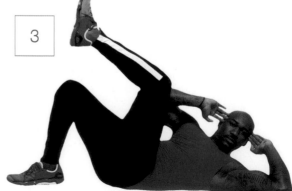

day 2

morning motivation:

Mind Over Body.

Tell your mind to get out of your body's way. Fear will stop you long before physical limitations do. And there's no better feeling than trying a workout or a particular move you think you "can't do," only to realize you can. Yes, you can. Doing a move with modifications is still doing the move. Even if your body says "enough" after one or two repetitions, that's OK. You still gave it your best, and you didn't let your mind hold you back from getting a great workout.

honor

36 MINUTES

WARM UP FOR 5 MINUTES

This workout is called Honor in honor of all of you who keep coming back, day after day. Losing weight and getting strong isn't easy, but what counts most is respecting the program, trusting the process, and showing up on the gym floor (aka your living room) when you least want to.

"Why do we only believe our worst reviews? It's crazy how we fixate on the negative. You would never believe these comments about your friends and family, so why are you believing them about yourself? Focus on the positive. What awesome things are you doing? You've decided to change your future—focus on that!"
—*The Biggest Loser* trainer Jennifer Widerstrom

THE WORKOUT

2 ROUNDS

1 High Knees X 30 seconds

2 Jogging X 30 seconds

3 Air Jump Rope X 30 seconds

4 Walking X 1 minute

— Jogging X 30 seconds

— Air Jump Rope X 30 seconds

5 Skater Jumps X 1 minute

— Walking X 1 minute

6 High Knees with Torso Twist X 1 minute

7 Rear-Stepping Lunges with Woodchops X 30 seconds

8 Jumping Jacks X 30 seconds

— Air Jump Rope X 1 minute

— Jogging X 30 seconds

— High Knees X 30 seconds

9 Traveling Squats X 30 seconds

— Air Jump Rope X 1 minute

— Rear-Stepping Lunges with Woodchops X 30 seconds

— Jumping Jacks X 30 seconds

— Walking X 1 minute

Repeat for Round 2

COOL DOWN FOR 5 MINUTES

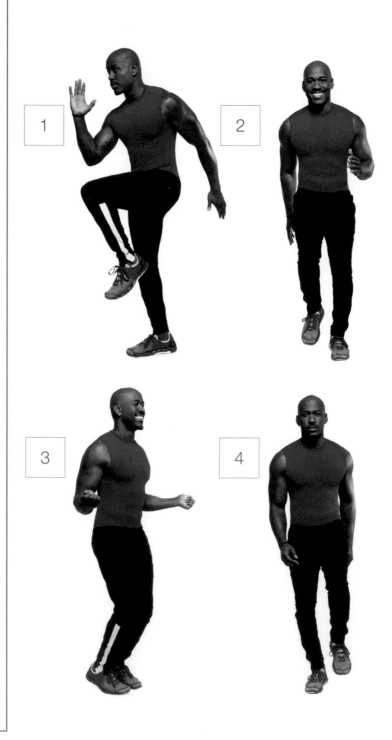

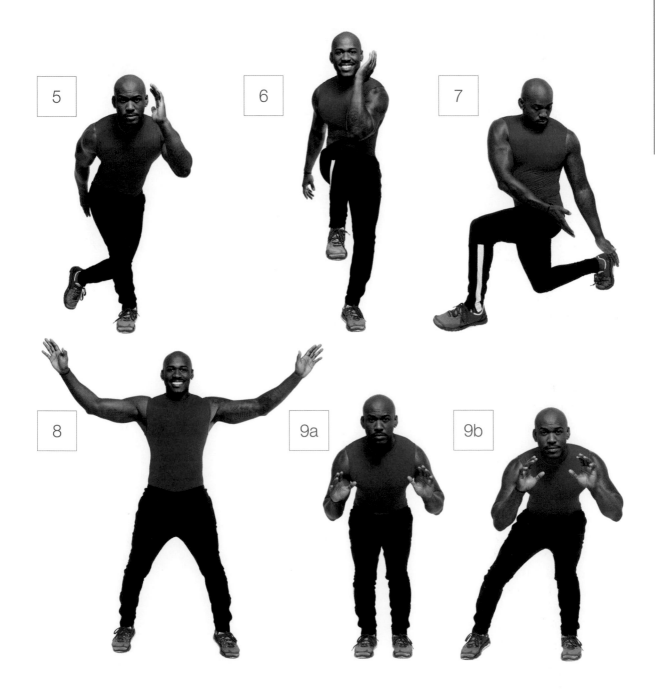

5

6

7

8

9a

9b

MEALS

BREAKFAST
egg white scramble
See recipe on page 100.

LUNCH
bahn mi salad

Serve with 1 oz. cooked brown rice noodles. Combine ½ cup each thinly sliced cucumbers, radishes, and carrots in a bowl with a pinch of salt and sugar and 1 tsp. rice vinegar. Set aside. Meanwhile, shred 3 oz. cooked pork tenderloin and place atop 3 cups salad greens. Drain the veggies, reserving the vinegar and mixing it with 1 Tbsp. reduced-fat mayonnaise. Drizzle the dressing on the salad, and add jalapeño slices (optional) and a handful of chopped cilantro.

VEGETARIAN OPTION Sub in 3 oz. cooked tofu or tempeh for the pork.

NUTRITION INFO: *Calories 234, Fat (g) 5, Sat fat (g) 2, Protein (g) 23, Carbs (g) 21, Fiber (g) 8, Sodium (mg) 475*

DINNER
cheesy quinoa & broccoli

In a small pot, stir together 2 oz. shredded reduced-fat cheddar cheese, ¼ cup each plain fat-free Greek yogurt and skim milk, and plenty of black pepper. Add 2 cups cooked quinoa and 4 cups cooked broccoli. Heat until the sauce has thickened.

NOTE You'll save half for lunch tomorrow.

NUTRITION INFO: *Calories 358, Fat (g) 7, Sat fat (g) 2, Protein (g) 22, Carbs (g) 54, Fiber (g) 9, Sodium (mg) 212*

SNACKS
Choose up to 300 calories of snacks to reach your calorie goal for the day. See the lists in Chapter 3 for snack ideas.

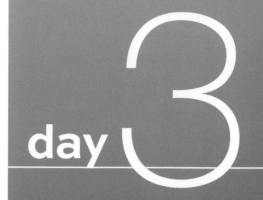

day 3

check-in:

So, It's the Middle of the Week.

How are you doing this week? What's working? What isn't? When the going gets tough, look at your goal for the week to remind yourself why you're doing this—and hit up your inner circle for some extra support. You've got this!

WORKOUT

do your own workout (dyow)

Just like last week, you get to choose the workout you do today. Go for a walk, take a kickboxing class, or do some yoga.

If you're stuck for ideas, simply repeat or flip ahead to one of the other workouts from this week.

It's OK to take this workout as an extra rest day, but only if your body needs it.

> **❝**Keep your power. We live a hectic, non-stop, fast-paced everything. We give to our spouses, kids, bosses, family, and friends. This is a friendly reminder to keep some of your amazing power for yourself. You are worth it, you deserve it, and most of all you need it.**❞**
> —*The Biggest Loser* trainer Jessie Pavelka

MEALS

BREAKFAST

slim bagel sandwich

Serve with 1 orange and 1 cup skim milk. Toast 1 thin whole-grain bagel. Spread on 1 Tbsp. reduced-fat herb and garlic cream cheese, and top with 3 oz. lean lower-sodium deli turkey, 1 slice tomato, 1 slice red onion, and a few slices of cucumber.

VEGETARIAN OPTION Sub 2 Tbsp. hummus for the cream cheese and turkey.

NUTRITION INFO: *Calories 210, Fat (g) 4, Sat fat (g) 2, Protein (g) 17, Carbs (g) 34, Fiber (g) 5, Sodium (mg) 433*

LUNCH

cheesy quinoa & broccoli

Last night's leftovers become today's lunch!

DINNER

parsley & lemon fish

See recipe on page 102.

Serve with 2 cups roasted or steamed cauliflower and 1 cup skim milk.

DESSERT

s'more stuffed banana

Preheat oven to 350°. Place 1 small banana on a piece of aluminum foil. Slice it down the middle almost all the way through. Fill with 1 tsp. each mini chocolate chips and mini marshmallows. Seal the foil around the banana, and bake for 10 minutes. Top with ¼ graham cracker sheet, crumbled.

NUTRITION INFO: *Calories 123, Fat (g) 2, Sat fat (g) 1, Protein (g) 2, Carbs (g) 35, Fiber (g) 3, Sodium (mg) 15*

SNACKS

Choose up to 300 calories of snacks to reach your daily goal. See the lists in Chapter 3 for snack ideas. Don't forget to include your dessert in your food journal (dessert gets included with your snack calories).

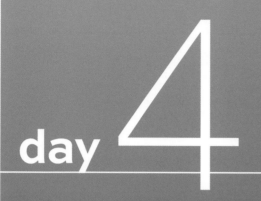

day 4

morning motivation:

Make It Happen.

Don't wait for it to happen. Make it happen. No one will do this for you. We are here to guide you, but at the end of the day, you're the only person who can make it happen. You have it within you. We know you do.

no challenge, no change

30 MINUTES
WARM UP FOR 5 MINUTES

That's the rule of fitness: no challenge, no change. It's the principle behind "body confusion," and it's also why each week of your program includes new moves or subtle changes to keep you challenged physically and mentally. That's how you get great results! Note that there are two sets of cardio intervals you will repeat at various times during the workout.

THE WORKOUT

INTERVAL A

1 Jogging X 30 seconds
2 High Knees X 30 seconds
3 Traveling Squats X 30 seconds

Then do

4 Squats X 1 minute or 15 reps
5 Forward Lunges X 1 minute or 6 reps per side

INTERVAL B

1 High Knees with Torso Twist X 30 seconds
2 Rear-Stepping Lunges with Woodchops X 30 seconds
3 Jumping Jacks X 30 seconds

Then do

4 Chest Presses X 1 minute

(CONTINUES)

INTERVAL A

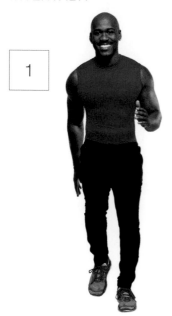

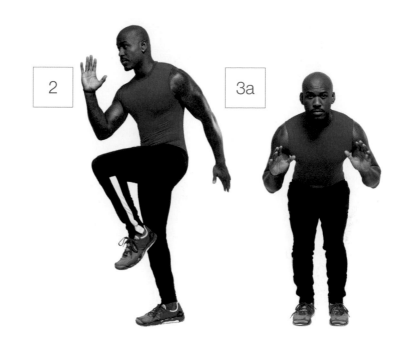

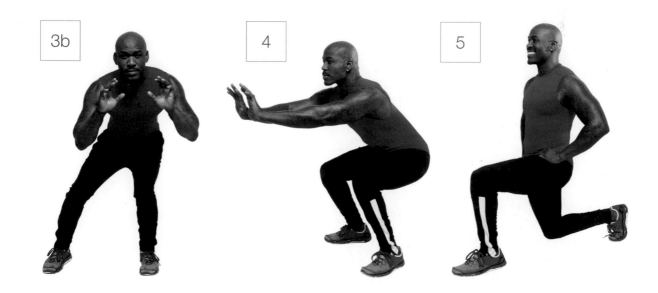

INTERVAL B

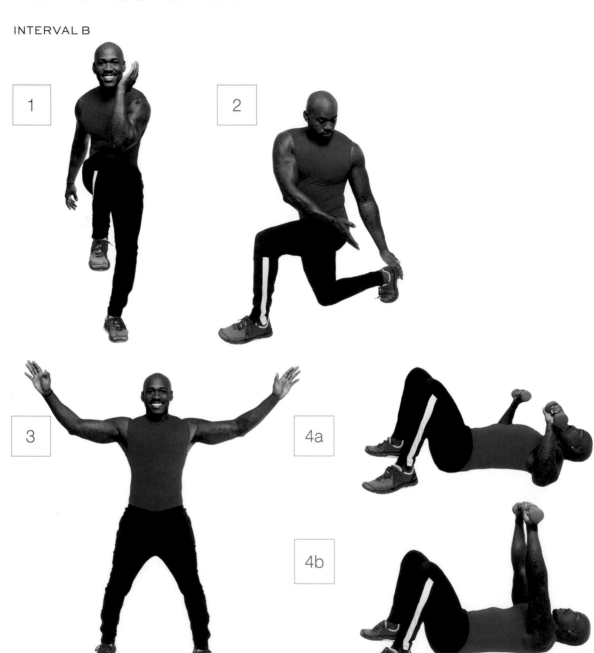

Repeat Interval A, then do

1 Curtsies X 1 minute

2 Side Lunges X 1 minute

Repeat Interval B, then do

3 Two-Arm Rows X 1 minute

Repeat Interval A, then do

4 Rear Lunges X 1 minute

— Squats X 1 minute

Repeat Interval B, then do

5 Russian Twists X 1 minute

COOL DOWN FOR 5 MINUTES

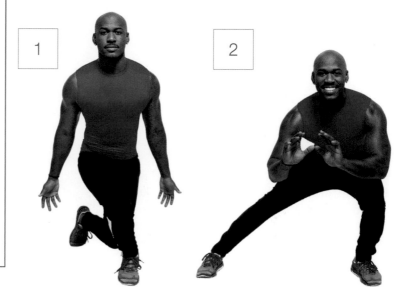

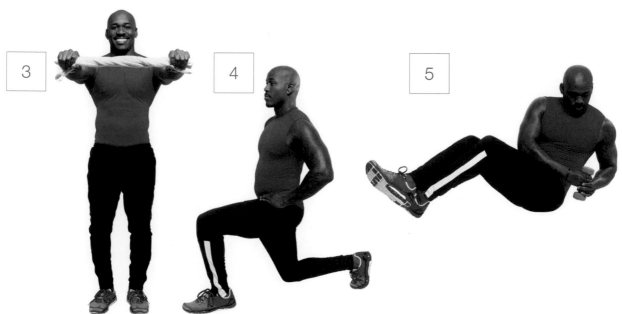

MEALS

BREAKFAST

peanut butter toast

Serve 2 slices whole-wheat bread, 1 Tbsp. peanut butter (or another nut butter), and 1 medium piece of fruit with 1 cup skim milk.

NUTRITION INFO: *Calories 395, Fat (g) 10, Sat fat (g) 1, Protein (g) 20, Carbs (g) 59, Fiber (g) 7, Sodium (mg) 390*

LUNCH

open-face turkey & swiss melt

Spread Dijon mustard on 2 slices whole-wheat bread. Divide 3 oz. lower-sodium deli turkey between the bread, then top each with ½ slice reduced-fat Swiss cheese. Broil until the cheese melts. Serve with 1 cup carrot and celery sticks with 2 Tbsp. fat-free salad dressing.

VEGETARIAN OPTION Skip the turkey and add a sliced hard-boiled egg.

NUTRITION INFO: *Calories 330, Fat (g) 5, Sat fat (1g), Protein (g) 27, Carbs (g) 48, Fiber (g) 4, Sodium (mg) 418*

DINNER

mark's bbq sauce with chicken

Serve 3 oz. cooked chicken breast with 1 serving Mark's BBQ Sauce (see recipe page 101), 1 small sweet potato, and 2 cups green beans.

VEGETARIAN OPTION Sub in 3 oz. grilled tofu or tempeh for the chicken.

NUTRITION INFO: *Calories 340, Fat (g) 1, Sat fat (g) 0, Protein (g) 31, Carbs (g) 46, Fiber (g) 8, Sodium (mg) 201*

SNACKS

Choose up to 300 calories of snacks to reach your calorie goal for the day. See the lists in Chapter 3 for snack ideas.

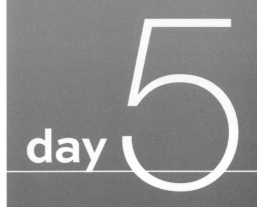

day 5

nutrition bite:

Healthier Favorites.

If you're battling the desire for a favorite comfort or snack food, try negotiating with yourself. Would a healthy smoothie satisfy your craving for ice cream? Would baked chips with a tasty salsa help satisfy your desire for that salty crunch? Make a habit of asking yourself: "How can I satisfy this craving in a healthier way?"

WORKOUT don't hate us for it

33 MINUTES | WARM UP FOR 5 MINUTES

In today's workout, we introduce an intense move new to this Bootcamp: burpees. That also explains the title of this workout (if you don't know what we mean now, you will 10 minutes into your workout—but you'll still be back tomorrow, right?).

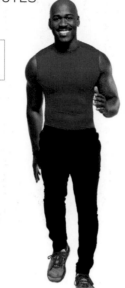

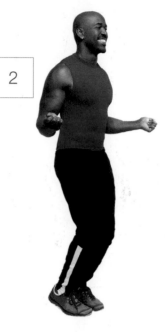

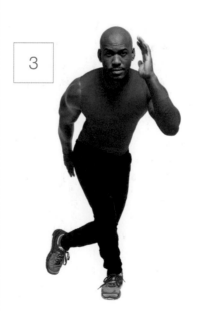

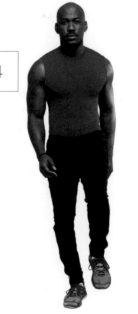

THE WORKOUT

2 ROUNDS

1   Jogging X 30 seconds
2   Air Jump Rope X 30 seconds
3   Skater Jumps X 30 seconds
4   Walking X 1 minute
—   Skater Jumps X 30 seconds
5   High Knees with Torso Twist X 30 seconds
6   Quick Feet X 30 seconds
—   Walking X 1 minute
—   Jogging X 30 seconds
7   High Knees X 30 seconds
8   Traveling Squats X 30 seconds

(CONTINUES)

THE WORKOUT
CONTINUED

— Air Jump Rope X 1 minute

9   Curtsies X 30 seconds

10 Burpees X 30 seconds

11 Forward Lunges X 30 seconds

— Air Jump Rope X 1 minute

— Jogging X 30 seconds

— High Knees X 30 seconds

— Traveling Squats X 30 seconds

— Walking X 1 minute

Repeat for Round 2

COOL DOWN FOR 5 MINUTES

5

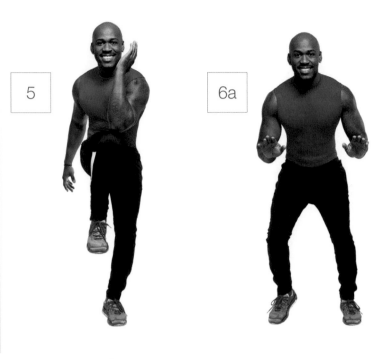

6a

6b

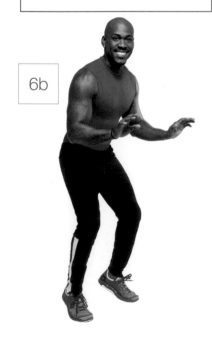

7

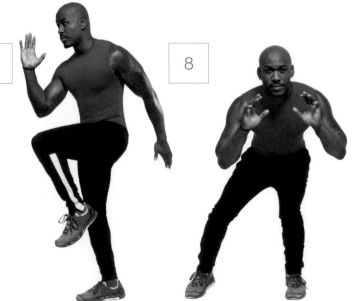

8

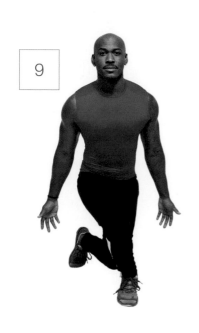

9

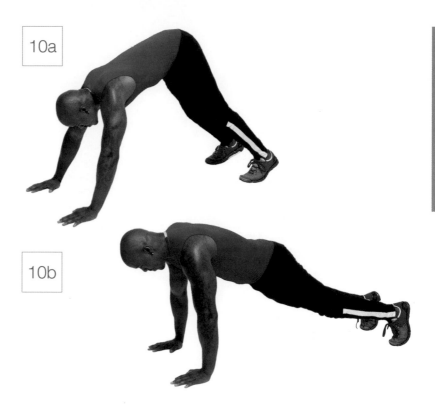

10a

10b

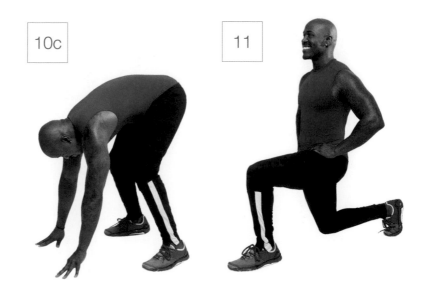

10c

11

91

MEALS

BREAKFAST

breakfast quinoa bowl

Reheat 1 cup cooked quinoa with ½ cup skim milk and ½ cup blueberries. Top with 2 Tbsp. sliced almonds and 1 tsp. brown sugar.

NUTRITION INFO: *Calories 416, Fat (g) 12, Sat fat (g) 1, Protein (g) 17, Carbs (g) 63, Fiber (g) 8, Sodium (mg) 79*

LUNCH

bbq chicken pizza

See recipe on page 100.

Serve with 2 cups green vegetables or a side salad with 2 Tbsp. fat-free vinaigrette.

VEGETARIAN OPTION Skip the chicken.

DINNER

egg white scramble

See recipe on page 100, swapping in different vegetables if you prefer.

Serve with 2 slices whole-wheat toast and 2 Tbsp. natural peanut butter, plus 1 orange.

SNACKS

Choose up to 300 calories of snacks to reach your calorie goal for the day. See the lists in Chapter 3 for snack ideas.

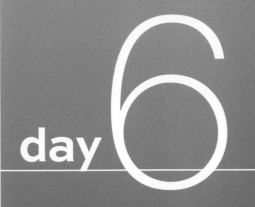

day 6

last chance:

Isn't it funny how Saturday seems to come around so quickly each week?

You know what time it is: your Last-Chance Workout. Make it count. We don't expect you to love these workouts. What you will love is the benefits they bring.

WORKOUT last-chance workout—patrick

45 MINUTES | WARM UP FOR 5 MINUTES

Today's last chance workout is dedicated to Season 10 winner Patrick House. Shout out to Patrick after you rock this workout. This father of two arrived on the Ranch weighing 400 pounds. At just 28 years old, he had high cholesterol, sleep apnea, and other health issues. Patrick lost 181 pounds and now works to help kids make better food choices. He did it—and so can you!

THE WORKOUT

2 ROUNDS

1 Squats X 1 minute
2 Rear Lunges X 1 minute
3 Skater Jumps X 1 minute

(CONTINUES)

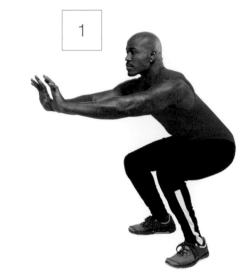

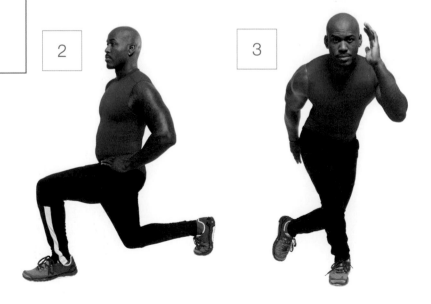

93

THE WORKOUT
CONTINUED

4 Push-Ups X 1 minute
5 Chest Presses X 1 minute
6 Jogging X 30 seconds
7 High Knees X 30 seconds
8 Traveling Squats X 30 seconds
9 Plank X 1 minute
10 Hip Bridge X 1 minute
11 Curtsies X 30 seconds

(CONTINUES)

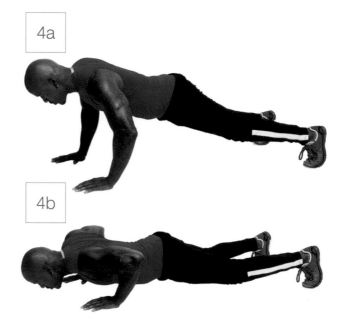

4a

4b

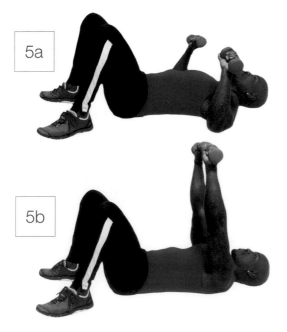

5a

5b

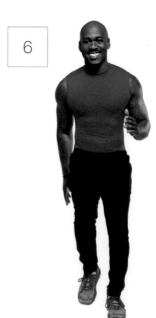

6

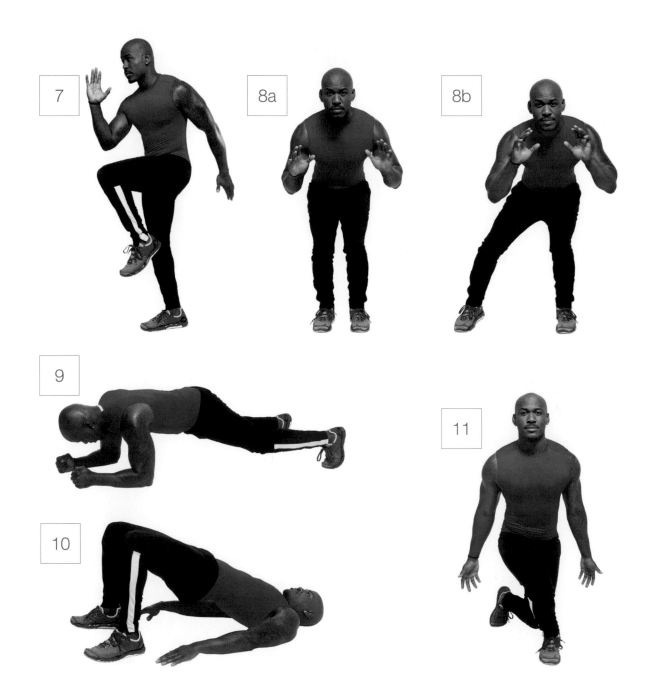

THE WORKOUT
CONTINUED

12 Burpees X 30 seconds

13 Forward Lunges X 30 seconds

14 Lat Pulldowns X 1 minute

15 Two-Arm Rows X 1 minute

16 Jumping Jacks X 1 minute

17 Forward Lunges X 1 minute

18 Side Lunges X 1 minute

19 Walking X 1 minute

Repeat for Round 2

COOL DOWN FOR 5 MINUTES

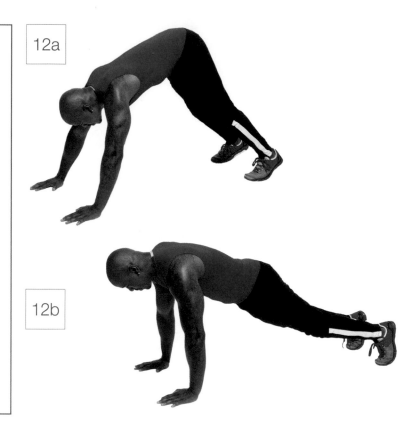

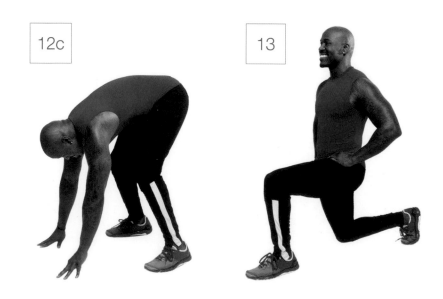

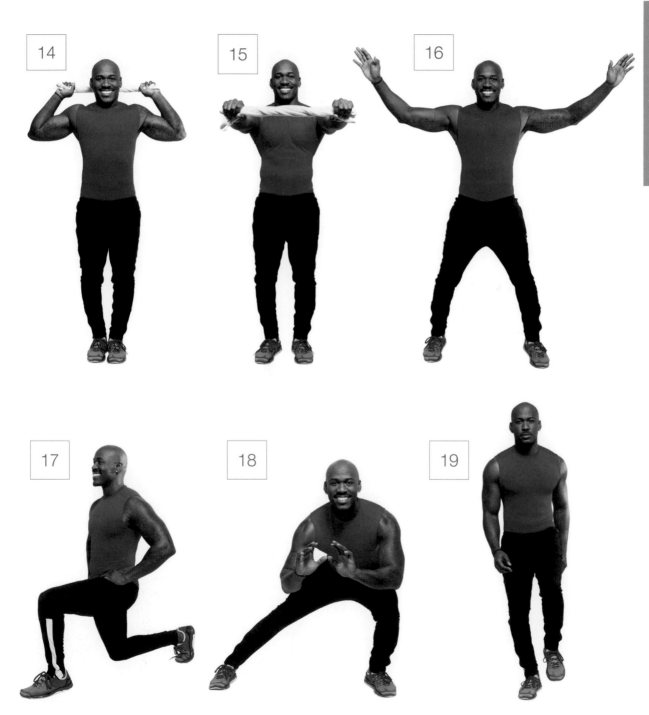

MEALS

BREAKFAST

breakfast bacon & egg grilled cheese

Serve with 1 orange and 1 cup skim milk.
Spread 1 tsp. margarine on 1 slice whole-wheat bread.
Toast the bread on 1 side in a skillet, then top with
2 cooked egg whites, 1 slice crumbled turkey bacon,
½ cup chopped fresh spinach, and 2 Tbsp. shredded
reduced-fat cheddar cheese. Continue cooking over
low heat until the cheese has melted.

VEGETARIAN OPTION: Sub in 1 slice tempeh bacon or
omit the bacon entirely.

NUTRITION INFO: *Calories 221, Fat (g) 11, Sat fat (g) 3, Protein (g)
19, Carbs (g) 14, Fiber (g) 2, Sodium (mg) 460*

LUNCH

grown-up pbj

Serve with 1 cup skim milk.
Mix 2 Tbsp. nut butter (cashew, sunflower seed, or
almond) with a pinch of sea salt and dried ginger.
Spread onto 2 slices whole-wheat bread. Top with ½
cup sliced strawberries.

NUTRITION INFO: *Calories 336, Fat (g) 18, Sat fat (g) 1, Protein
(g) 13, Carbs (g) 39, Fiber (g) 9, Sodium (mg) 231*

DINNER

sesame salmon with rice noodles

See recipe on page 102.

VEGETARIAN OPTION Sub in 3 oz. tempeh or tofu for
the salmon.

SNACKS

Choose up to 300 calories of snacks to reach your
calorie goal for the day. See the lists in Chapter 3 for
snack ideas.

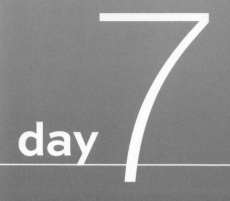

day 7

morning motivation:

You Gotta Work For It!

You might be new to working out,
but we suspect you're no stranger
to working hard. And you know
that in life, just like with your
health, everything takes work—at
least everything good, that is. We
like to say that if it doesn't challenge you, it doesn't change you.
You're feeling challenged, and
you're working hard. In return,
you're seeing results. Every bur-
pee, every healthy meal, and
every day, you're changing!

Today, you have to go out there
and work for it. Do your best, try
your hardest, and you will see
your work pay off.

WORKOUT

active rest day

You've made it through another week!

Congratulations. We are SO proud of you, and you should be, too. Give your body the rest it deserves so you'll be ready to start another week tomorrow. Remember that if you feel up for it, today is a great day to do some gentle stretching (such as yoga) or take a walk. You could even do some housework or gardening!

MEALS

BREAKFAST

spicy turkey breakfast quesadilla

Serve with 1 orange.
Sauté 2 oz. extra-lean ground turkey with ½ tsp. ground cumin, a pinch of chili powder, and ¼ cup each onions and peppers. Drain any excess grease, then add 1 egg and 1 egg white, scrambled. Heat 1 whole-grain tortilla in a skillet. Top with 1 Tbsp. shredded reduced-fat cheddar cheese and the turkey-egg mixture. Cut into wedges, and serve with 1 Tbsp. each plain fat-free Greek yogurt and low-sodium salsa for dipping.

VEGETARIAN OPTION Sub in ½ cup black or pinto beans for the turkey or omit it.

NUTRITION INFO: *Calories 342, Fat (g) 9, Sat fat (g) 3, Protein (g) 33, Carbs (g) 34, Fiber (g) 5, Sodium (mg) 489*

LUNCH

roast beef lettuce pocket with horseradish mayonnaise

Serve with 2 medium carrots and 2 Tbsp. hummus. Mix ¼ tsp. horseradish (or to taste) with 1 Tbsp. reduced-fat mayonnaise, and spread inside half of a whole-wheat pita. Add 3 oz. lean deli roast beef, 1 cup salad greens, and 3 slices tomato.

VEGETARIAN OPTION Sub in ½ cup mashed white beans for the beef.

NUTRITION INFO: *Calories 259, Fat (g) 8, Sat fat (g) 2, Protein (g) 22, Carbs (g) 29, Fiber (g) 4, Sodium (mg) 458*

DINNER

tempeh vegetable stir-fry

See recipe on page 103.

Serve with 1 cup brown rice or brown rice noodles.

DESSERT

baked apple

See recipe on page 103.

SNACKS

Choose up to 300 calories of snacks to reach your daily goal. See the lists in Chapter 3 for snack ideas. Don't forget to include your dessert in your food journal (dessert gets included with your snack calories).

WEEKLY RECIPES

BREAKFASTS

egg white scramble

Packed with protein but light enough for an everyday breakfast, you'll love this veggie-packed egg scramble. Use any veggies you like, but be sure to include at least a cup.

SERVES 1   PREP TIME 5 minutes   COOK TIME 7 minutes

- 2 Tbsp. chopped mushrooms
- 1½ cups spinach
- 2 Tbsp. chopped onions
- ¼ cup chopped bell peppers
- 3 egg whites

Spray cooking spray in a nonstick pan and heat over medium heat. Sauté the vegetables over medium heat until soft, about 5 minutes.

Whisk egg whites together and pour into the pan, cooking for 2 minutes or until set. Season with black pepper.

NUTRITION INFO: *Calories 81, Fat (g) 2, Sat fat (g) 0, Protein (g) 13, Carbs (g) 7, Fiber (g) 2, Sodium (mg) 202*

LUNCHES

bbq chicken pizza

This recipe, from The Biggest Loser Resorts Niagara, is a hit at lunchtime. We use Chef Mark's low-sugar, low-sodium BBQ sauce to keep this as healthy as it is delicious.

SERVES 2   PREP TIME 25 minutes   COOK TIME 15 minutes

- 4 oz. organic boneless, skinless chicken breast
- 3 Tbsp. Mark's BBQ Sauce (see recipe on page 101)
- 1 gluten-free pizza crust
- ¼ cup chopped tomatoes
- ¼ cup julienne red onion
- ¾ oz. (¼ cup) reduced-fat cheddar cheese, shredded
- ¾ oz. (¼ cup) Monterey Jack cheese, shredded

Preheat oven to 350°. Bake chicken on a baking pan until cooked, about 15 minutes. Let cool and cut into small pieces. Mix the cooked chicken with 2 Tbsp. of the BBQ sauce to coat. Brush remaining 1 Tbsp. of the BBQ sauce over pizza crust. Top pizza crust evenly with chopped chicken and the chopped tomatoes, onion, and cheeses. Bake at 350° for approximately 10 to 12 minutes. Refrigerate half for a snack, or serve to a guest.

VEGETARIAN OPTION Omit the chicken or sub in ½ cup black beans.

NUTRITION INFO: *Calories 258, Fat (g) 8, Sat fat (g) 3, Carbs (g) 23, Protein (g) 23, Fiber (g) 6, Sodium (mg) 405*

mark's bbq sauce

This tangy BBQ sauce is courtesy of The Biggest Loser Resorts Niagara. It is far lower in sugar and salt than commercial versions. It's an easy way to dress up grilled chicken and other lean protein.

SERVES 6 PREP TIME 5 minutes

- 7 oz. cider vinegar
- ½ Tbsp. black pepper
- 5 oz. ketchup
- 3 tsp. honey
- 2 Tbsp. molasses
- ¼ tsp. Tabasco sauce
- 2 tsp. granulated onion
- 1 Tbsp. Worcestershire sauce
- ⅛ tsp. chipotle pepper, (optional)
- 2 tsp. mustard

Combine all ingredients until well blended. Refrigerate leftovers for up to 2 weeks.

NUTRITION INFO: *Calories 48, Fat (g) 0, Sat fat (g) 0, Protein (g) 0, Carbs (g) 12, Fiber (g) 0, Sodium (mg) 42*

DINNERS

egg fried rice

This Chinese favorite is ready in less time than it takes to order takeout.

SERVES 1 PREP TIME 5 minutes COOK TIME 10 minutes

- 1 large egg
- 1 egg white
- ½ tsp. sesame oil
- ½ tsp. grated fresh ginger
- 1 (8-oz.) package frozen mixed vegetables
- ½ cup cooked brown rice
- 1 tsp. lower-sodium soy sauce

Break the egg and egg white into a small bowl and season with a dash of salt and pepper.

Heat a small nonstick skillet. Pour in the eggs and cook for 2 minutes on each side, until set. Slide the egg out of the pan, roughly chop into strips, and set aside.

Wipe the pan with a paper towel and place back on the heat. Add the sesame oil, ginger, and vegetables, and stir-fry for 3 minutes. Add a splash of water to help the vegetables cook, if required.

Mix in the rice and soy sauce. Cook for 2 minutes, stirring occasionally.

Toss the egg strips through the rice and continue heating until warmed through.

NUTRITION INFO: *Calories 380, Fat (g) 7, Sat fat (g) 0, Protein (g) 20, Carbs (g) 55, Fiber (g) 8, Sodium (mg) 414*

sesame salmon with rice noodles

Oodles of rice noodles and veggies are the perfect match for this savory salmon.

SERVES 1   PREP TIME 10 minutes   COOK TIME 15 minutes

- ¼ cup uncooked brown rice noodles
- 4 oz. salmon
- 1 cup snow peas
- 1 cup fresh green beans
- ½ zucchini, sliced
- ½ tsp. sesame seeds
- ½ tsp. grated fresh ginger
- 1 tsp. lower-sodium soy sauce
- 1½ Tbsp. honey
- ½ lemon, juiced
- ½ cup cilantro

Prepare noodles according to package directions.

Heat a nonstick skillet over medium heat. Season the salmon with a dash of salt and pepper, and cook for 2 minutes on each side, or until golden and cooked to your liking. Remove from heat and place in a warm area to rest. (The salmon will continue to cook from the residual heat while resting.)

Spray the same pan with cooking spray and add snow peas, green beans, and zucchini. Stir-fry for 2 to 3 minutes over medium heat, adding a dash of water if needed to help cook the vegetables through.

In a separate bowl, mix together the sesame seeds, ginger, soy sauce, honey, and lemon juice to create the dressing. Mix well until combined.

Pour the noodles into the pan with the vegetables, and toss for a minute to warm. Place in a serving bowl, and top with the salmon and cilantro. Drizzle with the dressing, and serve warm.

NOTE If you can't find fresh snow peas, replace them with 1 cup frozen peas, thawed. Soba noodles taste great in this recipe, so if you can find them, use them!

VEGETARIAN OPTION Sub in ½ cup cooked lentils, 3 oz. tofu, or ½ cup shelled edamame for the salmon.

NUTRITION INFO: *Calories 457, Fat (g) 5, Sat fat (g) 1, Protein (g) 32, Carbs (g) 69, Fiber (g) 8, Sodium (mg) 359*

parsley & lemon fish

This is a fresh and tasty way to serve fish.

SERVES 1   PREP TIME 10 minutes   COOK TIME 20 minutes

- 1 small sweet potato
- 2 Tbsp. fresh parsley
- ¼ tsp. black pepper
- 1 tsp. lemon zest
- 1 (4-oz.) fillet orange roughy
- ½ lemon, juiced
- 3 cups mixed salad greens
- 1 Tbsp. fat-free ranch dressing
- 10 raw almonds

Boil the potato. Once cooked, drain and set aside to cool. Dice the potato into ½-inch cubes.

Coat a nonstick pan with cooking spray and heat over medium heat. Press the parsley, pepper, and lemon zest onto the fish. Drizzle with lemon juice and place in the pan to cook for 2 to 3 minutes on each side or until cooked through.

Meanwhile, prepare a salad with the greens and ranch dressing, and add the cooled and cubed potato. Chop the almonds, and mix into the salad. Serve the fish alongside the salad.

NUTRITION INFO: *Calories 328, Fat (g) 7, Sat fat (g) 1, Protein (g) 15, Carbs (g) 51, Fiber (g) 10, Sodium (mg) 302*

tempeh vegetable stir-fry

Tempeh is a high-protein food made from fermented soybeans or other legumes. It has a nutty flavor and is easily digestible.

SERVES 1 PREP TIME 10 minutes COOK TIME 15 minutes

- ½ Tbsp. lower-sodium soy sauce
- ½ Tbsp. sherry vinegar or rice vinegar
- ¼ tsp. raw sugar
- ¼ tsp. cornstarch
- ½ tsp. dark sesame oil
- 2 oz. tempeh, cubed
- ½ cup broccoli
- ¼ carrot, sliced into coins
- ⅛ medium-size red bell pepper, chopped
- ¾ oz. mushrooms, caps only, sliced
- ¼ tsp. grated fresh ginger
- ½ clove garlic, chopped
- ½ cup fresh bean sprouts
- 2 Tbsp. sliced green onions

Combine first 4 ingredients in a small bowl; set aside.

Heat oil in a large nonstick skillet or wok over medium-high heat until hot. Add tempeh; stir-fry 3 minutes or until light brown. Add broccoli, carrot, and bell pepper; stir-fry 2 minutes. Add mushrooms, ginger, and garlic; stir-fry 1 minute.

Stir soy sauce mixture into tempeh mixture; bring to a boil. Stir in sprouts and green onions.

NUTRITION INFO: *Calories 197, Fat (g) 5, Sat fat (g) 1, Protein (g) 15, Carbs (g) 21, Fiber (g) 8, Sodium (mg) 385*

DESSERTS
baked apple

This comforting, healthy dessert elevates the humble apple to something you'll look forward to eating all day!

SERVES 1 PREP TIME 5 minutes COOK TIME 20 minutes

- 1 apple
- 1 tsp. mixed dried fruit
- 1 tsp. brown sugar
- ½ tsp. heart-healthy margarine

Preheat oven to 350°.

Core apple and make a shallow incision around the middle.

Mix fruit and brown sugar together, and stuff apple with mixture. Place margarine on top of mixture.

Place apple in a small ovenproof dish, and add a dash of water. Bake at 350° for 15 to 20 minutes or until apple is just tender.

Remove from oven and allow to cool for a couple of minutes before serving.

NUTRITION INFO: *Calories 124, Fat (g) 1, Sat fat (g) 0, Protein (g) 1, Carbs (g) 30, Fiber (g) 5, Sodium (mg) 18*

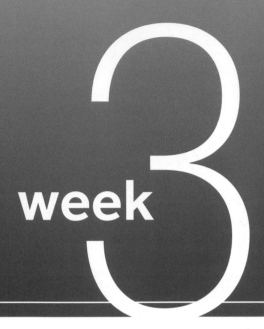

week 3

congratulations

for making it to Week 3 of Bootcamp! You are doing great, and we are really proud of you for putting in the work and committing to yourself in this way.

You probably didn't know this, but coaching you and hearing from *The Biggest Loser* fans fuels and inspires us to keep giving everything to our work; it motivates us to stay healthy!

We are going to start this week like every other week: Set a small, achievable goal you can conquer in Week 3. It could be a repeat of last week's goal, or something you've struggled with over the past few weeks. You can write down your goal in your notebook or online.

Some days will be harder than others. Some aspects of the program will be more challenging than others. That's OK. It's normal.

Do your best, both with the workouts and the meal plan. Remember: Your eating habits have been a long time in the making, so it might take more than a few weeks to change them completely. Keep your eye on the prize, and it will get easier. You can do this!

would you talk to your friend like that?

It is very eye-opening to notice the exact language that you use when you "talk" to yourself, especially when you feel like you came up short in one way or another. You might notice that your choice of words or your tone is negative or condescending. That sort of negative self-talk undermines your power to change. If you have noticed negative self-talk, use this week's exercise to help you cultivate more kindness with yourself.

Think of a time recently when your inner dialogue criticized something you did or didn't do. Recall the words you said to yourself and how you felt as a result. Then think about a dear friend and imagine that he or she has done the EXACT same thing under the EXACT same circumstances. Take a moment to see it play out in your mind.

Pretend that he or she has shared the details with you by e-mail and is clearly upset by it. Write an e-mail back to your friend with the intention of being compassionate and supportive. What would you say to help him or her let it go?

How might that same language help you if you applied it to your self-talk? The next time you need some self-compassion, start your self-talk with "Dear friend…"

WEEKLY WORKOUTS

MONDAY	Courage
TUESDAY	Rise and Grind
WEDNESDAY	DYOW
THURSDAY	Smash Up
FRIDAY	Yes, You Can
SATURDAY	Last-Chance Workout—Fernanda
SUNDAY	Active Rest Day

tip

FOOD IS FUEL Though we might have a complicated relationship with food, to our bodies, it is nothing more than energy units. And it only knows how to do two things with them—burn them or store them.

Every pound of body fat represents 3,500 calories of excess energy that your body has stored because it wasn't burned through your natural metabolism or exercise. That's the equivalent of 25 cans of soda, which is quite a lot of calories to "pay back," when you think about it. So as you make your food choices and work to "balance" your calorie target each day, consider that your body has a choice: Burn calories or store them. Staying on track with your eating and exercise will help you burn calories, shed body fat, and still have energy for whatever life throws your way.

WEEK 3 MEALS

MONDAY
B Egg White Scramble
L Hummus & Veggie Sandwich
D Chicken & Almond Stir-Fry

TUESDAY
B Quick Breakfast Couscous
L Crunchy Tuna Salad Stuffed Pepper
D Chicken, Lemon & Orzo Soup

WEDNESDAY
B Greek Breakfast Pita
L Chicken, Lemon & Orzo Soup
D Warm Chicken & Quinoa Salad

THURSDAY
B Peanut Butter Toast
L Warm Chicken & Quinoa Salad
D Portobello & Black Bean Quesadilla

FRIDAY
B Banana Yogurt Smoothie
L Chicken Caesar Collard Wrap
D Salsa Verde Smothered Turkey Burger

SATURDAY
B Spinach Feta Cups
L Chicken, Lemon & Orzo Soup
D Thai Lettuce Wraps

SUNDAY
B Chocolate, Banana, Peanut Butter Smoothie
L Korean BBQ Cabbage Bowl
D Japanese Shrimp Salad

day 1

nutrition bite:

Fill Up Without Filling Out.

How do you eat healthy at a buffet or potluck? Fill your plate mostly with salad and veggies, and sample only small portions of high-calorie dishes. You'll control your calories better, without calling attention to your weight-control plans. Instead of standing at the buffet table nibbling nonstop, fill your plate and then go sit down somewhere to eat. Follow the same rules you do at home: Half your plate should be fruits and vegetables, with ¼ lean protein and ¼ whole grains. And limit yourself to just one trip—maybe two if you decide to have a salad separately from your main course.

WORKOUT
courage

34 MINUTES | WARM UP FOR 5 MINUTES

It takes a lot of courage to take responsibility for your weight and health. Now bring that same courage to this new week of workouts. We turned up the heat last week with some challenging new moves. This week we amp it up even more with the optional introduction of weights. Note that there are two sets of cardio intervals you will repeat at various times during the workout. Moves marked with an asterisk (*) mean you can add optional weights.

You'll do four sets of exercises in this workout, with a few new moves inserted here and there to keep you on your toes.

tip

KEEP USING YOUR DIARY

At the beginning of Bootcamp, you learned just how important it is to track your food intake, but it's easy to get off track when you get busy. It only takes a few minutes a day, but tracking your food can have a huge effect on your success. Studies have shown that most people underestimate how many calories they consume by between 25 and 40 percent. If you're not following the meal plan, you're at greater risk of being a statistic.

If you want the best possible results, log every meal, snack, and drink at least four days a week. No one but you can see your diary, so you can tell it the truth, the whole truth, and nothing but the truth.

THE WORKOUT

INTERVAL A

1 Jogging X 30 seconds

2 High Knees X 30 seconds

3 Traveling Squats X 30 seconds

4 Squats* X 1 minute

INTERVAL B

5 High Knees with Torso Twist X 30 seconds

6 Rear-Stepping Lunges with Woodchops X 30 seconds

7 Jumping Jacks X 30 seconds

8 Lat Pulldowns* X 1 minute

INTERVAL C

9 Lunge Twists X 30 seconds

10 Traveling Squats with Pivot X 30 seconds

11 Skater Jumps X 30 seconds

12 Mountain Climbers X 30 seconds

13 Bicycle Crunches X 1 minute

(CONTINUES)

INTERVAL A

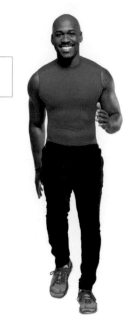

1

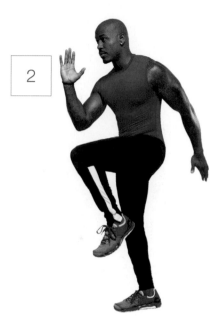

2

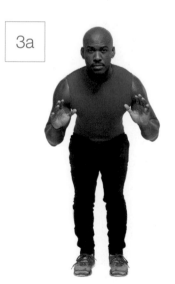

3a

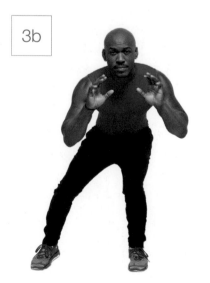

3b

107

INTERVAL B

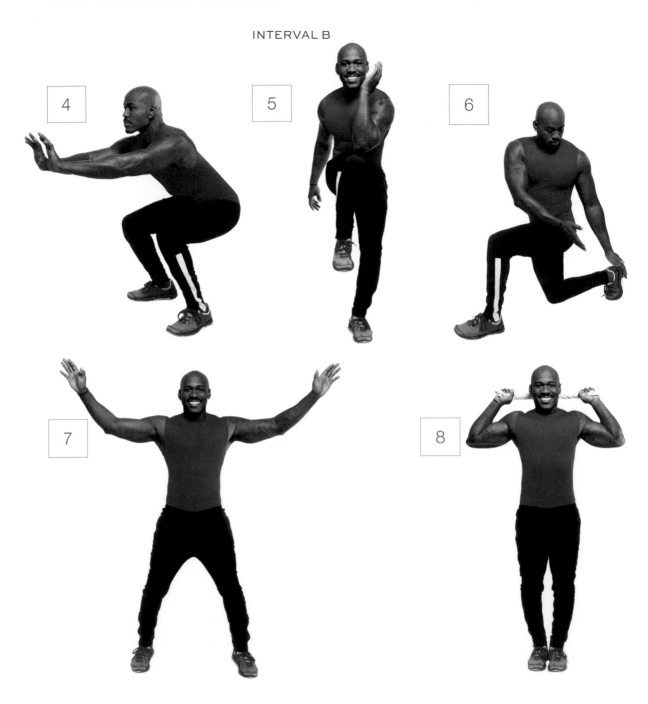

INTERVAL C

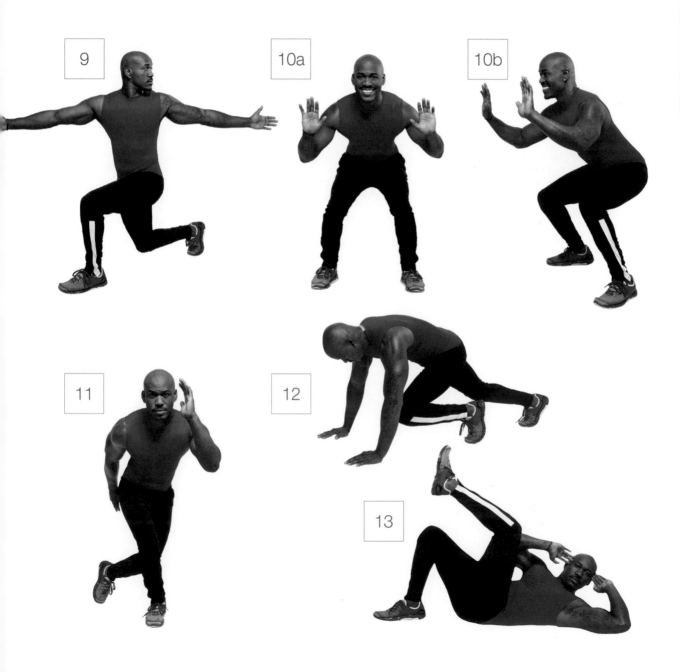

THE WORKOUT

CONTINUED

INTERVAL D

1. Curtsies X 30 seconds
2. Jogging X 30 seconds
3. Forward Lunges X 30 seconds
4. Burpees X 30 seconds
5. Chest Presses* X 1 minute

Repeat Interval C, then do

6. Squats X 1 minute

Repeat Interval D, then do

7. Lat Pulldowns* X 1 minute

Repeat Interval A, then do

8. Crunches X 1 minute

Repeat Interval B, then do

— Chest Presses* X 1 minute

COOL DOWN FOR 5 MINUTES

INTERVAL D

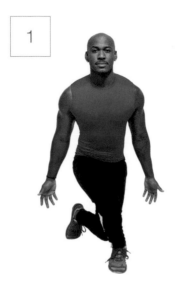

1

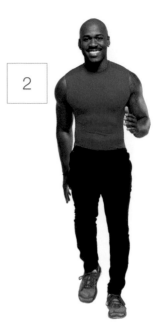

2

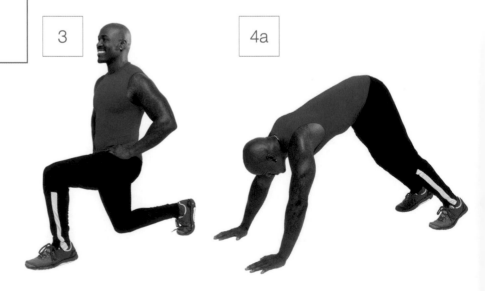

3

4a

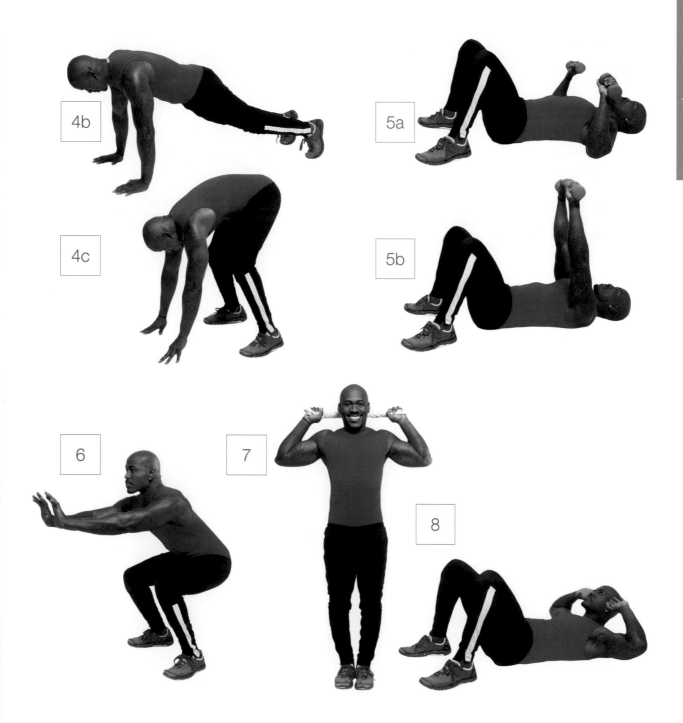

MEALS

BREAKFAST
egg white scramble
See recipe on page 100.

Serve with 2 slices whole-wheat toast and 2 Tbsp. natural peanut butter, plus 1 orange.

LUNCH
hummus & veggie sandwich
See recipe on page 135.

Serve with 1 (6-oz.) container plain fat-free Greek yogurt with 1 cup pineapple.

DINNER
chicken & almond stir-fry
See recipe on page 136.

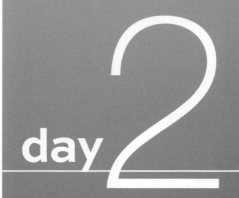

day 2

morning motivation:

Keep Aiming High.

Never lower your standards. We've seen so many contestants on *The Biggest Loser* who, before coming to the Ranch, had never pushed their own limits. They had no idea how much strength and possibility they had inside them. Refuse to lower your own standards. We want you to rise up to the high standards that you deserve to reach—that we know you can reach during your workouts and in the rest of your life. Now that's a recipe for greatness!

WORKOUT rise and grind

40 MINUTES | WARM UP FOR 5 MINUTES

Get up and give it your all today! Every day, even if you don't want to, rise and grind through your workout. You'll always feel better for it.

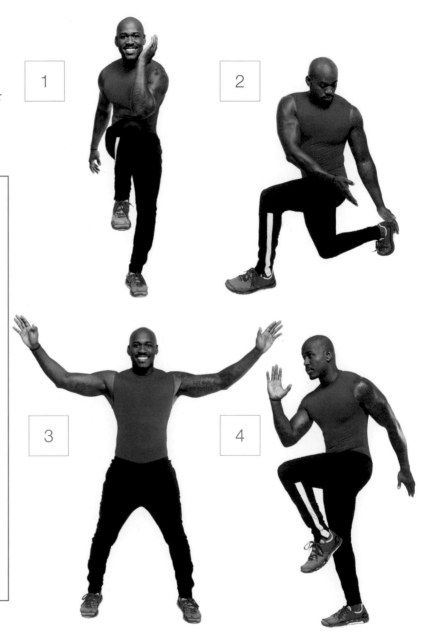

THE WORKOUT

2 ROUNDS

1. High Knees with Torso Twist X 30 seconds
2. Rear-Stepping Lunges with Woodchops X 30 seconds
3. Jumping Jacks X 30 seconds
4. High Knees X 1 minute
— Jumping Jacks X 30 seconds
— High Knees with Torso Twist X 30 seconds
5. Lunge Twists X 30 seconds
6. Air Jump Rope X 30 seconds
— Lunge Twists X 1 minute

(CONTINUES)

THE WORKOUT
CONTINUED

— High Knees X 1 minute

— Lunge Twists X 30 seconds

7   Traveling Squats with Pivot X 30 seconds

8   Skater Jumps X 30 seconds

9   Mountain Climbers X 30 seconds

— Air Jump Rope X 1 minute

— High Knees X 1 minute

Repeat for Round 2

COOL DOWN FOR 5 MINUTES

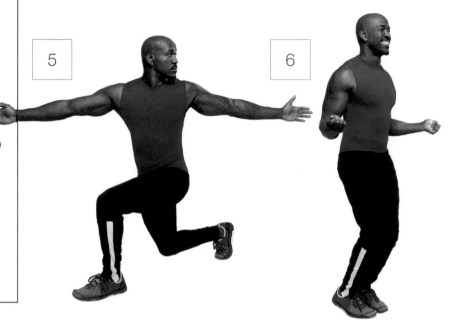

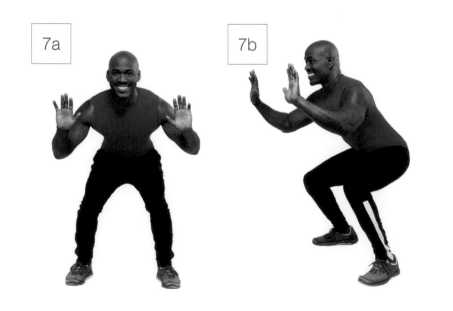

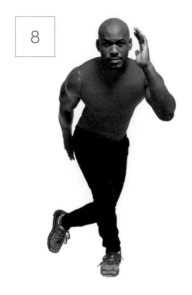

8

MEALS

BREAKFAST
quick breakfast couscous
See recipe on page 134.

LUNCH
crunchy tuna salad stuffed pepper

Combine 3 oz. tuna packed in water (drained) with 1 Tbsp. each chopped walnuts, celery, and onions. Add a squeeze of lemon juice, ¼ tsp. tarragon, and 1 Tbsp. plain fat-free Greek yogurt and 1 tsp. reduced-fat mayonnaise, plus plenty of black pepper. Pack into 1 red bell pepper with the top and seeds removed. Serve with ½ cup grapes.

VEGETARIAN OPTION Sub in ½ cup chopped chickpeas for the tuna.

NUTRITION INFO: *Calories 417, Fat (g) 22, Sat fat (g) 2, Protein (g) 30, Carbs (g) 34, Fiber (g) 7, Sodium (mg) 229*

DINNER
chicken, lemon & orzo soup
See recipe on page 135.

You'll save leftovers for later in the week.

SNACKS
Choose up to 300 calories of snacks to reach your calorie goal for the day. See the lists in Chapter 3 for snack ideas.

9

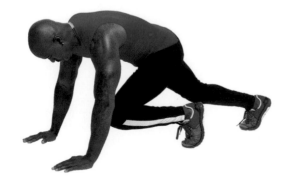

day 3

weekly check-in:

How's It Going, Friend?

This is your mid-week check-in. This week's motivation exercise focused on treating yourself as you would a friend. So tell us: How are you treating yourself today? Some days, you will feel like you've crashed and burned. That's just part of life. You'll be soaring high again soon. It's all part of the process. Keep working and keep reaching for your goals. You'll get there!

WORKOUT
do your own workout (dyow)

It's Wednesday, and you know what that means: Do Your Own Workout! You can't go wrong, as long as you get up and get moving. If you need ideas, consult the list in Chapter 3.

"Is who you *are* who you are *being*? Look inside and be you—the you that is amazing, fantastic, kind, caring, motivated, and driven. I know you are in there!**"**
—*The Biggest Loser* trainer Jennifer Widerstrom

MEALS

BREAKFAST

greek breakfast pita

Serve with 1 apple and 1 cup skim milk.
Sauté ½ cup red bell peppers and onions with a pinch
of oregano, then add 1 egg and 1 egg white, scrambled.
Stir in 2 Tbsp. reduced-fat feta. Toast half of a whole-
wheat pita and fill with 1 cup arugula or spinach, 2
slices tomato, and the egg mixture.

NUTRITION INFO: *Calories 270, Fat (g) 7, Sat fat (g) 2, Protein (g)
19, Carbs (g) 36, Fiber (g) 6, Sodium (mg) 461*

LUNCH

chicken, lemon & orzo soup

Serve 1 portion leftover soup from last night.

DINNER

warm chicken & quinoa salad

See recipe on page 138.

You'll save half for tomorrow's lunch.

SNACKS

Choose up to 300 calories of snacks to reach your
calorie goal for the day. See the lists in Chapter 3 for
snack ideas.

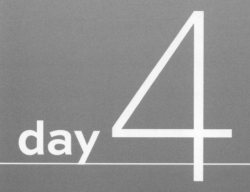

day 4

morning motivation:

Choices Or Excuses.

The only excuses you have are the
excuses you make. Excuses are the
opposite of choices. It is OK if you
"choose" to skip the occasional
workout because of a deadline at
work, but it is not OK if your busy
job is always an excuse. If you try
hard enough, you can always come
up with an excuse. We want to challenge you to start busting through
your excuses and putting yourself
first! We know you can do it.

WORKOUT smash up

36 MINUTES | WARM UP FOR 5 MINUTES

If you're not feeling sore at the end of the Bootcamp workouts, you're not working hard enough! Like the Courage workout earlier this week, today we have a great mix of moves that can be made more intense by adding weights. (Of course, you can still use your trusty towel for resistance or just your body weight.) The optional weights can be added to the moves marked with an asterisk (*). You do not need any equipment for the remaining moves. As you have seen before, you'll repeat two sets of intervals with other moves interwoven.

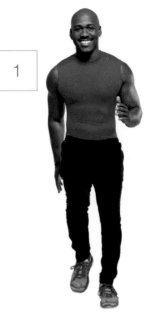

THE WORKOUT

1 Jogging X 30 seconds

2 High Knees X 30 seconds

3 Traveling Squats X 30 seconds

4 Squats* X 1 minute

INTERVAL A

5 Curtsies X 30 seconds

— Jogging X 30 seconds

6 Forward Lunges X 30 seconds

7 Burpees X 30 seconds

8 Bent-Over One-Arm Rows* X 1 minute

INTERVAL B

9 Lunge Twists X 30 seconds

— Traveling Squats with Pivot X 30 seconds

10 Skater Jumps X 30 seconds

11 Mountain Climbers X 30 seconds

12 Plank X 1 minute

(CONTINUES)

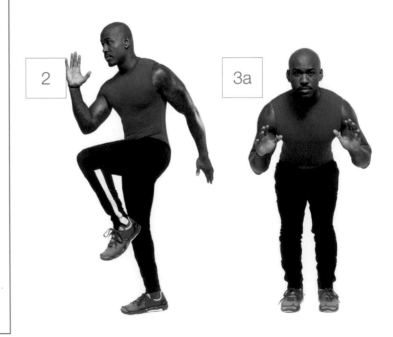

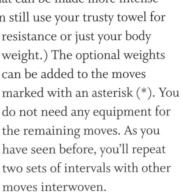

INTERVAL A

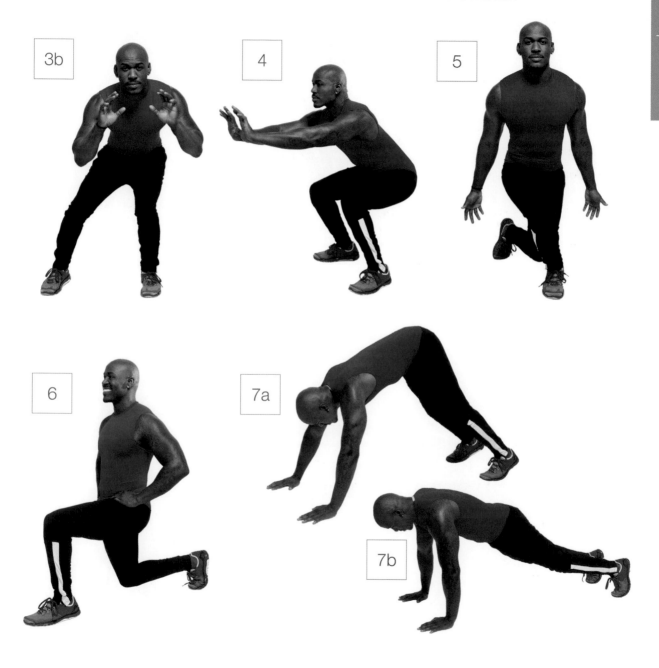

3b

4

5

6

7a

7b

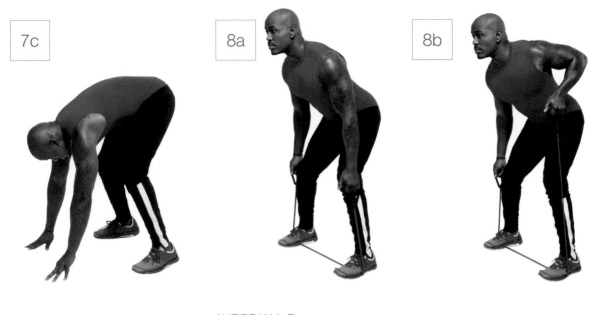

INTERVAL B

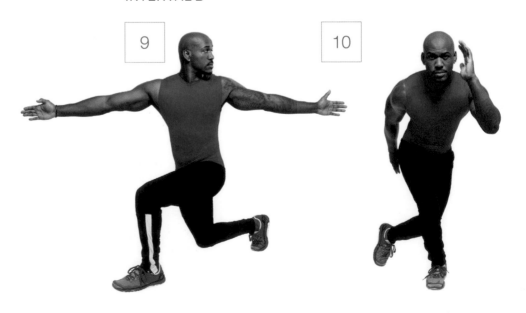

THE WORKOUT
CONTINUED

Repeat Interval A, then do

1   Overhead Presses* X 1 minute

Repeat Interval B, then do

—   Squats* X 1 minute

Repeat Interval A, then do

—   Bent-Over One-Arm Rows X 1 minute

Repeat Interval B, then do

2   Russian Twists* X 1 minute

3   High Knees with Torso Twist X 30 seconds

4   Rear-Stepping Lunges with Woodchops X 30 seconds

5   Air Jump Rope X 30 seconds

—   Overhead Presses X 1 minute

COOL DOWN FOR 5 MINUTES

11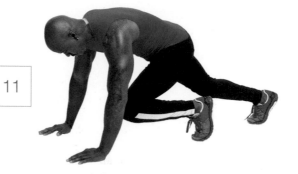

12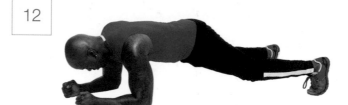

1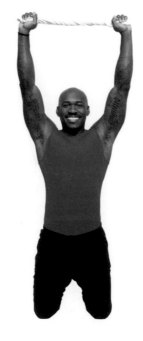

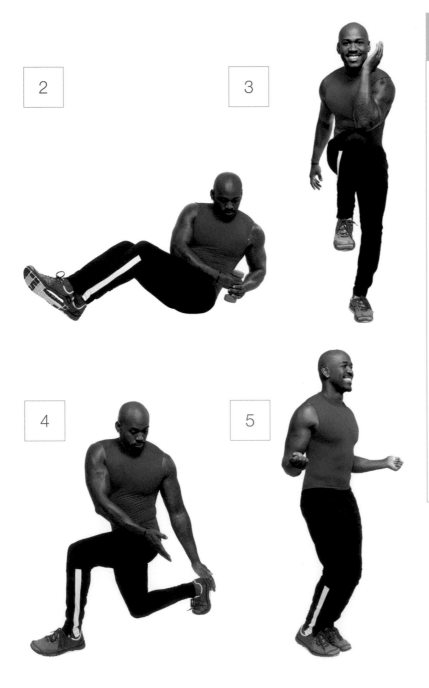

2

3

4

5

tip

THE ENERGY EQUATION The energy equation is the indisputable law of weight loss. Everything you eat and drink provides energy, which is measured in calories. Your body can only do two things with energy: burn it, or store it. When you consume more energy through food and drinks than you burn through exercise and your natural metabolism, your body turns that excess energy into fat.

To lose weight, you need to burn more energy than you consume. If you're not losing weight or inches, your energy equation is not in balance. You're either consuming too many calories or not doing enough exercise in most cases.

MEALS

BREAKFAST

peanut butter toast

Serve 2 slices whole-wheat bread, 1 Tbsp. peanut butter, and 1 orange with 1 cup skim milk.

NUTRITION INFO: *Calories 395, Fat (g) 10, Sat fat (g) 1, Protein (g) 20, Carbs (g) 59, Fiber (g) 7, Sodium (mg) 390*

LUNCH

warm chicken & quinoa salad

Serve last night's leftovers.

DINNER

portobello & black bean quesadilla

See recipe on page 137.

Serve with 2 Tbsp. each plain fat-free Greek yogurt and low-sodium salsa, 1 cup of grape tomatoes, and 1 orange.

DESSERT

apple-berry crumble

See recipe on page 139.

SNACKS

Choose up to 300 calories of snacks to reach your daily goal. See the lists in Chapter 3 for snack ideas. Don't forget to include your dessert in your food journal (dessert gets included with your snack calories).

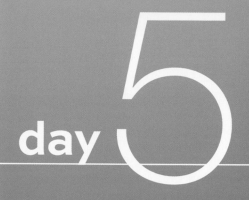

day 5

nutrition bite:

Water Matters.

How much better do you feel when you are well hydrated? Find out. Commit to your own one-week water experiment. For instance, you might set a goal of drinking two glasses of water between breakfast and lunch, then another two between lunch and dinner. That will get you halfway to your hydration goal of eight glasses a day right there! Write down what you notice about how you feel and your energy level when you're properly hydrated. Are you able to forgo the afternoon cup of coffee? Do you find yourself snacking less? Do you feel less cranky? You won't believe the effect that proper hydration can have on your life!

WORKOUT yes, you can

40 MINUTES | WARM UP FOR 5 MINUTES

There's no better feeling than when you do a move you think you "can't do." Your body is capable of much more than you imagine. Whenever you feel fear limiting you in a workout, remind yourself: Yes I can, yes I can, yes I can.

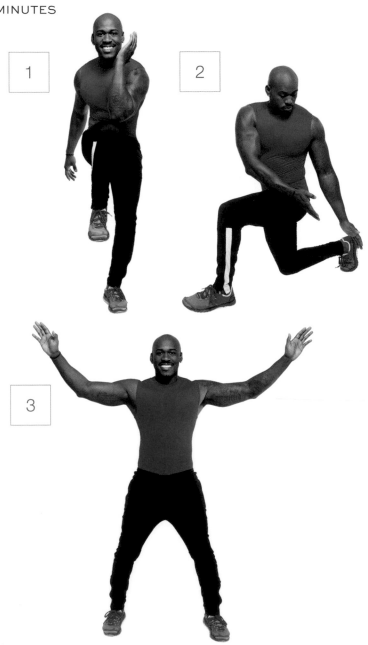

THE WORKOUT

2 ROUNDS

1   High Knees with Torso Twist X 30 seconds

2   Rear-Stepping Lunges with Woodchops X 30 seconds

3   Jumping Jacks X 30 seconds

4   High Knees X 1 minute

—   Jumping Jacks X 30 seconds

—   High Knees with Torso Twist X 30 seconds

5   Lunge Twists X 30 seconds

6   Air Jump Rope X 1 minute

—   Lunge Twists X 30 seconds

7   Traveling Squats with Pivot X 30 seconds

(CONTINUES)

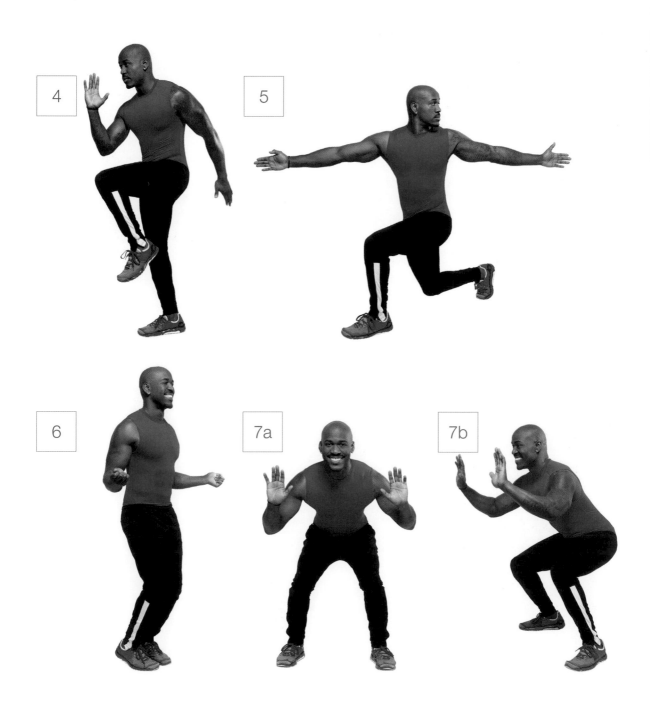

125

THE WORKOUT

CONTINUED

8 Skater Jumps X 30 seconds

9 Mountain Climbers X 30 seconds

— High Knees X 1 minute

10 Curtsies X 30 seconds

11 Jogging X 30 seconds

12 Forward Lunges X 30 seconds

13 Burpees X 30 seconds

— High Knees X 1 minute

Repeat for Round 2

COOL DOWN FOR 5 MINUTES

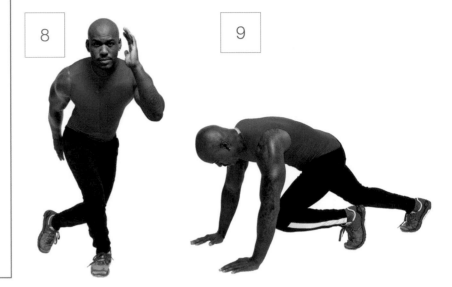

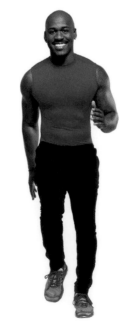

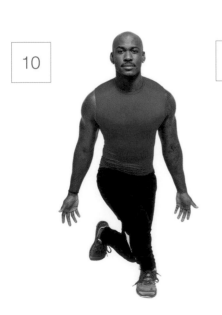

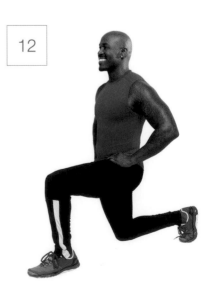

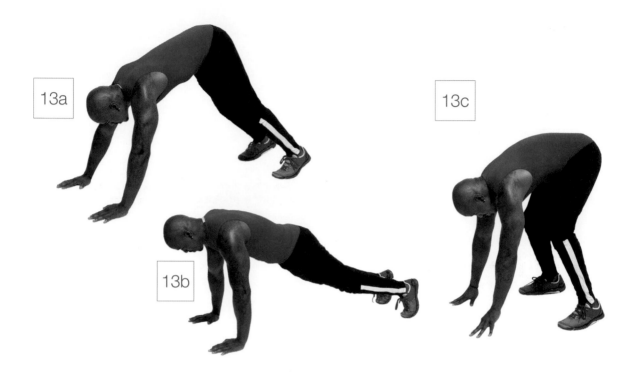

13a

13b

13c

127

MEALS

BREAKFAST

banana yogurt smoothie

See recipe on page 134.

Serve with 16 almonds (1 oz.) or walnuts.

LUNCH

chicken caesar collard wrap

Serve with 1 apple, sliced, with cinnamon. Remove the stems from 2 large collard leaves. Microwave for 30 seconds to soften, if desired. Combine 6 oz. cooked chicken with 2 Tbsp. low-fat Caesar dressing, 1 cup chopped tomatoes, and 2 tsp. grated Parmesan cheese. Season with plenty of black pepper; place in the center of the wrap, and roll like a burrito.

VEGETARIAN OPTION Sub in ½ cup chopped chickpeas for the chicken.

NUTRITION INFO: *Calories 328, Fat (g) 6, Sat fat (g) 2, Protein (g) 49, Carbs (g) 18, Fiber (g) 3, Sodium (mg) 203*

DINNER

salsa verde smothered turkey burger

Top 1 (3-oz.) cooked turkey burger with 1 oz. reduced-fat Monterey Jack cheese, 3 slices red onion, and ¼ cup salsa verde. Place in an oven-safe dish and broil until the cheese melts. Serve with ½ cup brown rice, 1 cup bell pepper strips, and ¼ avocado.

NUTRITION INFO: *Calories 416, Fat (g) 12, Sat fat (g) 3, Protein (g) 36, Carbs (g) 44, Fiber (g) 11, Sodium (mg) 334*

SNACKS

Choose up to 300 calories of snacks to reach your calorie goal for the day. See the lists in Chapter 3 for snack ideas.

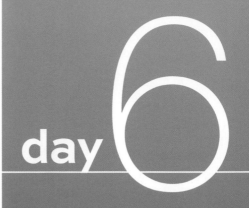

day 6

last chance:

It's that day of the week already: The Last-Chance Workout is here again! When you're sweating it out today, ask yourself: "Am I giving this workout everything I've got?" If not, why not? Make it count.

WORKOUT last-chance workout—fernanda

46 MINUTES | WARM UP FOR 5 MINUTES

This workout goes out to one of our favorite Biggest Loser ladies: Fernanda Abarca. She inspired us all in Season 15, and then she joined the first online Bootcamp to motivate and inspire more people. So get your sweat on and shout out to Fernanda once you finish this workout! Remember that the moves marked * can use optional weights for more of a challenge.

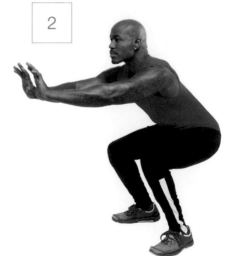

THE WORKOUT

2 ROUNDS

1. Jogging X 1 minute
2. Squats* X 1 minute
3. Quick Feet X 1 minute
4. Lat Pulldowns* X 1 minute
5. Skater Jumps X 1 minute
6. Chest Presses* X 1 minute
— Jogging X 1 minute
7. Plank X 1 minute
8. Air Jump Rope* X 1 minute
9. Forward Lunges* X 1 minute
10. Jumping Jacks X 1 minute
11. Bent-Over One-Arm Rows* X 1 minute
— Jogging X 1 minute
12. Russian Twists* X 1 minute
13. High Knees with Torso Twist X 1 minute
14. Overhead Presses* X 1 minute

Repeat for Round 2

COOL DOWN FOR 5 MINUTES

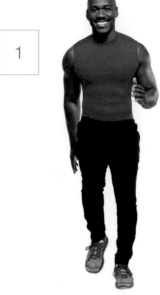

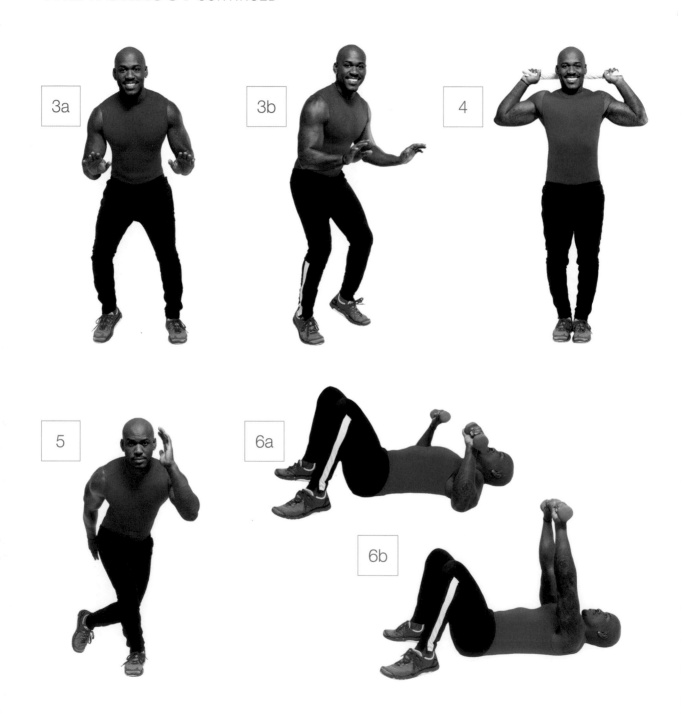

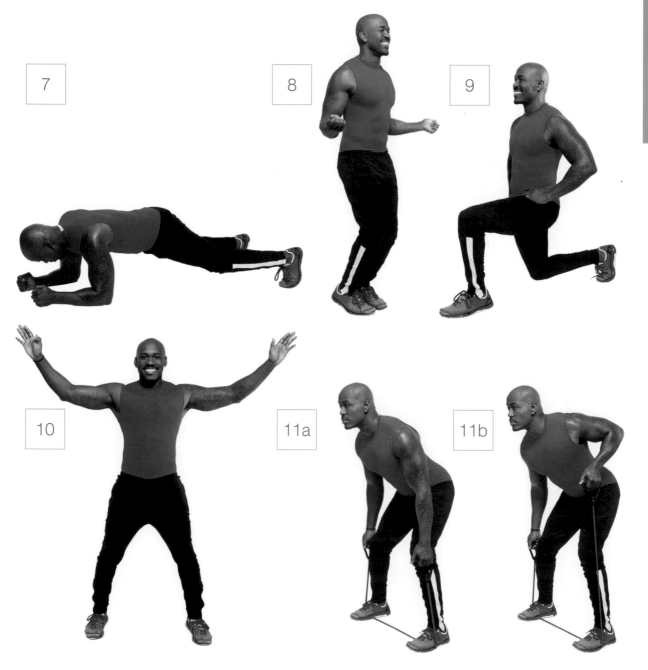

7

8

9

10

11a

11b

THE WORKOUT CONTINUED

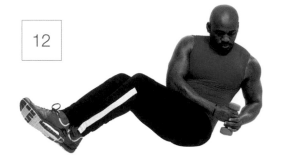

12

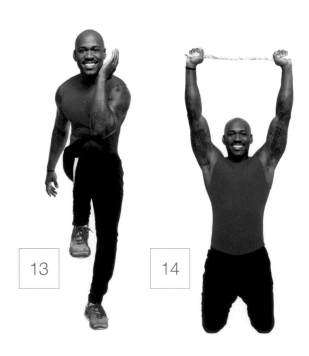

13

14

MEALS

BREAKFAST

spinach feta cups

Preheat oven to 350°. Combine 1 cup chopped spinach, ½ tsp. minced garlic, 2 Tbsp. reduced-fat feta cheese, and 1 egg plus 1 egg white. Season with a pinch of nutmeg and black pepper. Pour into 3 wells of a greased muffin tin. Bake for about 15 minutes, until the eggs have set. Serve with 1 slice whole-wheat toast, 1 cup skim milk, and 1 cup grape tomatoes.

NUTRITION INFO: *Calories 191, Fat (g) 8, Sat fat (g) 3, Protein (g) 17, Carbs (g) 16, Fiber (g) 3, Sodium (mg) 460*

LUNCH

chicken, lemon & orzo soup

Serve 1 portion leftover soup from earlier this week.

DINNER

thai lettuce wraps

See recipe on page 137.

SNACKS

Choose up to 300 calories of snacks to reach your calorie goal for the day. See the lists in Chapter 3 for snack ideas.

day 7

morning motivation:

Fight The Fear.

You need fear to become fearless! You might be afraid to lose weight, to go after your dreams, or to step into the spotlight. But don't let fear stop you.

Let your fear motivate you. You might still have fears, but you will learn to face them head-on and overcome them! It will only make you stronger. You don't have to fight them all day, and you don't have to overcome them all at once—some of them will take years and maybe even your whole life. But you do have to try to fight!

WORKOUT

active rest day

Three weeks down, five to go. Way to go! How do you feel? No matter what, you should be proud of yourself. Enjoy this rest day!

"When you make decisions in your day that make you feel good, you're going to look great! Making conscious healthy decisions in the kitchen and being consistent at the gym mean you can hit your goals. Your overall health goals and lifestyle changes are the foundation of the future you.**"**
—*The Biggest Loser* trainer Jennifer Widerstrom

MEALS

BREAKFAST
chocolate, banana, peanut butter smoothie

See recipe on page 67.

LUNCH
korean bbq cabbage bowl

Serve with ½ cup brown rice noodles.
Start with 1 cup cooked shredded cabbage. Top with 3 oz. extra-lean beef and ½ cup each carrots and onions sautéed in 2 Tbsp. Korean BBQ sauce. Sprinkle with ½ tsp. sesame seeds (optional) and hot sauce.

VEGETARIAN OPTION Sub in 3 oz. tempeh or ½ cup cooked lentils for the beef.

NUTRITION INFO: Calories 284, Fat (g) 8, Sat fat (g) 3, Protein (g) 24, Carbs (g) 26, Fiber (g) 5, Sodium (mg) 450

DINNER
japanese shrimp salad

See recipe on page 136.

DESSERT
honey pistachio dip

See recipe on page 139.

Serve with 1 sliced apple.

SNACKS

Choose up to 300 calories of snacks to reach your daily goal. See the lists in Chapter 3 for snack ideas. Don't forget to include your dessert in your food journal (dessert gets included with your snack calories).

WEEKLY RECIPES

BREAKFASTS
banana yogurt smoothie

This simple smoothie is perfect on busy mornings.

SERVES 1 **PREP TIME** 2 minutes

- 1 cup unsweetened soy milk
- 1 medium-size banana
- ¼ tsp. ground cinnamon
- ¼ cup plain fat-free Greek yogurt
- 1 Tbsp. ground flaxseed

Place 3 ice cubes, soy milk, banana, cinnamon, yogurt, and flaxseed into a blender. Blend until smooth and combined. Pour into a glass and serve.

NUTRITION INFO: Calories 279, Fat (g) 8, Sat fat (g) 1, Protein (g) 16, Carbs (g) 40, Fiber (g) 9, Sodium (mg) 162

quick breakfast couscous

Change up your normal oatmeal or granola with this quick and easy-to-make couscous breakfast.

SERVES 1 **PREP TIME** 2 minutes **COOK TIME** 5 minutes

- ¼ cup whole-wheat couscous
- ¼ tsp. ground cinnamon
- 1 tsp. orange peel
- 1 oz. orange juice
- 1 Tbsp. pumpkin seeds
- 1 Tbsp. raisins
- ½ oz. dried apricots
- ¼ cup plain fat-free Greek yogurt

Place couscous in a heatproof bowl and stir in the cinnamon. Cover with boiling water, and stir to coat the grains. Set aside for 5 minutes to absorb. Using a fork, fluff the grains to separate.

Add the orange peel and juice, and mix well. Add the pumpkin seeds, raisins, and apricots, and stir to combine. Serve topped with yogurt.

NUTRITION INFO: *Calories 323, Fat (g) 6, Sat fat (g) 1, Protein (g) 14, Carbs (g) 55, Fiber (g) 5, Sodium (mg) 39*

LUNCHES

hummus & veggie sandwich

Use hummus in place of mayo for a delicious and healthy addition to any sandwich!

SERVES 1 PREP TIME 5 minutes

- 2 Tbsp. hummus
- 2 slices whole-wheat bread
- 1 cup mixed salad greens

Spread the hummus on the bread, and top with greens.

TIP Boost the protein content of your hummus by using half chickpeas and half shelled edamame.

NUTRITION INFO: *Calories 200, Fat (g) 5, Sat fat (g) 0, Protein (g) 10, Carbs (g) 34, Fiber (g) 7, Sodium (mg) 422*

DINNERS

chicken, lemon & orzo soup

This quick chicken soup is soothing for the belly and the soul.

SERVES 4 PREP TIME 15 minutes COOK TIME 20 minutes

- 1 tsp. olive oil
- 1 onion, chopped
- 2 cloves garlic, chopped
- 2 tsp. grated fresh ginger
- 16 oz. cooked chicken breast, cubed
- ¼ tsp. black pepper
- 4 cups low-sodium chicken broth
- 1 cup whole-wheat orzo
- 1 (8-oz.) package mixed frozen vegetables
- 1 tsp. sugar
- 2 tsp. fish sauce (or lower-sodium soy sauce)
- ½ lemon, juiced
- 1 tsp. lemon zest
- ¼ cup cilantro, chopped

Heat the oil in a large saucepan over medium heat. Add onion, garlic, and ginger, and cook for 1 to 2 minutes. Mix in the chicken and pepper, and cook for another 2 to 3 minutes.

Stir in the broth and orzo, and simmer 10 minutes. Add the vegetables, sugar, and fish sauce, and simmer another 6 to 8 minutes, until the vegetables are cooked.

Mix in the lemon juice, lemon zest, and cilantro, and serve.

Reserve two servings for lunch later in the week, then freeze the remaining portion for up to 1 month.

NUTRITION INFO: *Calories 400, Fat (g) 3, Sat fat (g) 0, Protein (g) 36, Carbs (g) 54, Fiber (g) 4, Sodium (mg) 264*

chicken & almond stir-fry

Almonds add crunch to this simple stir-fry.

SERVES 1　PREP TIME 10 minutes　COOK TIME 10 minutes

- ½ cup brown rice noodles
- ½ Tbsp. olive oil
- 4 oz. chicken breast, sliced
- 1 clove garlic, chopped
- 1 tsp. grated fresh ginger
- 2 cups broccoli florets
- ½ oz. chopped almonds
- 1 tsp. lower-sodium soy sauce
- ½ tsp. oyster sauce (or additional soy sauce)

Prepare noodles according to package directions.

Meanwhile, heat the oil in a wok or nonstick skillet. Add the chicken, garlic, and ginger, and stir-fry for 2 minutes. Add the broccoli and continue to cook for another 2 minutes. Add a dash of water if needed.

Stir in the noodles, almonds, and soy and oyster sauces.

VEGETARIAN OPTION　Sub in 3 oz. firm tofu for the chicken.

NUTRITION INFO: *Calories 500, Fat (g) 13, Sat fat (g) 2, Protein (g) 37, Carbs (g) 60, Fiber (g) 7, Sodium (mg) 498*

japanese shrimp salad

With an exotic twist, this flavor-packed dish is sure to win you over. It gets its signature flavor from miso paste, a rich and salty condiment made from soybeans or other legumes.

SERVES 1　PREP TIME 10 minutes　COOK TIME 10 minutes

- 1 oz. soba noodles
- 1 tsp. miso paste (or lower-sodium soy sauce)
- 1 tsp. rice vinegar
- 1 tsp. sugar
- 1 tsp. sesame oil
- 4 oz. medium-size shrimp, peeled and deveined
- 1 large cucumber, sliced
- ¼ avocado, sliced

Prepare noodles according to package directions.

Meanwhile, prepare the dressing in a large bowl by mixing together the miso paste, rice vinegar, sugar, and sesame oil using a whisk to ensure that there are no lumps. Set aside.

Season the shrimp with a dash of salt and pepper. Grill in a nonstick pan for 2 minutes on each side, until they just turn pink.

Toss the cucumber, avocado, and noodles in the dressing. Place in a serving bowl and top with the shrimp.

VEGETARIAN OPTION　Sub in ½ cup shelled edamame for the shrimp.

NUTRITION INFO: *Calories 477, Fat (g) 17, Sat fat (g) 3, Protein (g) 28, Carbs (g) 60, Fiber (g) 10, Sodium (mg) 390*

portobello & black bean quesadilla

Quesadillas are a quick and easy dinner that everyone will love.

SERVES 1   PREP TIME 4 minutes   COOK TIME 7 minutes

1 (8-inch) whole-wheat tortilla
1 portobello mushroom, sliced
¼ (14.5-oz.) can black beans, drained and rinsed
¼ green bell pepper, sliced
3 Tbsp. reduced-fat cheddar cheese, shredded
1 Tbsp. sliced green onions
1 Tbsp. low-sodium salsa
½ Tbsp. chopped cilantro (optional)

Microwave the tortilla at HIGH 1 minute. Leave in microwave to keep warm while preparing filling.

Heat a large nonstick skillet over medium-high heat. Coat pan with cooking spray. Add mushroom; sauté 2 minutes or until tender. Add beans and pepper; cook 1 to 2 minutes, stirring constantly, or until liquid evaporates. Mash bean mixture slightly with a potato masher.

Spoon the bean mixture onto the tortilla. Sprinkle evenly with cheese and onions. Fold tortilla in half.

Wipe skillet with paper towels; heat over medium heat. Coat pan with cooking spray. Place quesadilla in pan; cook 2 to 3 minutes on each side or until golden and cheese melts. Cut quesadilla into 3 wedges. Serve immediately with salsa and cilantro, if desired.

NUTRITION INFO: *Calories 263, Fat (g) 6, Sat fat (g) 3, Protein (g) 13, Carbs (g) 38, Fiber (g) 9, Sodium (mg) 391*

thai lettuce wraps

Wrapping this sweet and savory pork in lettuce means you won't waste a single drop of the delicious sauce.

SERVES 1   PREP TIME 15 minutes   COOK TIME 8 minutes

DRESSING
1 tsp. lime juice
½ tsp. sesame oil
½ tsp. lower-sodium soy sauce
¼ tsp. sambal oelek (ground fresh chile paste, or sub red chili flakes)
¼ tsp. fish sauce (or use additional lower-sodium soy sauce)
FILLING
⅛ tsp. canola oil
2 oz. extra-lean ground pork
1 tsp. grated fresh ginger
TO SERVE
¼ cup grated (peeled and seeded) cucumber
¼ cup grated carrot
1 Tbsp. cilantro leaves
1 Tbsp. chopped fresh mint
2 tsp. thinly sliced green onions
½ Tbsp. chopped dry-roasted peanuts
3 Boston lettuce leaves

To prepare dressing, combine all dressing ingredients in a small bowl; stir well.

To prepare filling, heat a large nonstick skillet over medium-high heat. Add oil to pan; swirl to coat. Add pork and ginger; cook 6 to 8 minutes or until pork is browned, stirring to crumble. Drain well; return to pan. Stir in 4 tsp. dressing.

Spoon the pork mixture, cucumber, carrot, cilantro, mint, onions, and peanuts into lettuce leaves; drizzle with dressing.

VEGETARIAN OPTION Sub in 3 oz. crumbled tempeh or ½ cup cooked lentils for the pork.

NUTRITION INFO: *Calories 249, Fat (g) 11, Sat fat (g) 3, Protein (g) 30, Carbs (g) 9, Fiber (g) 2, Sodium (mg) 468*

warm chicken & quinoa salad

Quinoa is high in protein, iron, and fiber, but that's not why we love it—we love it because it's delicious!

SERVES 2 PREP TIME 10 minutes COOK TIME 20 minutes

⅓ cup quinoa
1 red bell pepper, chopped
1 zucchini, chopped
1 cup green beans
1 medium-size carrot, chopped
12 oz. chicken breast
2 tsp. ground cumin
2 Tbsp. plain fat-free Greek yogurt
2 Tbsp. lemon juice
2 tsp. tahini (sesame paste) or peanut butter
2 tsp. honey
1 cup flat-leaf parsley, chopped
½ cup fresh mint, chopped

Preheat oven to 350°. Place quinoa in a pot and cover with 1½ cups of water. Place over medium-low heat and bring to a gentle simmer; cook for 12 to 14 minutes. Drain and set aside to cool.

Meanwhile, place the bell pepper, zucchini, green beans, and carrot on a baking sheet lined with parchment paper. Season with salt and pepper, and spray lightly with cooking spray. Bake for 12 to 14 minutes, or until just cooked through. Add the vegetables to the quinoa, and toss to combine. Set aside.

Lightly spray a nonstick skillet with cooking spray, and heat over medium heat. Sprinkle the chicken with cumin and a dash of salt to coat. Cook chicken for 3 minutes on each side or until cooked through. Thinly slice into strips.

Stir the yogurt, lemon juice, tahini, and honey in a small bowl to combine. Add the parsley and mint to the quinoa salad, and toss to combine. Place half the salad in a serving bowl and the other half in a storage container for tomorrow's lunch. Top each portion with chicken and drizzle with yogurt dressing.

Refrigerate the second portion.

VEGETARIAN OPTION You don't have to include the chicken; quinoa has enough protein for a light vegetarian meal.

NUTRITION INFO: *Calories 377, Fat (g) 6, Sat fat (g) 1, Protein (g) 43, Carbs (g) 39, Fiber (g) 9, Sodium (mg) 149*

DESSERTS

apple-berry crumble

This recipe has double the fruit and double the flavor!

SERVES 1   PREP TIME 10 minutes   COOK TIME 45 minutes

1 medium-size apple, peeled and cored
1 tsp. granulated sugar
½ tsp. ground cinnamon
2 Tbsp. oats
1 tsp. brown sugar
1 tsp. heart-healthy margarine
½ cup fresh or frozen berries, any variety

Preheat oven to 350°. Slice the apple; place apple slices in a saucepan with 2 Tbsp. water, granulated sugar, and cinnamon. Heat over high heat until the mixture boils. Reduce heat and simmer for 10 minutes.

Meanwhile, use clean fingers to combine the oats, brown sugar, and margarine in a bowl. Set aside.

Drain any excess water from the apple mixture. Add the berries and combine well. Place the fruit in a ramekin, and top with the crumble mixture. Place the ramekin in a deep baking tray filled with enough water to surround the base of the ramekin. Bake for 30 minutes or until the crumble is golden. Allow the crumble to rest for 5 minutes before serving.

NUTRITION INFO: *Calories 245, Fat (g) 5, Sat fat (g) 1, Protein (g) 2, Carbs (g) 53, Fiber (g) 8, Sodium (mg) 52*

honey pistachio dip

This slightly sweet dip is perfect with apple slices or whole-grain crackers. You could also use walnuts, if you don't have pistachios at home.

SERVES 1   PREP TIME 5 minutes

2 Tbsp. shelled pistachios, finely chopped
1 Tbsp. reduced-fat cream cheese
1 Tbsp. plain fat-free Greek yogurt
½ tsp. honey

Combine all ingredients in a small bowl. Refrigerate or serve immediately.

NUTRITION INFO: *Calories 78, Fat (g) 6, Sat fat (g) 2, Protein (g) 3, Carbs (g) 4, Fiber (g) 0, Sodium (mg) 141*

week 4

welcome to Week 4 of
Bootcamp. You're almost halfway there. You have one month of healthy habits under your belt. Whether you've done every workout or you still need a few extra rest days each week, that's OK.

You're still here, still reading, still focusing on your goals. It's never too late to set a new goal, readjust your expectations, and find success. We know that this can be a challenging time. Reality sets in, your body is getting tired, and some of you feel like you're losing steam. That is completely normal! The best way to work through these feelings of frustration and doubt is by setting goals, because motivation is sparked through achievement. We say it every week, because it works: Set one small, achievable goal that you will commit to this week. Don't worry about last week. It's in the past. Don't think about next week. It's not here yet. Just focus on your next healthy choice: your next workout, your next meal, and your next glass of water.

If you're feeling strong, this halfway point is the time to keep your eyes on the prize and avoid falling into familiar old habits. If you're struggling, hang in there. Do what you can, and remember: We're looking for progress, not perfection!

There have been and there will continue to be daily challenges along your road to healthy living. They might come in the form of food, friends, family, or life itself. You have a choice of how you respond. We hope that by showing up here daily, reading the weekly guides, doing the workouts (even when you don't want to), and staying accountable to your eight-week Bootcamp program, you will have the strength to continue. Dedication and a belief in yourself is what will get you to the next level. Regardless of the challenges that present themselves (and they will), you are here, you have it in you to push through, and you will keep going. If this program were easy, you would not take such pride in your weekly accomplishments.

If you need a little extra motivation this week, go back and read through your goals from the previous weeks. Look at your starting weight, too. Once you see how far you've come, you'll feel motivated to keep going.

We believe in you!

thank you, thank you!

When you focus on the positive aspects in your life, what you appreciate and consider to be "working" well RIGHT NOW, you will experience more positivity and see more possibilities in your life. Research has found that keeping a gratitude journal helps to increase the positivity in your life. This week, write down three things that you are grateful for or that went well that day, and do this at least two times this week. Take a moment to think about each one as you write it down and notice any positive emotions that show up. Continue to keep your journal for the rest of the week and throughout Bootcamp. Just as it takes time to strengthen a muscle, the gratitude journal will help you develop more positivity in your life when you do it consistently.

WEEKLY WORKOUTS

MONDAY	Honeymoon Is Over
TUESDAY	Cardio Crazy
WEDNESDAY	DYOW
THURSDAY	Duty for the Booty
FRIDAY	Hear Me Roar
SATURDAY	Last-Chance Workout—Lisa
SUNDAY	Active Rest Day

WEEK 4 MEALS

MONDAY
B Peanut Butter Toast
L Niçoise Salad with Ahi Tuna
D Quick Chicken Parmesan with Spaghetti Squash

TUESDAY
B Chocolate, Banana, Peanut Butter Smoothie
L Quick Chicken Parmesan with Spaghetti Squash
D Lisa Rambo's Baked Fish Packets with Fresh Salsa

WEDNESDAY
B Italian Omelette
L Chicken Salad with Golden Tomato Dressing
D Loaded Bacon Cheeseburger Pasta

THURSDAY
B Quick Breakfast Couscous
L Chicken & Avocado Wrap
D Santa Fe Chicken Enchiladas

FRIDAY
B Oatmeal, Your Way
L Santa Fe Chicken Enchilada over Zucchini Noodles
D Individual Flatbread Pizza

SATURDAY
B Banana Yogurt Smoothie
L Lemony Chicken Salad
D Spicy Chicken Sandwich with Sweet Potato Fries & Chipotle Aioli

SUNDAY
B Peanut Butter Toast
L Spicy Chicken Sandwich with Sweet Potato Fries & Chipotle Aioli
D Shrimp in a White Bean, Vegetable & Sundried Tomato Broth

day 1

nutrition bite:

The Tao Of Pizza.

Find balance and a meaningful life lesson with pizza. (Yes, pizza.) If you crave a slice, make a simple change so that you can still keep it on the menu. Make it a rule to have a large green salad with a low-fat dressing every time you have pizza. Eating a couple of servings of salad before the pizza arrives will make it much easier to feel satisfied after one or two slices instead of needing three or four. Pizza, like life, isn't all or nothing. You can have your pizza and eat it, too!

honeymoon is over

38 MINUTES | WARM UP FOR 5 MINUTES

It's Week 4: The honeymoon is over and now the "marriage" with your health and fitness truly begins. Even if it feels tough at times, a long and happy marriage is worth working for!

Optional weights can be added to the moves marked with an asterisk (*). You do not need any equipment for the remaining moves.

> **"** Get to cravings before they get to you. If you're craving for pizza or something sweet, it's OK—we are all human. Have a piece of pizza or grab a few squares of dark chocolate. If you don't listen to your cravings and feed them in a healthy way, they will get the best of you. **"**
> —*The Biggest Loser* trainer Jennifer Widerstrom

THE WORKOUT

INTERVAL A
2 ROUNDS

1 Squats with Biceps Curls* X 1 minute
2 Quick Feet X 1 minute
3 Lunge Twists X 1 minute
4 Air Jump Rope X 1 minute
5 Squats with Overhead Presses* X 1 minute
6 Jogging X 1 minute

Repeat for Round 2

INTERVAL B
2 ROUNDS

7 Rear-Stepping Lunges with One-Arm Rows* X 1 minute
8 Skater Jumps X 1 minute
9 Woodchops* X 1 minute
10 Mountain Climbers X 1 minute
11 Side Lunges with Single Arm Lateral Raises* X 1 minute
12 Jumping Jacks X 1 minute

Repeat for Round 2

COOL DOWN FOR 5 MINUTES

INTERVAL A

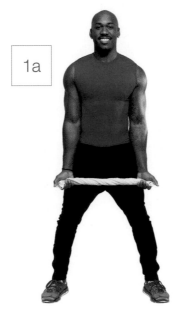
1a

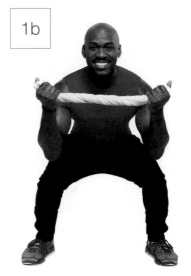
1b

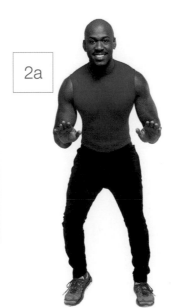
2a

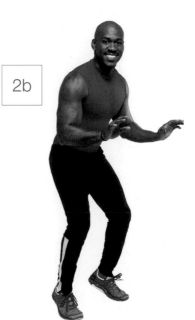
2b

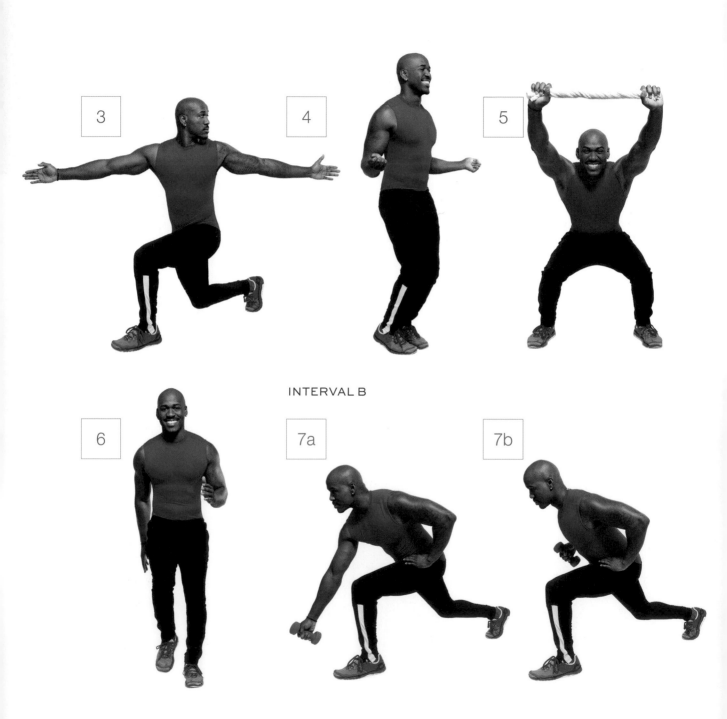

INTERVAL B

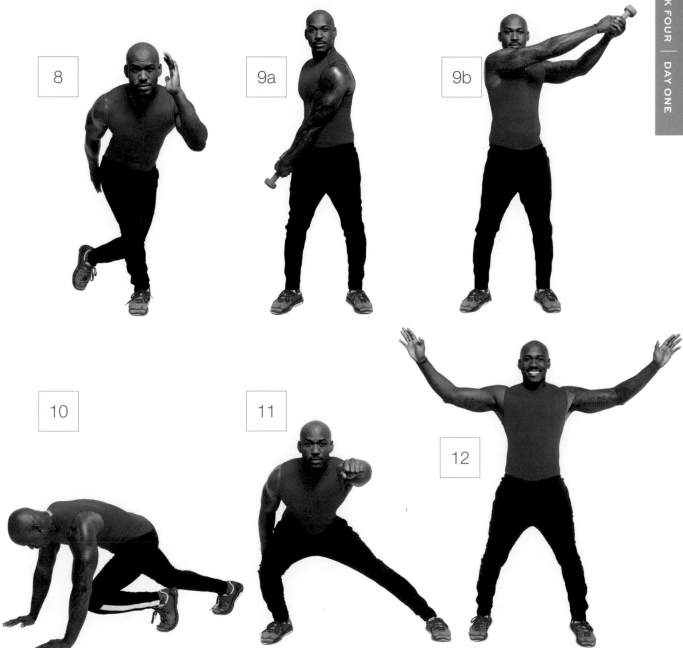

8

9a

9b

10

11

12

MEALS

BREAKFAST

peanut butter toast

Serve 2 slices whole-wheat bread, 1 Tbsp. peanut butter, and 1 medium-size piece of fruit with 1 cup skim milk.

NUTRITION INFO: *Calories 395, Fat (g) 10, Sat fat (g) 1, Protein (g) 20, Carbs (g) 59, Fiber (g) 7, Sodium (mg) 390*

LUNCH

niçoise salad with ahi tuna

See recipe on page 174.

DINNER

quick chicken parmesan with spaghetti squash

Serve with ½ cup plain fat-free Greek yogurt with ½ cup strawberries.

Top 2 cooked chicken breasts (3-oz. portions) with ¼ cup part-skim shredded mozzarella, 1 cup low-sodium pasta sauce, and 2 tsp. shredded Parmesan. Bake at 350° until bubbly, about 10 minutes (or microwave). Serve over 4 cups spaghetti squash with 2 cups sautéed mushrooms. Note that you'll save half of this for tomorrow's lunch.

VEGETARIAN OPTION Sub in a low-sodium veggie burger for the chicken.

NUTRITION INFO: *Calories 297, Fat (g) 6, Sat fat (g) 1, Protein (g) 33, Carbs (g) 18, Fiber (g) 3, Sodium (mg) 433*

SNACKS

Choose up to 300 calories of snacks to reach your calorie goal for the day. See the lists in Chapter 3 for snack ideas.

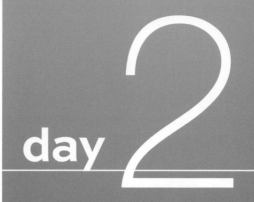

day 2

morning motivation:

What's It Worth?

Everything in life has a cost. Beyond the price tag, there is the opportunity cost to consider in every choice you make with regards to your journey. That is, what do you give up (beyond money) in exchange for these healthy choices?

If you start to waver in your dedication to this program, stop and think about what it's worth to you. What are you really sacrificing? Is it worth it? What will you give up now, for the rewards of health, fitness, and confidence that will come later? This journey is not easy, as you are discovering. But we think you see that the benefits are worth it.

WORKOUT cardio crazy

33 MINUTES | WARM UP FOR 5 MINUTES

Today we're going cardio crazy! That's right: We've got some of our longest, hardest intervals so far in Bootcamp, and we know you're going to love it!

THE WORKOUT

1. High Knees X 30 seconds
2. Jogging X 30 seconds
3. Air Jump Rope X 30 seconds
4. Lunge Twists X 1 minute
5. Walking X 1 minute
— Jogging X 30 seconds
— Air Jump Rope X 30 seconds
6. Skater Jumps X 30 seconds
7. Burpees X 1 minute
— High Knees X 1 minute
— Skater Jumps X 30 seconds
8. High Knees with Torso Twist X 30 seconds

(CONTINUES)

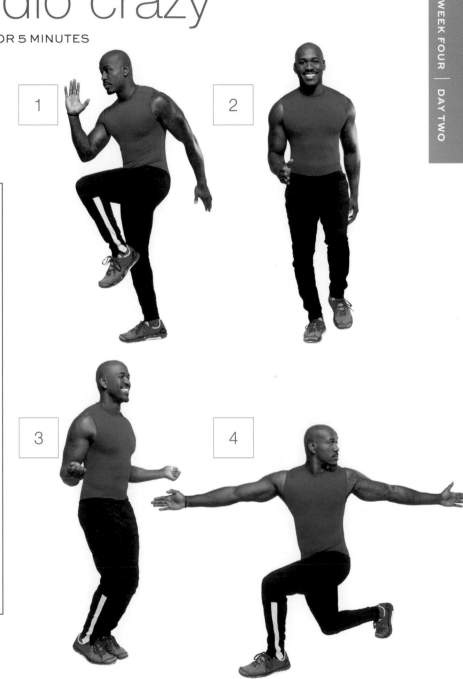

THE WORKOUT
CONTINUED

9   Quick Feet X 30 seconds

—   Jogging X 30 seconds

—   High Knees X 30 seconds

10   Traveling Squats X 30 seconds

—   Walking X 1 minute

—   High Knees with Torso Twist X 30 seconds

—   Quick Feet X 30 seconds

11   Jumping Jacks X 30 seconds

(CONTINUES)

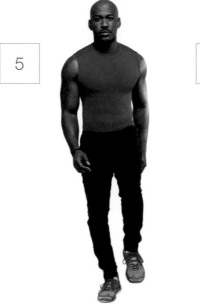

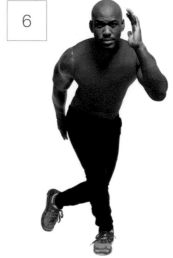

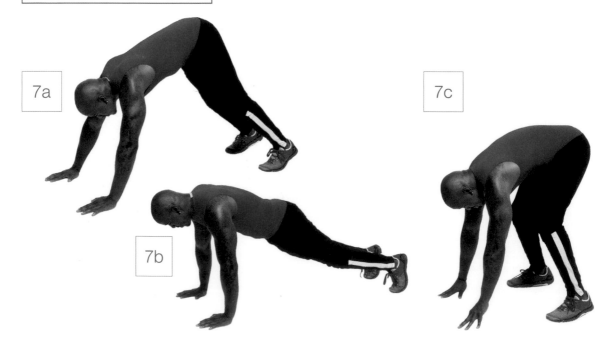

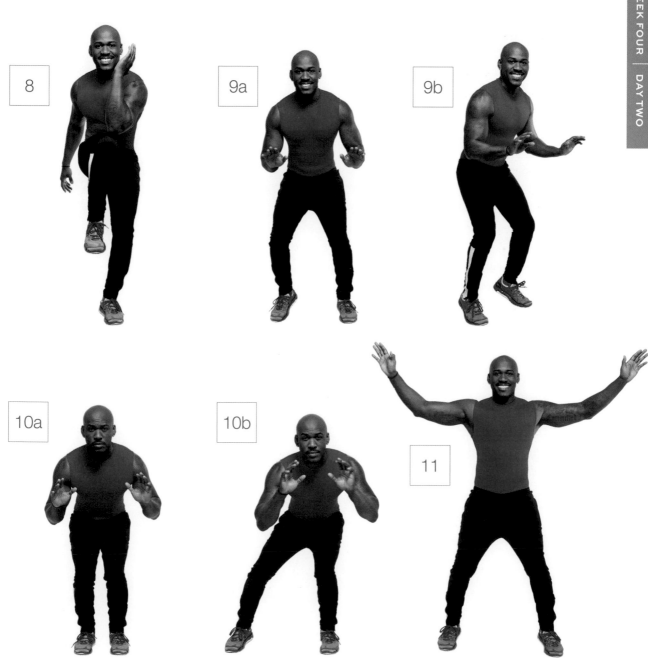

THE WORKOUT
CONTINUED

12 Traveling Squats with Pivot X 90 seconds

— High Knees X 1 minute

— Jogging X 30 seconds

13 Rear-Stepping Lunges with Woodchops X 30 seconds

— Jumping Jacks X 30 seconds

14 Mountain Climbers X 90 seconds

15 Curtsies X 30 seconds

— Burpees X 30 seconds

16 Forward Lunges X 30 seconds

— High Knees with Torso Twist X 30 seconds

— Quick Feet X 30 seconds

— Jumping Jacks X 30 seconds

— Walking X 1 minute

COOL DOWN FOR 5 MINUTES

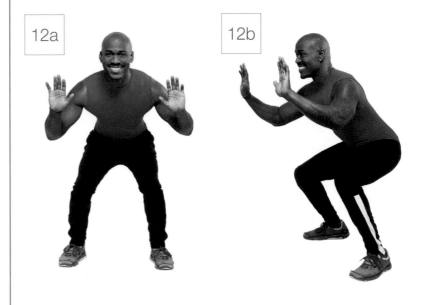

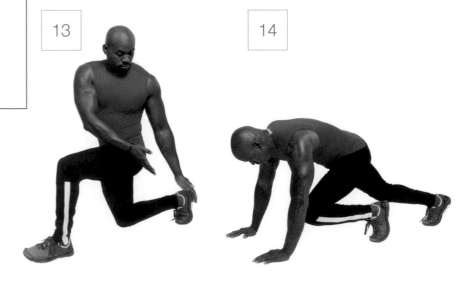

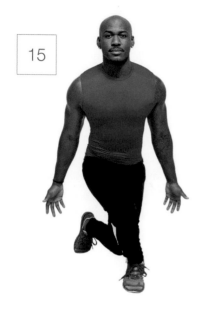

15

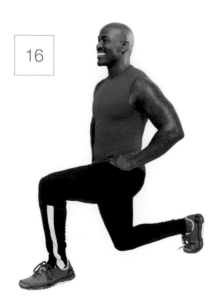

16

MEALS

BREAKFAST

chocolate, banana, peanut butter smoothie

See recipe on page 67.

LUNCH

quick chicken parmesan with spaghetti squash

Serve last night's leftovers. Serve with ½ cup plain fat-free Greek yogurt with ½ cup strawberries.

DINNER

lisa rambo's baked fish packets with fresh salsa

See recipe on page 175.

Serve with 1 cup brown rice or 3 corn tortillas and ¼ avocado.

SNACKS

Choose up to 300 calories of snacks to reach your calorie goal for the day. See the lists in Chapter 3 for snack ideas.

day 3

weekly check-in:

Ask The Tough Questions.

You know that for this to work, you've got to get real with yourself and start asking some tough questions. Here's some food for thought: What is the most painful thing about being overweight? What are you most ashamed of? What "baggage" are you still holding onto? You don't have to tell your answer, but you do have to think about it.

do your own workout (dyow)

It's Wednesday, and you know what that means: Do Your Own Workout! What'll it be this week? Now that you're more than halfway through the Bootcamp, consider trying something new: Swim laps, take a kickboxing class, or race your kids on the playground for an hour (yep, that counts).

"Tap into something greater than you. Think about where you can draw energy and strength from outside of yourself—for some it's community, for some it's nature, and for some it's spirit. Remember, you're not alone—there are powerful sources of strength and belonging just waiting for you to tap into.**"** —*The Biggest Loser* trainer Jessie Pavelka

MEALS

BREAKFAST
italian omelette

See recipe on page 173.

Serve with 1 cup skim milk and 1 orange.

LUNCH
chicken salad with golden tomato dressing

See recipe on page 174 for the dressing.

Combine 1 serving dressing with 3 cups kale (leaves only, chopped), 1 chopped cooked chicken breast (3 oz.), and 2 Tbsp. unsalted sunflower seeds.

NOTE You can toss the kale and dressing up to 1 day in advance; this will tenderize the kale.

VEGETARIAN OPTION Sub in ½ cup cooked chickpeas for the chicken.

NUTRITION INFO: *Calories 358, Fat (g) 12, Sat fat (g) 2, Protein (g) 37, Carbs (g) 26, Fiber (g) 6, Sodium (mg) 170*

DINNER
loaded bacon cheeseburger pasta

Serve with 3 cups mixed salad greens and 1 Tbsp. light vinaigrette.

Top 1 cup whole-wheat pasta with 3 oz. cooked lean ground beef, 1 slice crumbled turkey bacon, ¼ cup shredded reduced-fat cheddar cheese, 1 cup chopped spinach, and ½ cup chopped tomatoes, and heat through. Season with black pepper.

VEGETARIAN OPTION Sub in a low-sodium veggie burger for the beef.

NUTRITION INFO: *Calories 363, Fat (g) 8, Sat fat (g) 3, Protein (g) 31, Carbs (g) 39, Fiber (g) 5, Sodium (mg) 229*

DESSERT
trim tiramisu

Dip 2 vanilla wafer cookies into coffee. Top with ½ cup fat-free vanilla Greek yogurt and sprinkle with unsweetened cocoa powder.

NUTRITION INFO: *Calories 91, Fat (g) 2, Sat fat (g) 0, Protein (g) 8, Carbs (g) 12, Fiber (g) 0, Sodium (mg) 62*

SNACKS
Choose up to 300 calories of snacks to reach your daily goal. See the lists in Chapter 3 for snack ideas. Don't forget to include your dessert in your food journal (dessert gets included with your snack calories).

day 4

morning motivation:

Fight For Your Right To A Better You!

If you want this, you have to be willing to fight for it. Now, we don't want to condone violence. We simply mean that you have to be willing to do whatever it takes to reach your goals: You have to be willing to pack your lunches the night before, get your workout clothes ready to go for the morning, or sign up for that cycling class for DYOW Wednesday. These choices will become habits, and then they won't feel like a sacrifice. You won't even think about them. Sometimes the fight is internal. You can be your own worst enemy, so you have to fight yourself to get out of your own way. You can't just sit back and let life happen—you have to make it happen. So get out there and fight for what you want today!

WORKOUT
duty for the booty

38 MINUTES
WARM UP FOR 5 MINUTES

Think of today's workout as the duty you must fulfill for that strong booty you're getting in Bootcamp! Lunging, squatting, and squeezing are building a better posterior, which will help you in all major movements in life—not just in aesthetic ways.

Optional weights can be added to the moves marked with an asterisk (*). You do not need any equipment for the remaining moves.

❝ What should my plate look like? 70% of your plate should be grown and 30% should be animal, simple as that. Eating real food and lots of vegetables, fruit, and grains will keep you full and satisfied. Eating this way gives your body food that it can more easily digest which will nourish your body and help lean out your physique. ❞
—*The Biggest Loser* trainer Jennifer Widerstrom

THE WORKOUT

INTERVAL A
2 ROUNDS

1 Squats with Biceps Curls* X 1 minute

2 Skater Jumps X 1 minute

3 Lunge Twists X 1 minute or 6 reps per side

4 Jumping Jacks X 1 minute

5 Squats with Overhead Presses* X 1 minute

6 High Knees X 1 minute

Repeat for Round 2

INTERVAL B
2 ROUNDS

7 Rear-Stepping Lunges with One-Arm Rows X 1 minute

8 Burpees X 1 minute

9 Woodchops X 1 minute

10 Air Jump Rope X 1 minute

11 Side Lunges X 1 minute

12 Quick Feet X 1 minute

Repeat for Round 2

COOL DOWN FOR 5 MINUTES

INTERVAL A

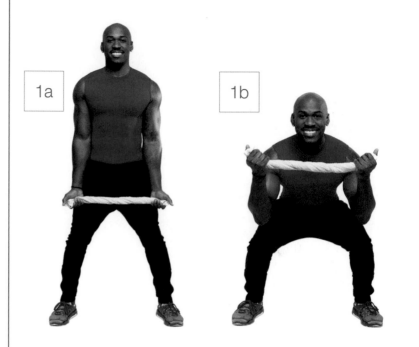

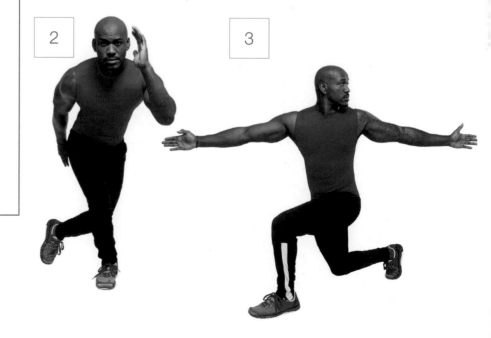

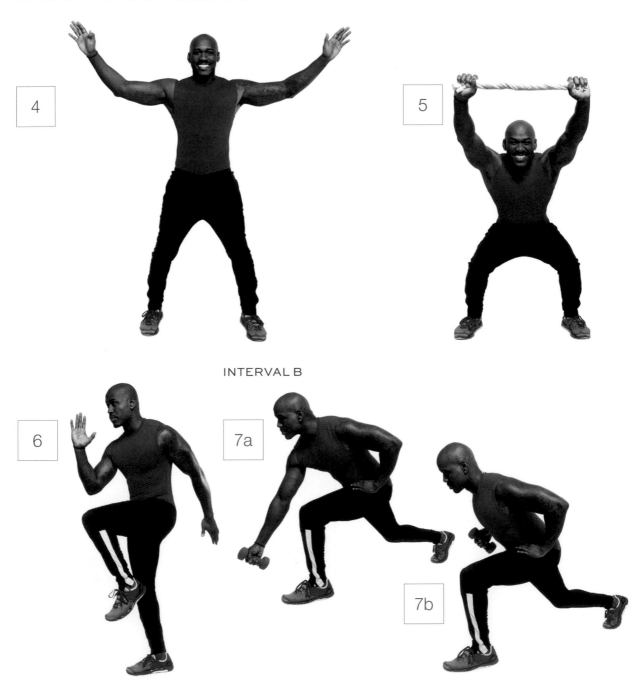

4

5

INTERVAL B

6

7a

7b

8a

8b

8c

9a

9b

10

THE WORKOUT CONTINUED

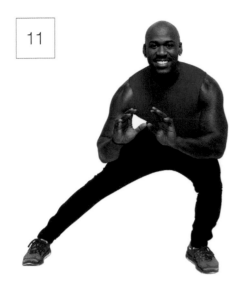

11

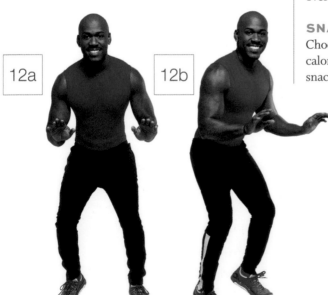

12a   12b

MEALS

BREAKFAST
quick breakfast couscous
See recipe on page 134.

Serve with 1 cup skim milk.

LUNCH
chicken & avocado wrap
See recipe on page 174.

Serve with 1 cup watermelon and 1 carrot with 2 Tbsp. hummus.

DINNER
santa fe chicken enchiladas
See recipe on page 176.

Serve with ½ cup black beans, 3 cups spinach, 2 Tbsp. low-sodium salsa, and ½ cup mango. You'll save leftovers for later in the week.

SNACKS
Choose up to 300 calories of snacks to reach your calorie goal for the day. See the lists in Chapter 3 for snack ideas.

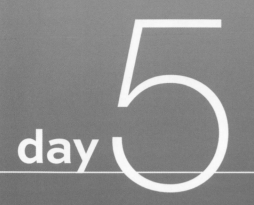

day 5

nutrition bite:

Make Temptation Less Tempting.

Studies have shown that when a person can reach a candy dish at work, he or she consumes 100 more calories per day than if the dish is 6 feet away. What are some of your temptation foods that you can make less convenient by moving them out of reach or out of sight? While you're at it, what are healthy choices that you can make more convenient, such as keeping fresh fruit in your kitchen, cutting up your favorite vegetables, or packing a small bag of unsalted nuts and an apple when you leave the house?

WORKOUT hear me roar

35 MINUTES | WARM UP FOR 5 MINUTES

On Tuesday we went cardio crazy, and today we want to HEAR YOU ROAR! Using exercise as an escape is a healthy way to deal with life's ups and downs, so let this be your chance to release any anger or frustration you've bottled up this week.

THE WORKOUT

1   Skater Jumps X 30 seconds
2   High Knees with Torso Twist X 30 seconds
3   Quick Feet X 30 seconds
4   Traveling Squats X 1 minute
5   Walking X 1 minute
—   High Knees with Torso Twist X 30 seconds
—   Quick Feet X 30 seconds
6   Jumping Jacks X 30 seconds
7   Mountain Climbers X 1 minute
—   Walking X 1 minute
8   Jogging X 30 seconds
9   High Knees X 30 seconds
—   Traveling Squats X 30 seconds
10 Burpees X 1 minute
—   Walking X 1 minute
—   High Knees with Torso Twist X 30 seconds

(CONTINUES)

THE WORKOUT
CONTINUED

11 Rear-Stepping Lunges with Woodchops X 30 seconds

— Jumping Jacks X 30 seconds

12 Lunge Twists X 1 minute

— High Knees X 1 minute

13 Curtsies X 30 seconds

— Burpees X 30 seconds

14 Forward Lunges X 30 seconds

15 Traveling Squats with Pivot X 90 seconds

— High Knees X 1 minute

— Lunge Twists X 30 seconds

— Traveling Squats with Pivot X 30 seconds

— Skater Jumps X 30 seconds

— Mountain Climbers X 30 seconds

— Walking X 1 minute

— Jumping Jacks X 30 seconds

— High Knees with Torso Twist X 30 seconds

— Lunge Twists X 30 seconds

16 Air Jump Rope X 30 seconds

— Walking X 1 minute

COOL DOWN FOR 5 MINUTES

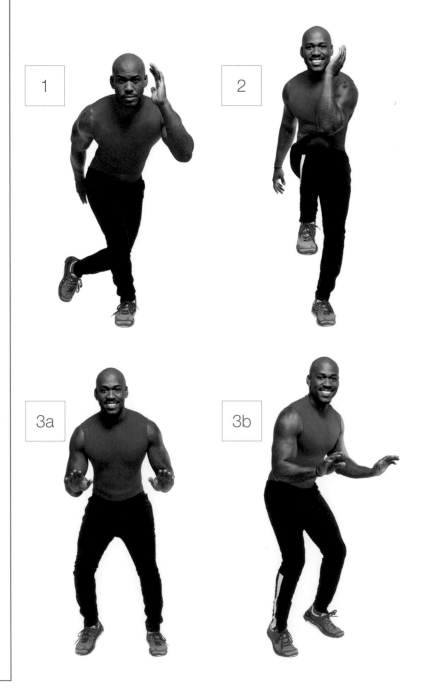

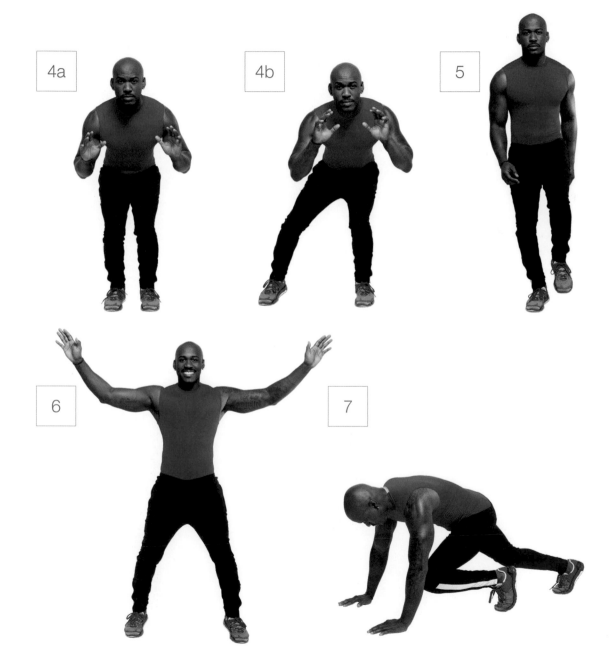

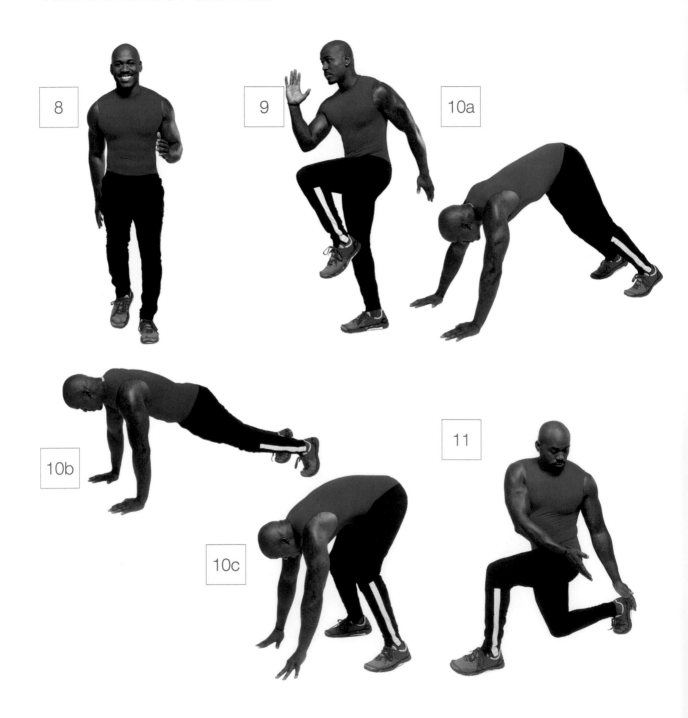

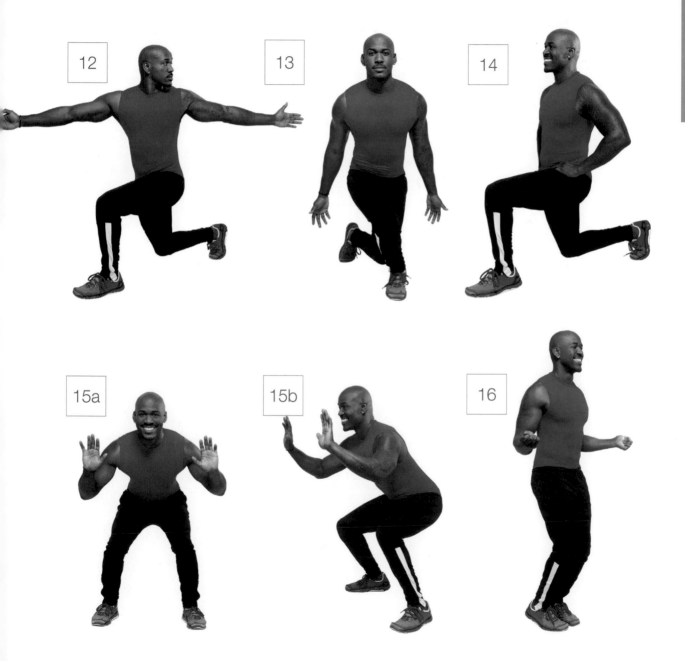

MEALS

BREAKFAST

oatmeal, your way

Prepare ½ cup oats with enough water (at least ½ cup) to achieve your desired consistency. Top your oatmeal with ½ cup fruit and ½ oz. nuts or 1 Tbsp. nut butter, and serve with 1 cup skim milk. The nutrition info will vary slightly depending on what you choose, but stick with the ratios provided, and this meal will fit into your plan.

NUTRITION INFO: *Calories 387, Fat (g) 12, Sat fat (g) 1, Protein (g) 17, Carbs (g) 58, Fiber (g) 7, Sodium (mg) 121*

LUNCH

santa fe chicken enchilada over zucchini noodles

Serve 1 leftover Santa Fe Chicken Enchilada atop 1 shredded or spiralized zucchini with 2 Tbsp. low-sodium salsa and ¼ avocado.

DINNER

individual flatbread pizza

See recipe on page 175.

Serve with 1 (6-oz.) container plain fat-free Greek yogurt and 1 cup strawberries.

SNACKS

Choose up to 300 calories of snacks to reach your calorie goal for the day. See the lists in Chapter 3 for snack ideas.

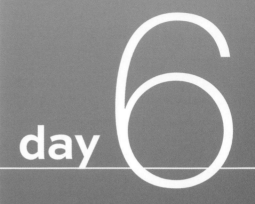

day 6

last chance:

We Know You Want It.

You know you want it. You've been waiting all week for it. Today is your last chance to chalk up one more workout for the week. Even if this is the only workout you do this week, no one is judging you. The past is the past, and it doesn't matter anymore. Get it done.

WORKOUT last-chance workout—lisa

41 MINUTES | WARM UP FOR 5 MINUTES

You met Lisa early in the book. Lisa Rambo inspired the nation during Season 14 of *The Biggest Loser*. What is even more of an inspiration is seeing how she's stayed fit and healthy away from the Ranch. So this workout goes out to Lisa—she inspires all of us to keep going! Note that there are two sets of cardio intervals you will repeat at various times during the workout. Optional weights can be added to the moves marked with an asterisk (*). You do not need any equipment for the remaining moves.

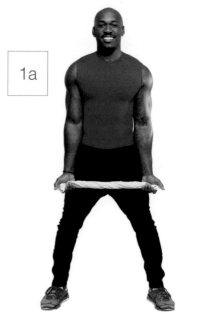

THE WORKOUT

INTERVAL A

1   Squats with Biceps Curls* X 1 minute

2   Squats with Overhead Presses* X 1 minute

(CONTINUES)

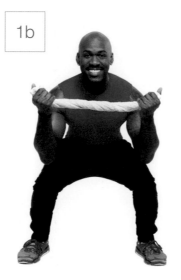

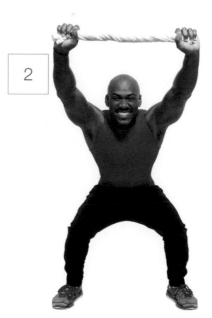

THE WORKOUT
CONTINUED

INTERVAL A

3 Jumping Jacks X 30 seconds

4 High Knees with Torso Twist X 30 seconds

5 Lunge Twists X 30 seconds

6 Air Jump Rope X 30 seconds

7 Push-Ups X 1 minute

8 Walking X 30 seconds

9 Woodchops* X 1 minute

10 Side Lunges X 1 minute

(CONTINUES)

INTERVAL A

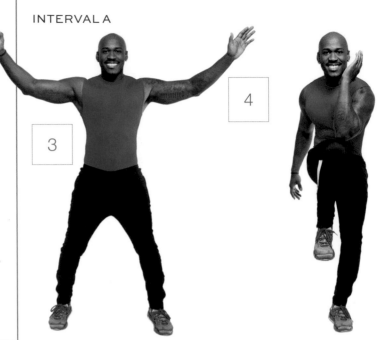

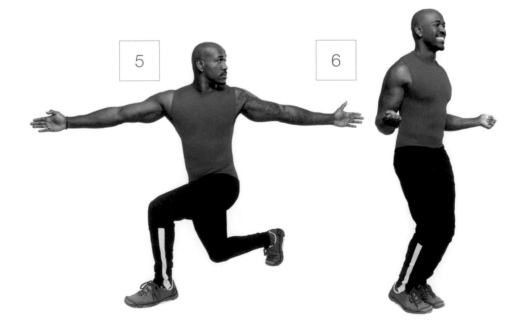

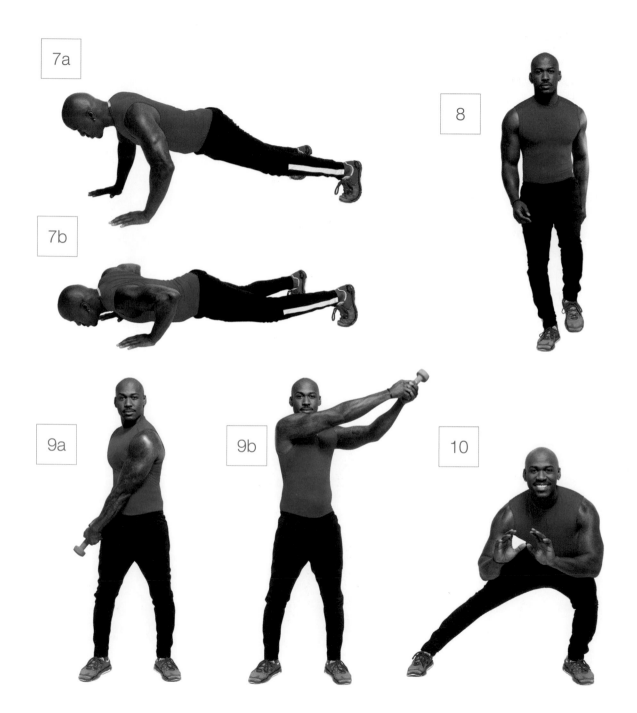

7a

7b

8

9a

9b

10

THE WORKOUT
CONTINUED

INTERVAL B

— Lunge Twists X 30 seconds

1 Traveling Squats with Pivot X 30 seconds

2 Skater Jumps X 30 seconds

3 Mountain Climbers X 30 seconds

4 Lat Pulldowns X 1 minute

— Walking X 30 seconds

5 Rear-Stepping Lunges with One-Arm Rows* X 1 minute

— Squats with Overhead Presses* X 1 minute

6 Curtsies X 30 seconds

— Jogging X 30 seconds

7 Forward Lunges X 30 seconds

8 Burpees X 30 seconds

9 Overhead Presses* X 1 minute

— Walking* X 30 seconds

— Squats with Biceps Curls* X 1 minute

— Woodchops* X 1 minute

(CONTINUES)

INTERVAL B

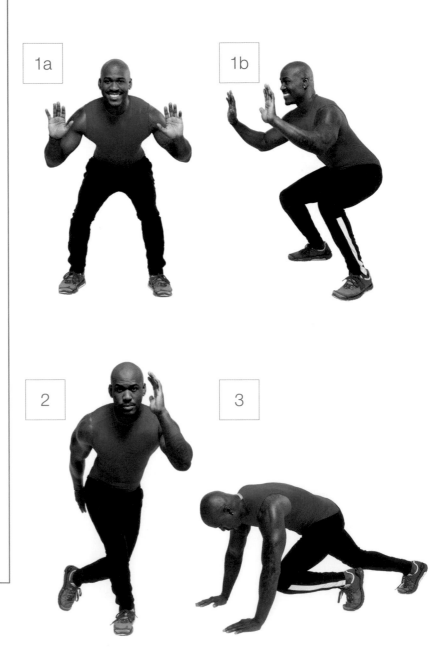

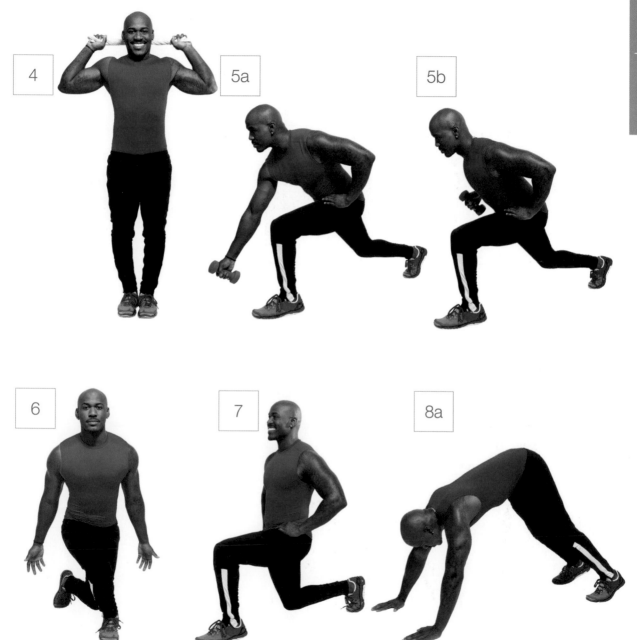

4

5a

5b

6

7

8a

THE WORKOUT

CONTINUED

Repeat Interval A, then do

10 Two-Arm Rows* X 1 minute

— Walking X 30 seconds

— Rear-Stepping Lunges with One-Arm Rows* X 1 minute

— Side Lunges X 1 minute

Repeat Interval B, then do

— Push-Ups X 1 minute or 10 reps

— Walking X 30 seconds

COOL DOWN FOR 5 MINUTES

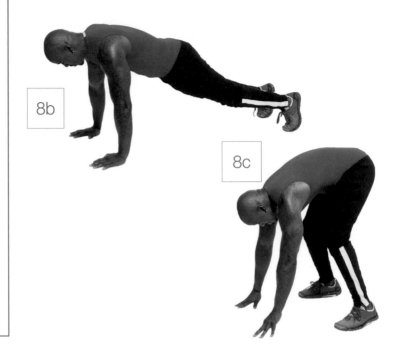

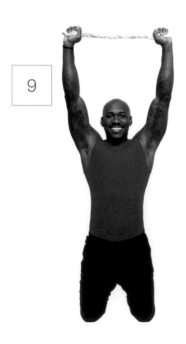

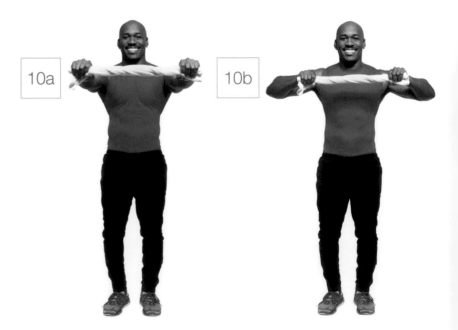

MEALS

BREAKFAST
banana yogurt smoothie
See recipe on page 134.

Serve with 1 slice whole-wheat toast with 1 Tbsp. natural peanut butter.

LUNCH
lemony chicken salad
Serve with ½ cup cooked quinoa.
Combine 3 oz. shredded chicken with 2 Tbsp. plain fat-free Greek yogurt, 2 Tbsp. reduced-fat feta, 1 Tbsp. lemon juice, ½ cup chopped cucumber, 2 Tbsp. chopped red onion, and a pinch each dried oregano, dill, and black pepper. Serve in 4 large Swiss chard leaves.

VEGETARIAN OPTION Sub in 3 oz. tofu or tempeh for the chicken.

NUTRITION INFO: *Calories 269, Fat (g) 4, Sat fat (g) 2, Protein (g) 49, Carbs (g) 7, Fiber (g) 2, Sodium (mg) 416*

DINNER
spicy chicken sandwich with sweet potato fries & chipotle aioli
Tonight you'll make an extra serving for tomorrow's lunch. Preheat oven to 425°. Slice 2 small sweet potatoes into wedges. Toss with 1 tsp. cornstarch, ½ tsp. each paprika, ground cumin, and black pepper, and a pinch of salt. Place on a baking sheet, and spray with nonstick spray. Bake 30 minutes, flipping halfway through. Mix 2 Tbsp. chipotle low-sodium salsa with 2 Tbsp. reduced-fat mayonnaise. To serve, place 1 cooked chicken breast on a whole-wheat bun and top with one slice each of tomato, onion, lettuce, plus 1 Tbsp. chipotle aioli. Serve an additional 1 Tbsp. of the aioli with half the fries.

Refrigerate the leftovers for the next day's meal.

NOTE Store the toppings separately from the rest of the meal until lunchtime tomorrow.

VEGETARIAN OPTION Sub in a low-sodium veggie burger for the chicken.

NUTRITION INFO: *Calories 369, Fat (g) 3, Sat fat (g) 0, Protein (g) 32, Carbs (g) 50, Fiber (g) 8, Sodium (mg) 379*

SNACKS
Choose up to 300 calories of snacks to reach your calorie goal for the day. See the lists in Chapter 3 for snack ideas.

day 7

morning motivation:

You Are Great.

For a lot of us, weight gain goes hand in hand with feeling down about ourselves. We're here to tell you that you are GREAT, no matter what the scale says or what anyone else says. Today, we want you to be great! We know that it's common to start your fitness journey feeling down on yourself. We know that you're going to have days when you get mad at yourself for getting tired or for making a decision you regret. It's easy to tell yourself "I'm not good enough." Today, be your own biggest champion, and don't let anyone—especially you—tell you that you're anything less than GREAT.

WORKOUT
active rest day

Can you believe you're halfway through the Bootcamp? Wow! Look back at all the workouts you've done. You're so much stronger, and you're just going to keep gaining strength as you lose weight and inches.

" We choose how we experience what happens to us. Has something upset you? A person? Is it really upsetting, or are you choosing to experience the event from a negative viewpoint? Take a deep breath and remember, little things can seemingly be big—if you let them. So don't."
—*The Biggest Loser* trainer Jennifer Widerstrom

MEALS

BREAKFAST

peanut butter toast

Serve 2 slices whole-wheat bread, 1 Tbsp. peanut butter, and 1 apple with 1 cup skim milk.

NUTRITION INFO: *Calories 395, Fat (g) 10, Sat fat (g) 1, Protein (g) 20, Carbs (g) 59, Fiber (g) 7, Sodium (mg) 390*

LUNCH

spicy chicken sandwich with sweet potato fries & chipotle aioli

Serve last night's leftovers.

DINNER

shrimp in a white bean, vegetable & sundried tomato broth

See recipe on page 176.

DESSERT

berry crisp

See recipe on page 177.

SNACKS

Choose up to 300 calories of snacks to reach your daily goal. See the lists in Chapter 3 for snack ideas. Don't forget to include your dessert in your food journal (dessert gets included with your snack calories).

WEEKLY RECIPES

BREAKFASTS

italian omelette

A hearty and satisfying breakfast that's quick enough for weekday meals.

SERVES 1   PREP TIME 5 minutes   COOK TIME 10 minutes

- ½ cup chopped onions
- 1 clove garlic, chopped
- 1 oz. low-sodium deli ham, chopped
- 3 egg whites
- 1 Tbsp. skim milk
- ½ tsp. dried oregano
- 2 Tbsp. fat-free ricotta cheese
- 1 Tbsp. sundried tomatoes (not packed in oil)

Lightly spray a small frying pan with cooking spray and heat over low heat. Gently cook the onions, garlic, and ham for a few minutes until the onions soften.

Combine the egg whites, milk, and oregano in a mixing bowl. Remove the onion mixture from the heat, allow to cool slightly, and fold into the eggs.

Spray the frying pan lightly with a little more cooking spray, and pour the mixture into the pan. Cook over medium heat until it begins to set. Sprinkle the ricotta and sundried tomatoes over one-half of the omelette, and use a spatula to fold the other side over to cover. Cook for another 5 minutes. Loosen the base and sides and gently slide out of the pan.

VEGETARIAN OPTION Sub ¼ cup sliced mushrooms for the ham.

NUTRITION INFO: *Calories 197, Fat (g) 6, Sat fat (g) 1, Protein (g) 21, Carbs (g) 17, Fiber (g) 2, Sodium (mg) 489*

chicken & avocado wrap

Avocado makes every sandwich or wrap better!

SERVES 1 **PREP TIME** 5 minutes

- ¼ avocado
- 1 (8-inch) whole-wheat tortilla
- 3 oz. cooked chicken, shredded
- 3 cups mixed salad greens

Spread avocado over tortilla. Fill with chicken and greens, and roll up tortilla. Cut into 2 pieces.

TIP If you dislike avocado or the one you bought isn't ripe yet, replace it with 2 Tbsp. hummus or light mayonnaise.

VEGETARIAN OPTION Sub 3 oz. tofu for the chicken.

NUTRITION INFO: *Calories 293, Fat (g) 13, Sat fat (g) 1, Protein (g) 30, Carbs (g) 28, Fiber (g) 20, Sodium (mg) 436*

golden tomato dressing

Sweet tomatoes create a thick, rich dressing with very little fat. Use on salads or grilled meats. This recipe is courtesy of The Biggest Loser Resorts Niagara.

SERVES 8 (serving size 2 Tbsp.) **PREP TIME** 2 minutes

- 1 Tbsp. extra-virgin olive oil
- 1½ cups golden tomatoes, roasted
- 1 clove garlic
- 1 Tbsp. fresh basil
- ¼ tsp. oregano
- 1½ Tbsp. honey
- 1½ oz. red wine vinegar
- Sea salt and coarsely ground black pepper, to taste

Combine all ingredients in a blender or food processor until smooth. Refrigerate for up to 2 weeks.

NUTRITION INFO: *Calories 22, Fat (g) 1, Sat fat (g) 0, Protein (g) 0, Carbs (g) 2, Fiber (g) 0, Sodium (mg) 2*

niçoise salad with ahi tuna

This recipe is quite easy to assemble, so don't let the lengthy ingredient list deter you. The salad, which comes from The Biggest Loser Resorts Niagara, is a bit fancier than most of our meals, but it perfectly illustrates how delicious and beautiful healthy food can be.

SERVES 1 **PREP TIME** 15 minutes **COOK TIME** 10 minutes

- 4 oz. ahi tuna steak
- 1 oz. Mango Vinaigrette (see recipe, page 212)
- 1 cup salad greens
- 2 Tbsp. diced beefsteak tomatoes
- 1 hard-boiled egg, cut into wedges
- 1½ Tbsp. chopped red onion
- 4 Niçoise olives
- ¼ small sweet potato, cooked and cut into wedges
- 1 artichoke heart, quartered
- ½ cup green beans, cooked

Sear the tuna rare. Dress the lettuce, and season to taste. This is a composed salad, so arrange the various vegetables and egg by color or texture. Slice tuna and fan across the salad.

NOTE If ahi tuna isn't in the budget, you can use a pouch of tuna, drained, or a piece of salmon.

VEGETARIAN OPTION Sub in ½ cup cooked chickpeas for the tuna.

NUTRITION INFO: *Calories 313, Fat (g) 9, Sat fat (g) 2, Protein (g) 38, Carbs (g) 19, Fiber (g) 6, Sodium (mg) 326*

DINNERS

lisa rambo's baked fish packets with fresh salsa

This recipe is a weekly staple at Lisa Rambo's house. "We eat at least three jars of fresh salsa a week," she says. "We put it on and in everything! It goes on our eggs, in our salads, on tacos, and we put it over fish and bake it!" We used store-bought salsa to save time, and it keeps fish moist and delicious, while the parchment makes for easy cleanup.

SERVES 1   PREP TIME 5 minutes   COOK TIME 12 minutes

3 oz. tilapia or other white fish
1 square parchment paper
½ cup fresh salsa

Preheat oven to 375°. Place the fish in the center of the parchment. Top with the salsa, and seal the edges. Place on a baking sheet to catch any drips. Bake for about 12 minutes, until the fish easily flakes.

You can also do this with chicken, but it will take longer to bake, about 30 minutes.

VEGETARIAN OPTION Serve fresh salsa on top of 3 oz. grilled tofu or mushrooms. So you know: Tofu gets mushy when baked in packets.

NUTRITION INFO: *Calories 128, Fat (g) 2, Sat fat (g) 1, Protein (g) 22, Carbs (g) 4, Fiber (g) 2, Sodium (mg) 280*

individual flatbread pizza

This quick pizza is our healthy spin on a bistro favorite.

SERVES 1   PREP TIME 15 minutes   COOK TIME 20 minutes

2 cups fresh spinach
½ tsp. balsamic vinegar
1 whole-wheat tortilla
1 clove garlic, sliced in half
1 oz. reduced-fat goat cheese or feta cheese
1 plum tomato, chopped
1 Tbsp. fresh basil, sliced into ribbons

Preheat oven to 400°.

Place spinach in a microwave-safe bowl. Cover and microwave at HIGH 2 to 3 minutes or until wilted; drain well. Combine spinach and vinegar; toss well.

Place tortilla on an ungreased baking sheet. Rub cut sides of garlic over top of the tortilla. Spread goat cheese evenly over tortilla. Top with spinach and tomato. Sprinkle with basil, salt, and pepper.

Bake at 400° for 10 to 12 minutes or until pizza is lightly browned and thoroughly heated. Cut into quarters, and serve immediately.

NUTRITION INFO: *Calories 190, Fat (g) 7, Sat fat (g) 3, Protein (g) 8, Carbs (g) 24, Fiber (g) 6, Sodium (mg) 345*

santa fe chicken enchiladas

Precooked chicken helps cut down cooking time on this delicious dinner. This 30-minute meal will feed you a few times this week, leaving more time for your other healthy habits.

SERVES 4   PREP TIME 10 minutes   COOK TIME 20 minutes

    1 cup cooked diced chicken breast
    3 Tbsp. chopped fresh cilantro, divided
    ¼ tsp. pepper
    1 (14.5-oz.) can chunky chili-style tomato sauce
    2 Tbsp. water
    4 (6-inch) corn tortillas
    1 (14.5-oz.) can black beans, drained, rinsed, and divided
    ⅓ cup (1⅓ oz.) Monterey Jack cheese, shredded, divided
    ¼ cup plain fat-free Greek yogurt

Combine chicken, 2 Tbsp. cilantro, and pepper in a small bowl; stir well.

Preheat oven to 375°.

Combine tomato sauce and water; pour into a plate. Set aside.

Microwave 2 tortillas, uncovered, at HIGH 10 seconds; dip each tortilla in sauce mixture. Spoon ¼ cup chicken mixture down center of each tortilla; top each with 2 Tbsp. black beans and 1 Tbsp. cheese. Roll up tortillas, and place seam sides down in an 8-inch square baking dish coated with cooking spray. Repeat procedure with remaining 2 tortillas, sauce mixture, chicken mixture, black beans, and cheese.

Pour any remaining tomato sauce mixture over enchiladas; top with remaining black beans and remaining cheese. Bake, uncovered, for 20 minutes or just until bubbly. Sprinkle with remaining 1 Tbsp. cilantro. Serve with yogurt.

Refrigerate 1 portion for tomorrow's lunch; freeze the other 2 for up to 1 month.

VEGETARIAN OPTION Add a second can of beans—black or pinto.

NUTRITION INFO: *Calories 239, Fat (g) 4.5, Sat fat (g) 2, Protein (g) 15, Carbs (g) 32, Fiber (g) 7, Sodium (mg) 460*

shrimp in a white bean, vegetable & sundried tomato broth

This recipe, from The Biggest Loser Resorts Niagara, is in the meal plan halfway through Bootcamp. We think this dinner is perfect for an active rest day—you'll have more time to spend making dinner, and you can get your loved ones in on the fun of healthy cooking!

SERVES 6   PREP TIME 20 minutes   COOK TIME 25 minutes

    1 Tbsp. extra-virgin olive oil
    ½ cup yellow onion, sliced very thin
    1 cup fennel bulb, sliced very thin
    1 Tbsp. saffron thread (optional)
    ¾ tsp. chopped garlic
    3 cups low-sodium vegetable broth
    ¾ cup Swiss chard, torn
    1½ cups asparagus, chopped
    1½ cups zucchini, diced
    ⅓ cup sundried tomatoes (not packed in oil), diced, drained
    1¼ cups canned cannellini beans
    2 Tbsp. chopped fresh basil
    ¼ tsp. orange zest
    ¾ cup red bell pepper, sliced very thin
    ⅛ tsp. sea salt, to taste
    ⅛ tsp. chili flakes
    1 Tbsp. lemon juice
    6 oz. no-salt-added tomato sauce
    18 oz. "sustainable choice" shrimp
    3 Tbsp. chopped Italian parsley

Heat 1 Tbsp. oil in a heavy-bottomed saucepan. Add onion, fennel, saffron (if using), and garlic. Cook 1 minute. Add the broth and remaining ingredients except for shrimp and parsley. Simmer for 10 minutes. Place shrimp in a 2-inch-deep pan, pour the vegetable mixture over the shrimp, and cover. Bake the shrimp for 7 to 10 minutes. Using a slotted spoon, gently remove the shrimp and place in a shallow serving bowl. Ladle the hot broth and vegetables over the shrimp.

Refrigerate in single serving portions for up to 3 days, or freeze for up to 1 month. Garnish with parsley.

NUTRITION INFO: *Calories 217, Fat (g) 5, Sat fat (g) 1, Protein (g) 23, Carbs (g) 18, Fiber (g) 8, Sodium (mg) 233*

DESSERTS

berry crisp

This berry crisp is as delicious with fresh berries as it is with frozen, so it's the perfect dessert any time of year. It comes to us from The Biggest Loser Resorts Niagara.

SERVES 1 PREP TIME 5 minutes COOK TIME 25 minutes

BERRY FILLING:
½ cup fresh berries
¼ tsp. fresh lemon juice
1 tsp. organic coconut palm sugar

CRISP TOPPING:
2 Tbsp. rolled oats
½ Tbsp. whole-wheat flour
½ Tbsp. organic coconut palm sugar
½ Tbsp. unsweetened coconut flakes
¼ tsp. ground cinnamon
⅛ tsp. ground ginger
½ Tbsp. coconut oil, melted
½ Tbsp. unsweetened almond milk

Preheat oven to 375°. Prepare the filling: Place berries in a small ovenproof dish. Drizzle lemon juice over fruit. Sprinkle fruit mixture with 1 tsp. sugar. For the topping, in a medium bowl, combine oats, flour, sugar, coconut, cinnamon, and ginger. Add coconut oil and almond milk; stir until crumbly. Sprinkle topping over fruit. Bake at 375° for 20 to 25 minutes until bubbly around edges and topping is browned.

Serve slightly warm or completely cooled.

NUTRITION INFO: *Calories 96, Fat (g) 5, Sat fat (g) 0, Protein (g) 2, Carbs (g) 13, Fiber (g) 2, Sodium (mg) 3*

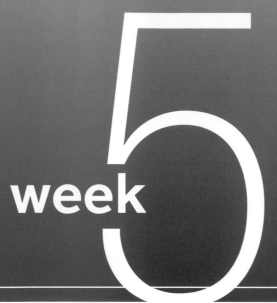

week 5

you're over the hump of Bootcamp. We set out on this journey together, and we're still in this together. We are extremely proud of you for getting out of your comfort zone and achieving so many goals.

Let's take a moment to reflect on the past four weeks, refocus on the next four weeks, and reignite the passion you have to change your life.

We know many of you have come a long way, but we also know you have plenty of hard work ahead. That's why you need to remind yourself of the positives. Again and again—each time you have a bad day or feel your motivation slip, tell yourself: "I can do this. Look what I've done already!"

We are here to help guide you to your goal, but we need you to keep your eyes on the road, stay committed to the journey, and remember to enjoy every twist, every bump, and every hill.

refocus

In life as well as in this Bootcamp, we use the past to improve our future. So, once you've reflected on all the good stuff that's happened over the past

four weeks, ask yourself: What can I do differently over the next four weeks to get better results? Some of you will answer, "Nothing, I just need to keep doing what I've been doing." Others will have some more specific areas to focus on.

Use these specifics in your weekly goals. Don't fall into the trap of trying to do everything at once: Focus on one area of improvement at a time. You've learned a lot about yourself, nutrition, and fitness over the past four weeks. And you're capable of a lot more than you think you are.

reignite

We all started Week 1 of Bootcamp pumped up and ready to go. Enthusiasm was off the charts and emotions were high. Over the weeks, that energy ebbs and flows, which is normal.

coaches' corner

YOU'RE MORE THAN A NUMBER: NON-SCALE victories. You know that you're on the right track, and yet sometimes the scale doesn't show the progress you are making. When you celebrate all of the positive changes, big or small, you'll feel more motivated to keep pushing.

At this halfway milestone, write down a list of all of the non-scale victories you've experienced since starting the Bootcamp. Think about EVERYTHING that has changed for the better. Examples might include how your clothes fit differently, how well you are sleeping, how easily you can walk flights of stairs, and how much better your mood has become.

- What can you do now that you couldn't do four weeks ago?

- Which aspects of your life are better than they were four weeks ago?

- How do you feel now compared with four weeks ago?

- How do your clothes fit now?

- How has your attitude changed?

- How much weight have you lost?

- How many inches have you lost?

Here are two big ones:

- You started this Bootcamp.

- You are still reading this book!

WEEK 5 MEALS

MONDAY

B Berry Green Smoothie

L Tex Mex Stuffed Sweet Potato

D Frittata with Whole-Wheat Spaghetti & Spinach

TUESDAY

B Frittata with Whole-Wheat Spaghetti & Spinach

L Kale Salad with Chicken & Mango Vinaigrette

D Bacon, Lentil & Tomato Soup

WEDNESDAY

B Morning Oatmeal

L Bacon, Lentil & Tomato Soup

D Spaghetti Squash Chicken Alfredo

THURSDAY

B Vegetarian Breakfast Stacks

L Confetti Quinoa

D Pesto Fish

FRIDAY

B Peanut Butter Toast

L Loaded Beans & Rice

D Zucchini Meatball "Sub"

SATURDAY

B Breakfast Quinoa Bowl

L Korean BBQ Cabbage Bowl

D Apricot Pork with Rice

SUNDAY

B Slim Bagel Sandwich

L Crunchy Tuna Salad Stuffed Pepper

D Barbecued Burger

Many of you are in the groove and now need less support than you did in the first week or two. But you might sometimes feel like you are slipping. If you're finding it hard to stay committed to this journey, use this week as a chance to reignite that spark from Week 1.

If you haven't completed as many workouts as you would have liked, that's OK. It's never too late to start. Every day is a new day. Every meal is a new opportunity to start again and be better.

You know that we start the week by setting a small, achievable goal. But what you might not know is that it's OK to repeat goals, or reuse the same one from the previous week. You don't have to come up with a new goal every time!

WEEKLY WORKOUTS

MONDAY	Game On
TUESDAY	Dolvett's Ladder
WEDNESDAY	DYOW
THURSDAY	Killin' It
FRIDAY	Cardio Arrest
SATURDAY	Last-Chance Workout—Craig
SUNDAY	Active Rest Day

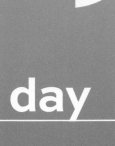

day 1
nutrition bite:

Is Coffee A Culprit?

Sugar lurks in all kinds of foods, but the sneakiest place you'll find sugar is in beverages. Raise your hand if you're a coffee drinker. That's OK—you're allowed a cup or two. Now, how do you take your coffee? If you said with sugar or artificial sweeteners, we want to challenge you to wean yourself off it. Start with one less spoonful or packet today, and each day or each week, cut back a bit more. Soon, you might find you actually like the taste of the coffee itself.

If you like creamer, what kind do you use? The flavored ones have just 10 to 15 calories a serving, but many of us use far more than one serving. If you're overdoing it, just like with the sugar, start cutting back one spoonful at a time.

WORKOUT
game on

39 MINUTES | WARM UP FOR 5 MINUTES

It's Week 5, and we're back at it. This week's workouts dial it up, and you'll find you have to push through it to get it done. Bootcamp is at half-time, and it's GAME ON!

Optional weights can be added to the moves marked with an asterisk (*). You do not need any equipment for the remaining moves.

THE WORKOUT
2 ROUNDS

1 Squats* X 30 seconds
2 Side Lunges X 30 seconds
3 Warrior 1 X 1 minute
4 Jogging X 1 minute
5 Chest Presses* X 30 seconds
6 Overhead Presses* X 30 seconds
7 Plank X 1 minute
8 Air Jump Rope X 1 minute
9 Walking X 30 seconds
10 Forward Lunges X 30 seconds
11 Curtsies X 30 seconds
— Warrior 2 X 1 minute
12 Skater Jumps X 1 minute
13 Lat Pulldowns X 30 seconds

(CONTINUES)

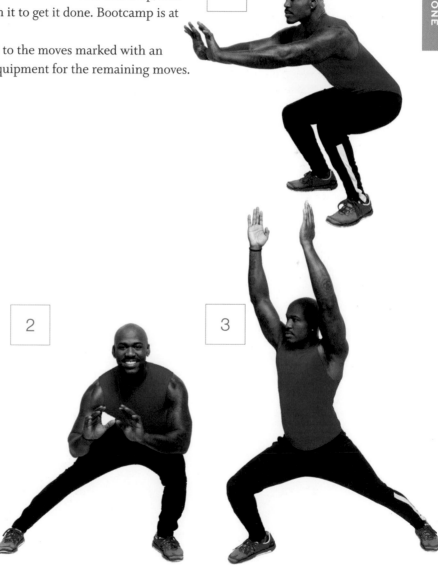

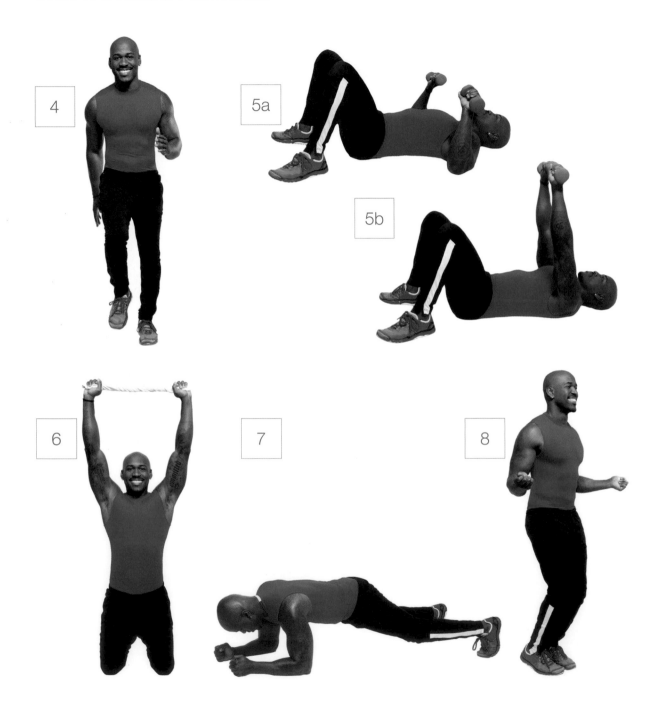

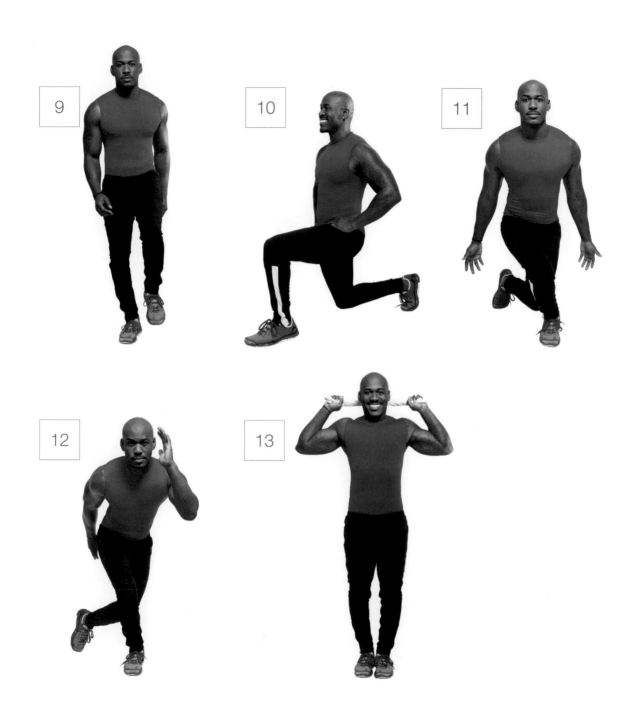

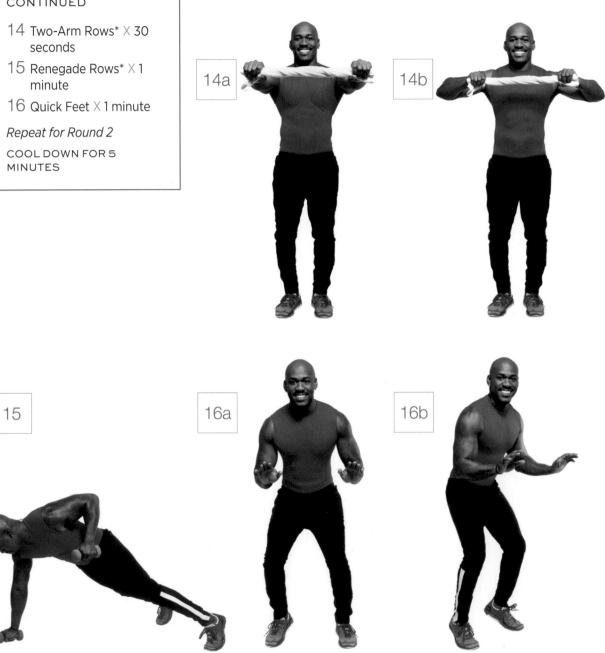

THE WORKOUT

CONTINUED

14 Two-Arm Rows* X 30 seconds

15 Renegade Rows* X 1 minute

16 Quick Feet X 1 minute

Repeat for Round 2

COOL DOWN FOR 5 MINUTES

14a

14b

15

16a

16b

MEALS

BREAKFAST

berry green smoothie

See recipe on page 211.

Serve with 1 slice whole-wheat toast and 1 Tbsp. natural peanut butter.

LUNCH

tex mex stuffed sweet potato

Serve with 1 cup bell pepper strips.
Microwave or bake 1 small potato. Split open and fill with 3 oz. ground turkey cooked with taco seasonings, ¼ cup low-sodium salsa, and 2 Tbsp. reduced-fat shredded cheese of your choice, and heat until the cheese melts. Top with 1 Tbsp. plain fat-free Greek yogurt, cilantro, hot sauce, and chopped cilantro.

VEGETARIAN OPTION Sub in ½ cup cooked black beans for the turkey.

NUTRITION INFO: *Calories 359, Fat (g) 4, Sat fat (g) 1, Protein (g) 30, Carbs (g) 47, Fiber (g) 7, Sodium (mg) 428*

DINNER

frittata with whole-wheat spaghetti & spinach

See recipe on page 214.

Serve with 1 cup grapes.

SNACKS

Choose up to 300 calories of snacks to reach your calorie goal for the day. See the lists in Chapter 3 for snack ideas.

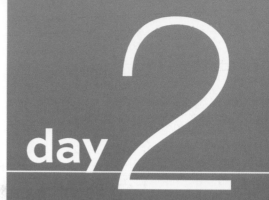

day 2

morning motivation:

Why Are You Doing This?

When you wake up in the morning and think about whether or not you should work out, ask yourself: Why am I doing this? Why do you want to work so hard? Back in Week 1, you set your intention and told yourself why you're here. In Week 4, you looked back at how far you've come. It's time to remind yourself again.

Focus on why you committed to this healthy lifestyle, and let your goal be your motivation to stick to your plan. Even the most successful among us need to keep returning to the "why" over and over. Don't take your eyes off that prize. It will make getting up early, doing these workouts, and eating healthier foods that much easier.

WORKOUT dolvett's ladder

34 MINUTES | WARM UP FOR 5 MINUTES

Today we have body confusion, cardio style. We're doing a "pyramid" workout that tests your mettle by "ascending" to a peak with cardio intervals that gradually increase in difficulty. We call it Dolvett's Ladder, and we want you to think of climbing up to something really high, earning your reward, then climbing back down with gradually decreasing intervals.

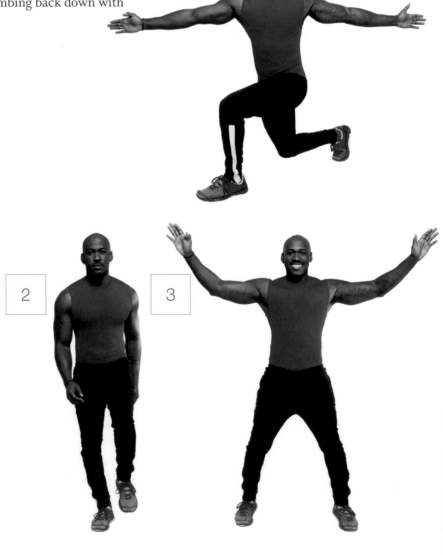

THE WORKOUT

DO IT ONCE, AND REPEAT THIS IF YOU'RE FEELING SPUNKY!

1 Lunge Twists X 30 seconds

2 Walking X 15 seconds

3 Jumping Jacks X 1 minute

4 High Knees X 1 minute

5 Jogging X 30 seconds

6 Air Jump Rope X 30 seconds

— Walking X 45 seconds

— Lunge Twists X 30 seconds

7 Traveling Squats with Pivot X 30 seconds

8 Skater Jumps X 30 seconds

(CONTINUES)

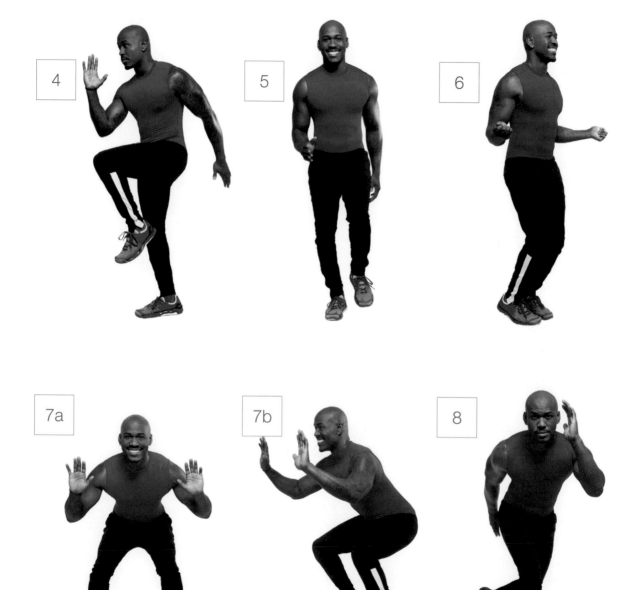

4

5

6

7a

7b

8

THE WORKOUT
CONTINUED

9   Mountain Climbers X 30 seconds

10 High Knees X 1 minute

—   Jumping Jacks X 30 seconds

11 Curtsies X 30 seconds

12 Forward Lunges X 30 seconds

—   Skater Jumps X 30 seconds

13 Burpees X 30 seconds

—   Walking X 1 minute

—   Air Jump Rope X 30 seconds

—   Lunge Twists X 30 seconds

—   Skater Jumps X 30 seconds

—   Jogging X 30 seconds

—   Traveling Squats with Pivot X 30 seconds

—   High Knees X 1 minute

—   Jumping Jacks X 30 seconds

—   High Knees with Torso Twist X 30 seconds

—   Lunge Twists X 30 seconds

—   Air Jump Rope X 30 seconds

—   Walking X 1 minute

—   Jogging X 30 seconds

—   Air Jump Rope X 30 seconds

—   Skater Jumps X 30 seconds

—   High Knees X 45 seconds

—   Mountain Climbers X 1 minute

—   Walking X 30 seconds

—   Burpees X 30 seconds

—   High Knees X 15 seconds

COOL DOWN FOR 5 MINUTES

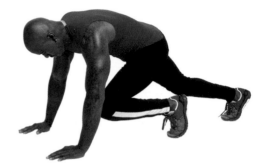

9

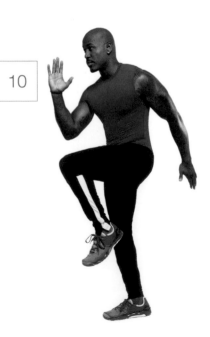

10

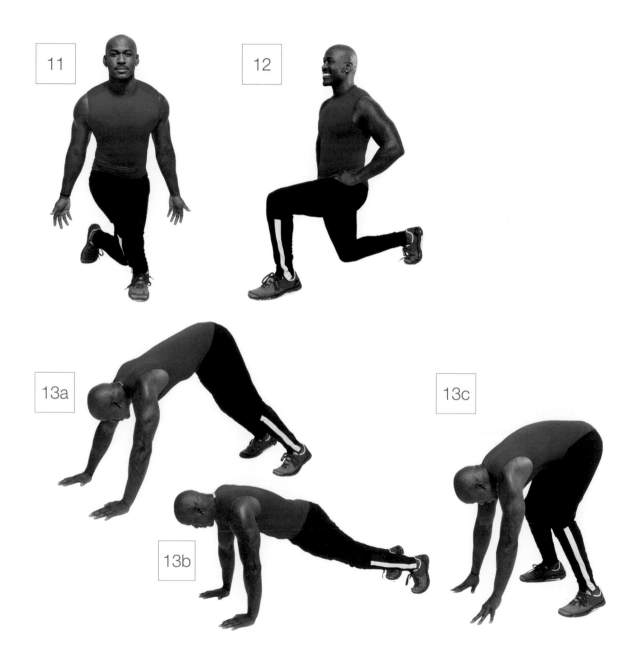

11

12

13a

13b

13c

MEALS

BREAKFAST

frittata with whole-wheat spaghetti & spinach

See recipe on page 214.

Serve leftovers from last night's dinner with 1 banana.

LUNCH

kale salad with chicken & mango vinaigrette

See recipe on page 212 for the dressing.

Combine 1 serving dressing with 3 cups kale (leaves only, chopped), 1 chopped cooked chicken breast (3 oz.), and 2 Tbsp. unsalted peanuts.

NOTE You can toss the kale and dressing up to 1 day in advance; this will tenderize the kale.

VEGETARIAN OPTION Sub in ½ cup cooked chickpeas for the chicken.

NUTRITION INFO: *Calories 347, Fat (g) 10, Sat fat (g) 2, Protein (g) 37, Carbs (g) 31, Fiber (g) 6, Sodium (mg) 170*

DINNER

bacon, lentil & tomato soup

See recipe on page 213.

Serve with 1 portion whole-wheat crackers and 1 apple. Save the leftovers for later in the week.

DESSERT

dessert nachos with fruit salsa

Slice half of a whole-wheat pita into wedges. Spritz with cooking spray, and sprinkle with ½ tsp. sugar and ¼ tsp. ground cinnamon. Toast. Top with 1 cup finely chopped fruit, a squeeze of lemon juice, and 2 Tbsp. vanilla fat-free Greek yogurt.

NUTRITION INFO: *Calories 146, Fat (g) 1, Sat fat (g) 0, Protein (g) 6, Carbs (g) 27, Fiber (g) 3, Sodium (mg) 181*

SNACKS

Choose up to 300 calories of snacks to reach your daily goal. See the lists in Chapter 3 for snack ideas. Don't forget to include your dessert in your food journal (dessert gets included with your snack calories).

day 3

weekly check-in:

How Are Things Going?

How has your week been? We're more than halfway through Bootcamp, so we want to know what you're going to do differently in the final weeks of this program than you did in the first half. What has worked? What hasn't? How are you going to use that feedback to move forward? This isn't a test; it's a challenge. Are you up for it?

WORKOUT

do your own workout (dyow)

Happy Wednesday, Bootcampers! Today's the day you get to Do Your Own Workout. If you missed one of the Bootcamp workouts, this is your chance to make it up. As long as you're up and moving, you can do whatever you want. Maybe today's the day you dance like no one's watching or run like someone's chasing you!

"Water is the elixir of life. Water suppresses your appetite, aids in digestion, and keeps away bloating. You can improve your skin, relieve fatigue, and improve your overall health. Drink more water!" —*The Biggest Loser* trainer Jessie Pavelka

MEALS

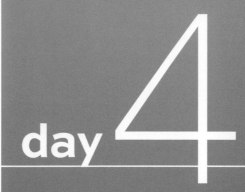

BREAKFAST
morning oatmeal

Prepare ½ cup oats with ½ to ¾ cup water. Top with 1 sliced peach and 7 chopped walnuts (½ oz.). Serve with 1 cup skim milk.

NUTRITION INFO: *Calories 387, Fat (g) 12, Sat fat (g), 1 Protein (g) 17, Carbs (g) 58, Fiber (g) 7, Sodium (mg) 121*

LUNCH
bacon, lentil & tomato soup

Serve 1 leftover portion of last night's dinner with 1 portion whole-wheat crackers and 1 apple.

DINNER
spaghetti squash chicken alfredo

Combine 2 Tbsp. plain fat-free Greek yogurt, 2 Tbsp. Parmesan cheese, ½ tsp. minced garlic, and plenty of black pepper. Toss with 1 cup cooked spaghetti squash and 3 oz. cooked chicken breast, and heat through.

VEGETARIAN OPTION Sub in ½ cup cooked white beans or 3 oz. tofu for the chicken.

NUTRITION INFO: *Calories 327, Fat (g) 5, Sat fat (g) 2, Protein (g) 48, Carbs (g) 14, Fiber (g) 3, Sodium (mg) 330*

SNACKS

Choose up to 300 calories of snacks to reach your calorie goal for the day. See the lists in Chapter 3 for snack ideas.

day 4

morning motivation:

Today Is The Day.

Everyone has rough days—even your Biggest Loser coaches and trainers. Everyone has days where they don't quite feel ready to take on the world (or even to get out of bed). But we do it anyway. Don't put off what you know you need to accomplish because you don't feel ready. If we all waited until we felt ready, chances are good that we'd never even get started.

We all have excuses: Wake up and tell yourself today is the day. Get out of bed, and set your sights on doing something today to make yourself better. If you're struggling, remember that something is always better than nothing. You've got this!

WORKOUT killin' it

39 MINUTES | WARM UP FOR 5 MINUTES

You are killing it! Since you started this journey, you've proved to yourself that you've got what it takes. Today we want you to kill it in this workout. When your mind says no, tell it to get out of your body's way and give more, more, more!

Optional weights can be added to the moves marked with an asterisk (*). You do not need any equipment for the remaining moves.

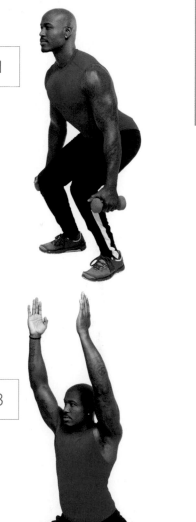

THE WORKOUT
2 ROUNDS

1   Weighted Squats X 30 seconds

2   Rear Lunges X 30 seconds

3   Warrior 1 X 1 minute

4   Skater Jumps X 1 minute

5   Push-Ups X 30 seconds

6   Overhead Presses* X 30 seconds

7   Front Press Hold X 1 minute

8   Air Jump Rope X 1 minute

9   Walking X 30 seconds

10 Curtsies X 30 seconds

11 Side Lunges X 30 seconds

—   Warrior 2 X 60 seconds

12 Quick Feet X 1 minute

(CONTINUES)

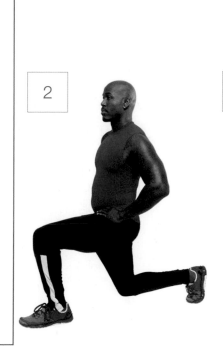

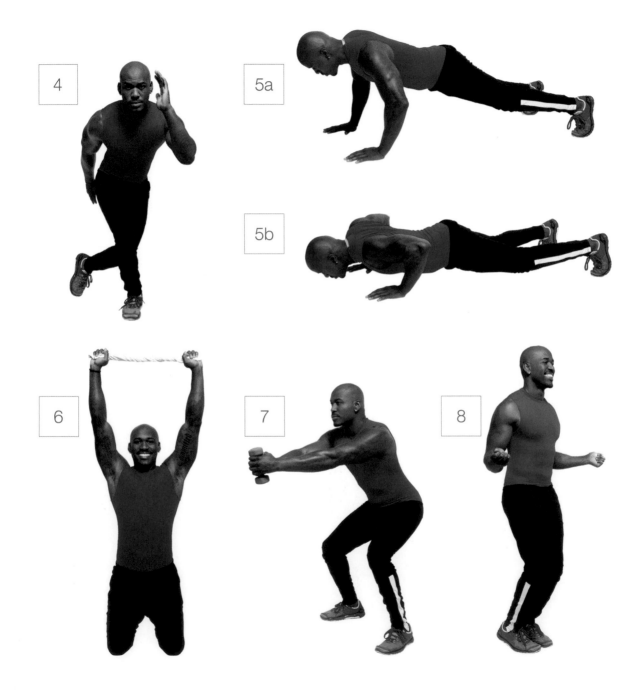

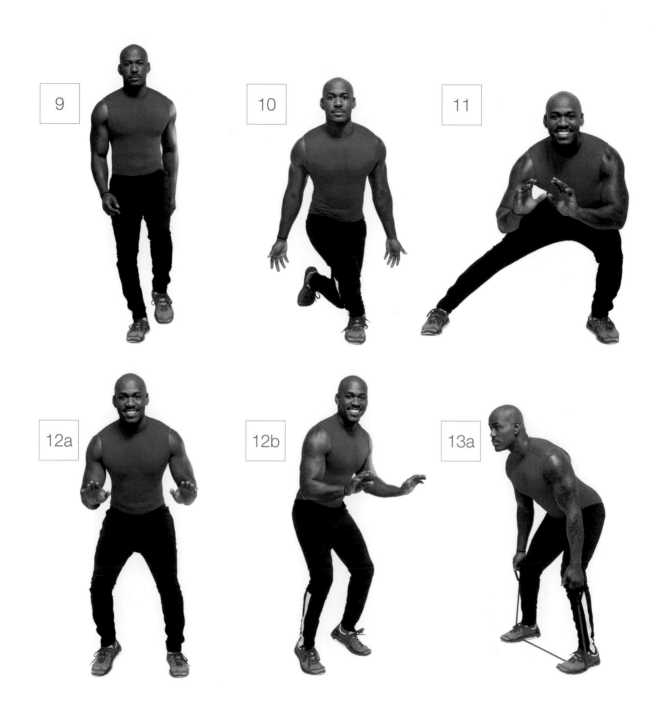

THE WORKOUT
CONTINUED

13 Bent-Over One-Arm Rows* X 30 seconds

14 Renegade Rows* X 30 seconds

15 Biceps Curls to Overhead Presses* X 1 minute

16 High Knees with Torso Twist X 1 minute

Repeat for Round 2

COOL DOWN FOR 5 MINUTES

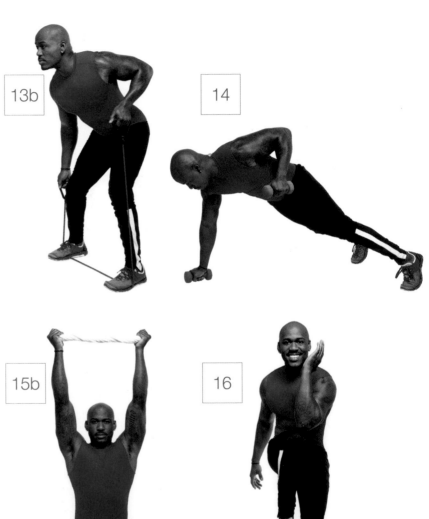

13b

14

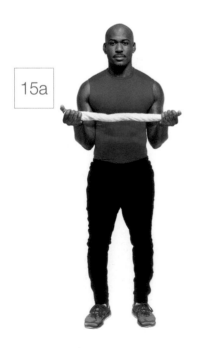

15a

15b

16

MEALS

BREAKFAST
vegetarian breakfast stacks
See recipe on page 211.

Serve with 1 cup skim milk.

LUNCH
confetti quinoa
Toss ½ cup cooked quinoa with ½ cup shelled edamame, ½ cup shredded carrots, ½ cup chopped yellow bell pepper, 2 Tbsp. chopped red onion, 1 Tbsp. dried cranberries, and 1 Tbsp. reduced-fat feta cheese. Drizzle on 2 Tbsp. fat-free balsamic vinaigrette.

NUTRITION INFO: *Calories 374, Fat (g) 9, Sat fat (g) 2, Protein (g) 21, Carbs (g) 56, Fiber (g) 10, Sodium (mg) 396*

DINNER
pesto fish
See recipe on page 215.

Serve with 1 cup cherries.

SNACKS
Choose up to 300 calories of snacks to reach your calorie goal for the day. See the lists in Chapter 3 for snack ideas.

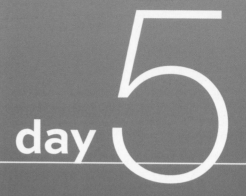

day 5

nutrition bite:

Stick With Sticky Notes.

Resisting the urge to snack, graze, or even binge isn't easy, especially as you're adjusting to a new eating plan. You're doing great, and we have a secret weapon to help you fight temptation. Write questions on sticky notes and post them on your snack cupboards and fridge to help remind you of your intentions.

Writing things like "Are you really hungry?," "Did you eat your veggies?," or "Why are you reaching for food?" can be a helpful reminder before selecting a snack.

WORKOUT cardio arrest

33 MINUTES | WARM UP FOR 5 MINUTES

This workout follows the same pyramid style as Tuesday's workout—Dolvett's Ladder. We're climbing up the cardio ladder, reaching a peak, then climbing back down.

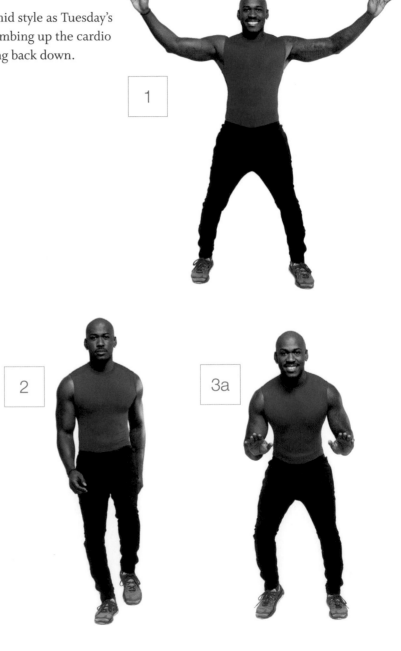

THE WORKOUT

1 Jumping Jacks X 30 seconds

2 Walking X 15 seconds

3 Quick Feet X 1 minute

4 High Knees X 30 seconds

5 Skater Jumps X 30 seconds

6 High Knees with Torso Twist X 30 seconds

— Quick Feet X 30 seconds

— Walking X 45 seconds

— Jumping Jacks X 30 seconds

— High Knees with Torso Twist X 30 seconds

7 Lunge Twists X 30 seconds

8 Air Jump Rope X 30 seconds

— High Knees X 1 minute

— Air Jump Rope X 30 seconds

— Lunge Twists X 30 seconds

— Skater Jumps X 30 seconds

(CONTINUES)

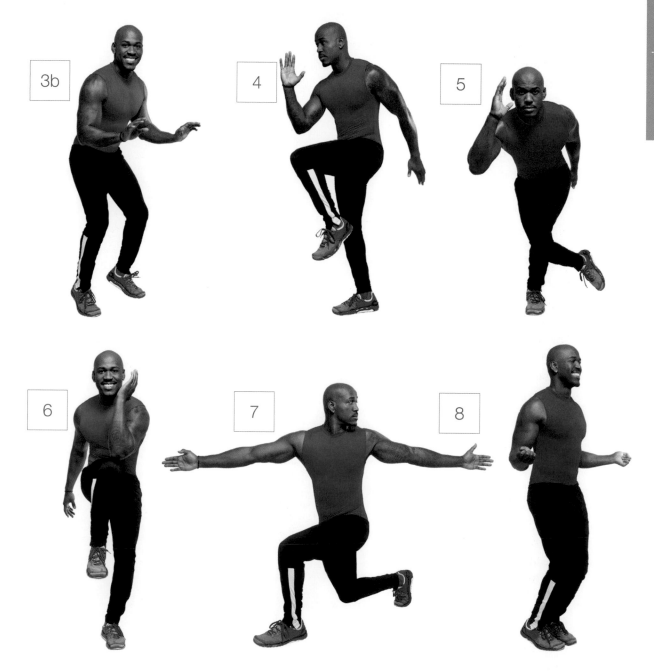

THE WORKOUT
CONTINUED

9   Jogging X 30 seconds

10 Traveling Squats with Pivot X 30 seconds

— Walking X 30 seconds

— Lunge Twists X 30 seconds

— High Knees with Torso Twist X 30 seconds

— Air Jump Rope X 30 seconds

11 Mountain Climbers X 30 seconds

— Traveling Squats X 30 seconds

— High Knees X 1 minute

12 Curtsies X 30 seconds

— Jogging X 30 seconds

13 Forward Lunges X 30 seconds

14 Burpees X 30 seconds

— Walking X 1 minute

— High Knees with Torso Twist X 30 seconds

— Quick Feet X 30 seconds

— Jumping Jacks X 30 seconds

— High Knees X 45 seconds

— Skater Jumps X 1 minute

— Walking X 30 seconds

— Jumping Jacks X 30 seconds

— High Knees X 15 seconds

COOL DOWN FOR 5 MINUTES

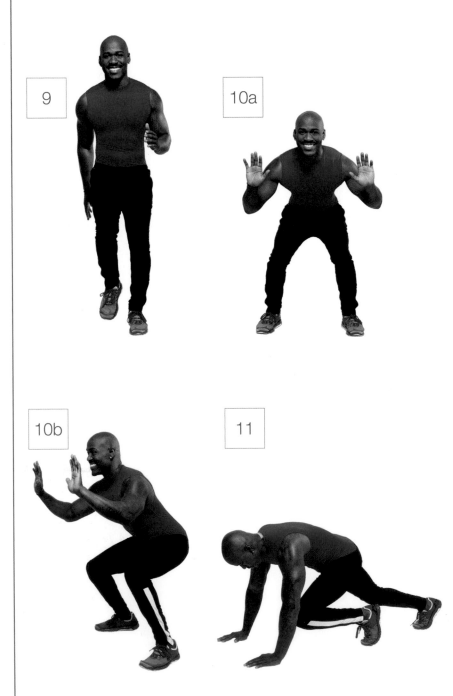

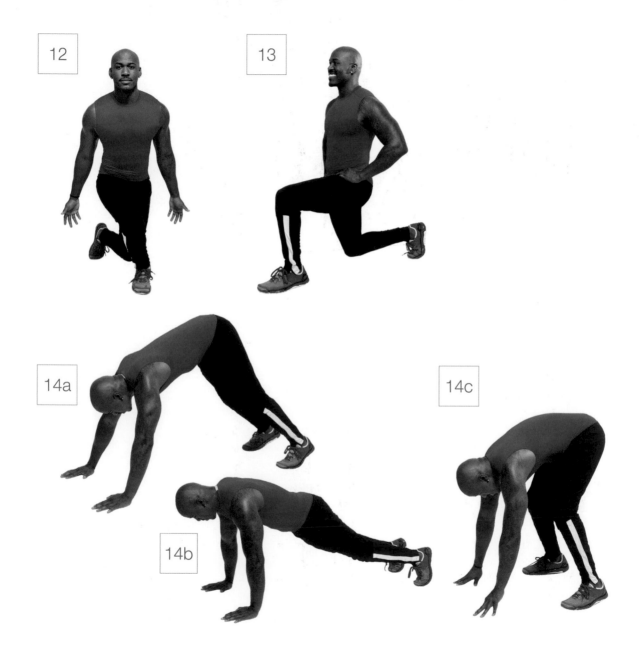

12

13

14a

14b

14c

MEALS

BREAKFAST

peanut butter toast

Serve 2 slices whole-wheat bread, 1 Tbsp. peanut butter, and 1 medium-size piece of fruit with 1 cup skim milk.

NUTRITION INFO: *Calories 395, Fat (g) 10, Sat fat (g) 1, Protein (g) 20, Carbs (g) 59, Fiber (g) 7, Sodium (mg) 390*

LUNCH

loaded beans & rice

See recipe on page 212.

Serve with 1 (6-oz.) container plain fat-free Greek yogurt and ½ cup pineapple.

DINNER

zucchini meatball "sub"

Serve with ½ cup cooked quinoa.
Slice 1 medium-size zucchini in half, then use a melon baller to remove the seeds. Bake at 400° for 10 minutes. Meanwhile, combine 4 oz. extra-lean ground turkey mixed with 2 Tbsp. each chopped onions and peppers, ½ tsp. Italian seasoning, and 1 Tbsp. bread-crumbs. Form into meatballs and stuff into the zucchini. Top with 1 Tbsp. shredded Parmesan, and bake for 20 minutes, until the meat is cooked through.

NUTRITION INFO: *Calories 218, Fat (g) 4, Sat fat (g) 1, Protein (g) 33, Carbs (g) 13, Fiber (g) 2, Sodium (mg) 174*

SNACKS

Choose up to 300 calories of snacks to reach your calorie goal for the day. See the lists in Chapter 3 for snack ideas.

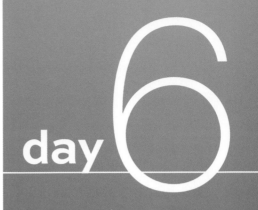

day 6

last chance:

Working Out, For Many Of Us, Is An Escape.

It's a time to forget the world and focus on you and on keeping yourself healthy. Find that same mind-set in today's Last-Chance Workout. Give in to it, and be grateful for it.

WORKOUT last-chance workout—craig

54 MINUTES | WARM UP FOR 5 MINUTES

Today's workout goes out to a Biggest Loser superstar and all-around great guy, Craig Arrington. He inspired us all by losing 162 pounds during Season 15 of The Biggest Loser, so celebrate him by getting your sweat on today!

Optional weights can be added to the moves marked with an asterisk (*). You do not need any equipment for the remaining moves.

THE WORKOUT

2 ROUNDS

1. Weighted Squats* X 30 seconds
2. Rear Lunges X 30 seconds
3. Warrior 1 X 1 minute
4. Lunge Twists X 30 seconds
5. Traveling Squats with Pivot X 30 seconds
6. Skater Jumps X 30 seconds
7. Mountain Climbers X 30 seconds
8. High Knees X 30 seconds
9. Push-Ups X 30 seconds
10. Overhead Presses* X 30 seconds
11. Front Press Hold* X 1 minute
12. Jumping Jacks X 30 seconds

(CONTINUES)

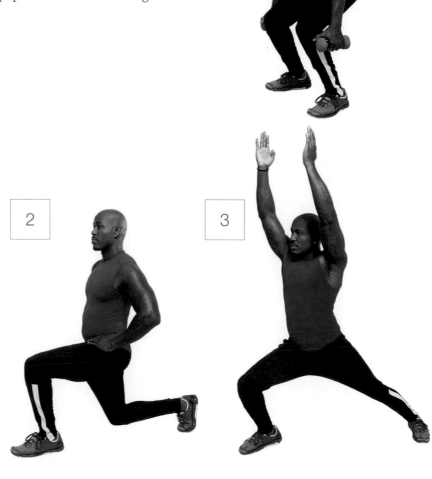

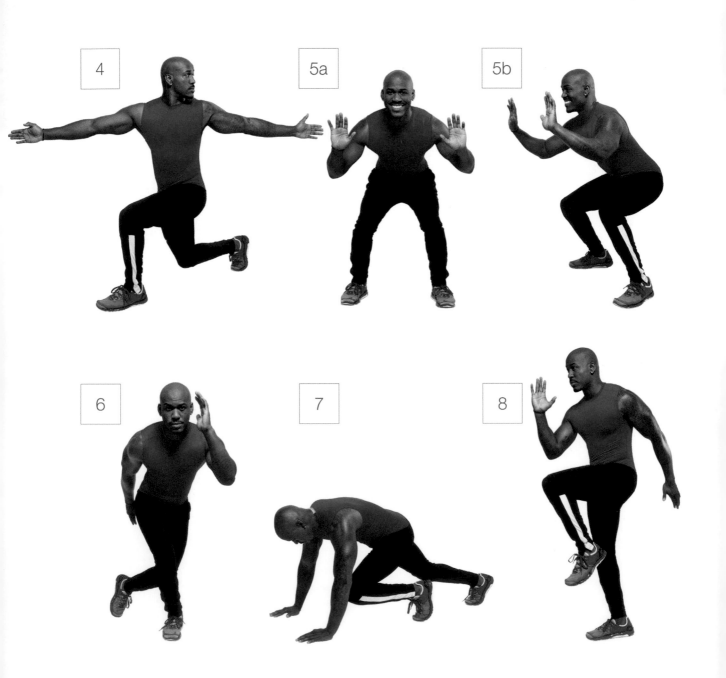

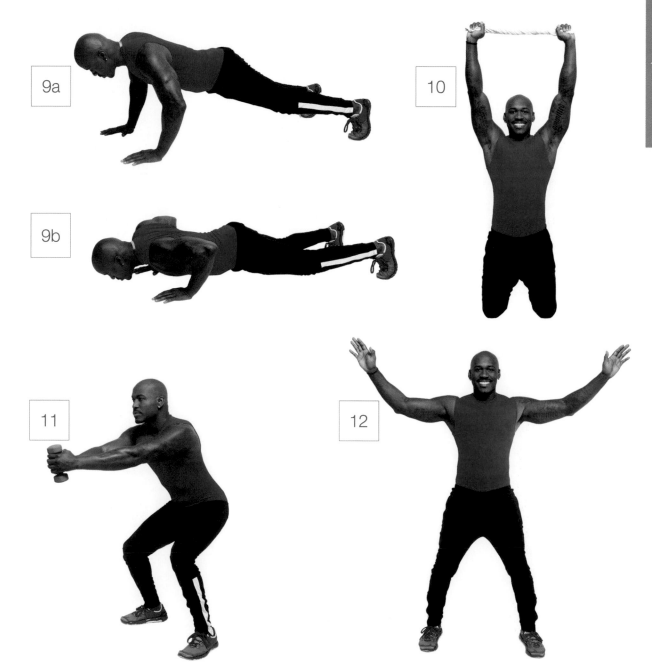

9a

9b

10

11

12

THE WORKOUT
CONTINUED

13 High Knees with Torso Twist X 30 seconds

— Lunge Twists X 30 seconds

14 Air Jump Rope X 30 seconds

15 Walking X 30 seconds

16 Curtsies X 30 seconds

17 Side Lunges X 30 seconds

18 Warrior 2 X 1 minute

— Curtsies X 30 seconds

19 Jogging X 30 seconds

20 Forward Lunges X 30 seconds

21 Burpees X 30 seconds

— High Knees X 30 seconds

22 Bent-Over One-Arm Rows* X 30 seconds

23 Renegade Rows* X 30 seconds

24 Biceps Curls to Overhead Presses* X 1 minute

— Air Jump Rope X 30 seconds

— Lunge Twists X 30 seconds

— Skater Jumps X 30 seconds

— Jogging X 30 seconds

— Traveling Squats with Pivot X 30 seconds

— Walking X 1 minute

Repeat for Round 2

COOL DOWN FOR 5 MINUTES

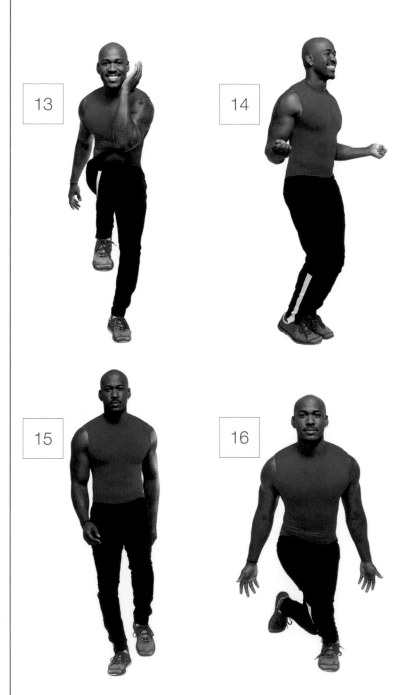

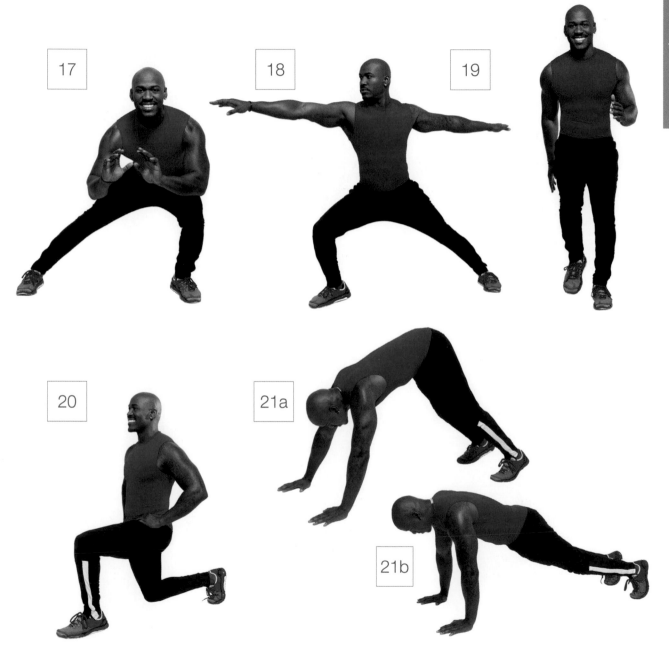

17

18

19

20

21a

21b

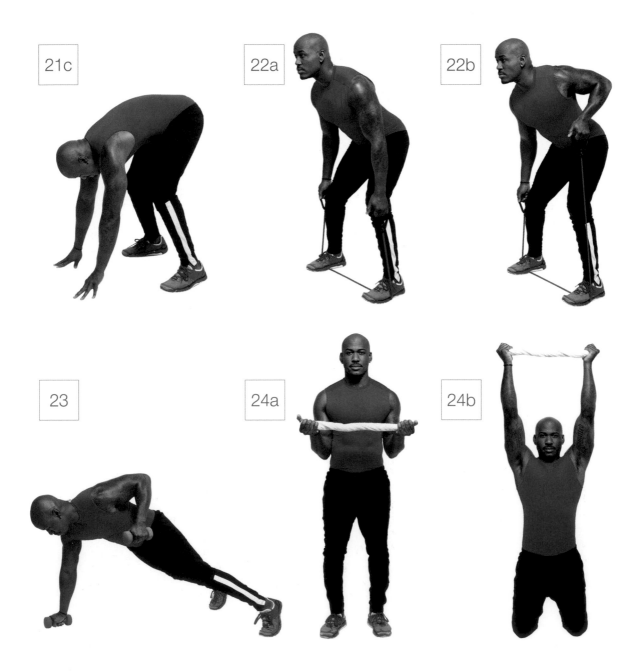

21c

22a

22b

23

24a

24b

MEALS

BREAKFAST

breakfast quinoa bowl

Reheat 1 cup cooked quinoa with ½ cup skim milk and ½ cup blueberries. Top with 2 Tbsp. sliced almonds and 1 tsp. brown sugar.

NUTRITION INFO: *Calories 416, Fat (g) 12, Sat fat (g) 1, Protein (g) 17, Carbs (g) 63, Fiber (g) 8, Sodium (mg) 79*

LUNCH

korean bbq cabbage bowl

Serve with ½ cup brown rice noodles.
Start with 1 cup cooked shredded cabbage. Top with 3 oz. extra-lean ground beef and ½ cup each carrots and onions sautéed in 2 Tbsp. Korean BBQ sauce. Sprinkle with ½ tsp. sesame seeds (optional) and hot sauce.

VEGETARIAN OPTION Sub in 3 oz. tempeh or ½ cup cooked lentils for the beef.

NUTRITION INFO: *Calories 284, Fat (g) 8, Sat fat (g) 3, Protein (g) 24, Carbs (g) 26, Fiber (g) 5, Sodium (mg) 450*

DINNER

apricot pork with rice

See recipe on page 213.

SNACKS

Choose up to 300 calories of snacks to reach your calorie goal for the day. See the lists in Chapter 3 for snack ideas.

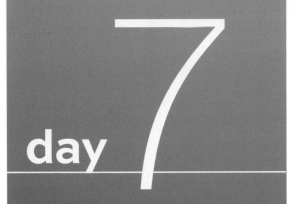

day 7

morning motivation:

Eyes On The Prize.

When you have a rough day, you often think of your goal, but today we want you to literally look at it. Take a few minutes to write down your goal or find photos of something that represents what you want to achieve. Now take those goal reminders and put them where you'll see them: on the bathroom mirror, on the lock screen of your phone, in your purse, or on the fridge. This, in addition to the sticky notes you posted to keep your snacking in check, will bolster your willpower like never before. The adage "out of sight, out of mind" works in reverse as well. Keeping your goals in sight keeps them on your mind!

active rest day

Another week down! Congratulations! You've earned today's rest day—remember that rest is an important part of your workout routine. Of course, rest is not the same as inactivity. Find something active to do today: Take your pup to the park, help a friend clean their garage, or walk laps at the mall while window shopping for clothes for your new body (or buy some to reward yourself).

MEALS

BREAKFAST
slim bagel sandwich

Serve with 1 orange and 1 cup skim milk.
Toast 1 thin whole-grain bagel. Spread on 1 Tbsp. reduced-fat cream cheese, and top with 3 oz. lean lower-sodium deli turkey, 1 slice tomato, 1 slice of red onion, and a few slices of cucumber.

VEGETARIAN OPTION Sub in hummus for the cream cheese and turkey.

NUTRITION INFO: *Calories 210, Fat (g) 4, Sat fat (g) 2, Protein (g) 17, Carbs (g) 34, Fiber (g) 5, Sodium (mg) 433*

LUNCH
crunchy tuna salad stuffed pepper

Combine 3 oz. tuna packed in water (drained) with 1 Tbsp. each chopped walnuts, celery, and onions. Add a squeeze of lemon juice, ¼ tsp. tarragon, 1 Tbsp. plain fat-free Greek yogurt, and 1 tsp. reduced-fat mayonnaise, plus plenty of black pepper. Pack into 1 red bell pepper with the top and seeds removed. Serve with ½ cup grapes.

VEGETARIAN OPTION Sub in ½ cup chopped cooked chickpeas for the tuna.

NUTRITION INFO: *Calories 417, Fat (g) 22, Sat fat (g) 2, Protein (g) 30, Carbs (g) 34, Fiber (g) 7, Sodium (mg) 229*

DINNER
barbecued burger

See recipe on page 214.

Serve with 2 cups sautéed kale.

DESSERT
orange & mango ice pops

See recipe on page 215.

SNACKS

Choose up to 300 calories of snacks to reach your daily goal. See the lists in Chapter 3 for snack ideas. Don't forget to include your dessert in your food journal (dessert gets included with your snack calories).

WEEKLY RECIPES

BREAKFASTS

berry green smoothie

This is a classic smoothie combo. It's so delicious that you won't even taste the spinach! Change it up by swapping in a different fruit each time.

SERVES 1   PREP TIME 5 minutes

- 3 cups raw spinach
- 1 cup strawberries
- ½ cup skim milk
- ½ cup plain fat-free Greek yogurt

Place all ingredients in a blender with ice cubes, and process until smooth (about 1 minute). Pour into a glass and serve.

NUTRITION INFO: *Calories 199, Fat (g) 1, Sat fat (g) 0, Protein (g) 19, Carbs (g) 31, Fiber (g) 6, Sodium (mg) 177*

vegetarian breakfast stacks

This recipe includes mushrooms, tomatoes, avocado, and spinach—it's a veggie lover's heaven.

SERVES 1   PREP TIME 5 minutes   COOK TIME 10 minutes

- ½ baked sweet potato
- 3 Tbsp. sliced mushrooms
- 1 large egg
- 1 small tomato
- ¼ avocado, sliced
- 1 cup spinach, washed
- 1 tsp. chopped sweet basil
- Black pepper to taste

Reheat half a baked sweet potato, then slice into 3 pieces.

Meanwhile, coat a large nonstick skillet with cooking spray and set over medium heat. Add the mushrooms and a dash of salt, and cook for 2 minutes, adding 1 Tbsp. of water if needed.

Push the mushrooms to the side of the pan, and add the egg, sliced tomato, and sliced potato next to each other. Cook for 3 to 4 minutes, or until the egg is just cooked.

On a serving plate, arrange sliced potato, avocado, and spinach, and top with mushrooms, 2 slices of tomato, and egg. Top with basil and pepper, and serve warm.

NUTRITION INFO: *Calories 329, Fat (g) 11, Sat fat (g) 1, Protein (g) 12, Carbs (g) 45, Fiber (g) 10, Sodium (mg) 164*

loaded beans & rice

Here's a filling, tasty, and healthy lunch that's super-quick to make.

SERVES 1   PREP TIME 2 minutes   COOK TIME 5 minutes

- 3 cups spinach
- ½ cup black or pinto beans, drained and rinsed
- ½ cup cooked brown rice
- 2 Tbsp. reduced-fat cheddar, shredded
- 2 Tbsp. salsa
- 1 Tbsp. chopped cilantro
- 1 green onion, sliced

Combine the spinach, beans, and rice. Warm in a bowl in the microwave or in a small pan over the stove.

Top with cheese and salsa, and garnish with cilantro and green onions.

NUTRITION INFO: *Calories 289, Fat (g) 5, Sat fat (g) 2, Protein (g) 16, Carbs (g) 47, Fiber (g) 11, Sodium (mg) 273*

mango vinaigrette

This tasty, fat-free dressing is as delicious on salads as it is on grilled chicken. Mango thickens and binds the dressing without any added fat! This recipe comes from The Biggest Loser Resorts Niagara. Be warned: It's sweet and sassy, thanks to the ginger.

SERVES 6 (serving size 2 Tbsp.)   PREP TIME 5 minutes

- 3½ Tbsp. rice vinegar
- 8 tsp. lime juice
- 1¼ Tbsp. shallots
- 1¼ Tbsp. grated fresh ginger
- 13 oz. mango
- 8 oz. coconut water

Puree all ingredients in a blender until smooth.

Refrigerate leftover dressing for up to 1 week.

NUTRITION INFO: *Calories 20, Fat (g) 0, Sat fat (g) 0, Protein (g) 1, Carbs (g) 4, Fiber (g) 0, Sodium (mg) 2*

DINNERS

bacon, lentil & tomato soup

This hearty soup is packed with fiber and flavor. You'll eat the leftovers throughout the week. If you have any uneaten servings, you can freeze them.

SERVES 4   PREP TIME 15 minutes   COOK TIME 75 minutes

- 2 medium-size onions, diced
- 2 cloves garlic, crushed
- 1 stalk celery, diced
- 4 slices reduced-sodium bacon
- 1 tsp. dried thyme
- ¾ cup lentils, rinsed and picked over
- 1 (14.5-oz.) can no-salt-added crushed tomatoes
- 2 bay leaves
- ¼ cup chopped cilantro

Coat a large saucepan with cooking spray and heat over low heat.

Add onions, garlic, and celery, and cook gently for a few minutes until soft. Add bacon and thyme, and cook for another 2 minutes.

Add lentils, tomatoes, 4¼ cups of water, and bay leaves, increase heat to high, and bring to a boil.

Reduce heat, cover, and simmer for 1 hour, stirring occasionally, until lentils are tender.

Remove bay leaves and serve topped with cilantro.

Freeze extra servings.

VEGETARIAN OPTION Sub in 1 oz. dried mushrooms for the bacon.

NUTRITION INFO: *Calories 185, Fat (g) 2, Sat fat (g) 1, Protein (g) 12, Carbs (g) 31, Fiber (g) 12, Sodium (mg) 226*

apricot pork with rice

All-fruit preserves are a great way to boost the flavor of a dish without any added fat.

SERVES 1   PREP TIME 15 minutes   COOK TIME 15 minutes

- 1 Tbsp. all-fruit apricot spread
- 2 tsp. Dijon mustard
- 4 oz. lean pork
- 1 cup frozen mixed vegetables
- ½ cup cooked brown rice

Combine the apricot spread and mustard, and spread over pork.

Coat a nonstick pan with cooking spray and heat over medium heat. Cook pork for approximately 3 minutes on each side, until the internal temperature reaches 160° (slightly pink). Steam vegetables, and serve alongside pork and rice.

VEGETARIAN OPTION Sub 3 oz. tofu for the pork.

NUTRITION INFO: *Calories 379, Fat (g) 7, Sat fat (g) 2, Protein (g) 30, Carbs (g) 48, Fiber (g) 9, Sodium (mg) 361*

barbecued burger

This simple burger is lean, juicy, and packed with flavor. You could use ground turkey or chicken, if you prefer.

SERVES 1   PREP TIME 10 minutes   COOK TIME 15 minutes

- 4 oz. extra-lean ground beef
- 1 Tbsp. low-sugar barbecue sauce, divided
- 1 Tbsp. whole-wheat panko
- ½ Tbsp. dried onion flakes
- ⅛ tsp. black pepper
- 1 slice red onion
- 1 whole-wheat bun

Combine ground beef, half the barbecue sauce, panko, onion flakes, and pepper; shape mixture into a patty.

Coat rack of a broiler pan with cooking spray. Place patty and onion slice on rack; broil 5½ inches from heat (with electric oven door partially open) 8 minutes, brushing occasionally with remaining barbecue sauce.

Place the patty and onion on bottom half of bun. Top with remaining half of bun.

NUTRITION INFO: *Calories 327, Fat (g) 6, Sat fat (g) 2, Protein (g) 30, Carbs (g) 39, Fiber (g) 7, Sodium (mg) 448*

frittata with whole-wheat spaghetti & spinach

This filling frittata makes a great breakfast or dinner. In our meal plan, you'll eat it for both, so breakfast-for-dinner fans, this one's for you!

SERVES 4   PREP TIME 15 minutes   COOK TIME 30 minutes

- 4 oz. whole-wheat spaghetti
- 1 tsp. unsalted butter, divided
- 1 onion, diced
- 2 cloves garlic, minced
- 3 eggs
- 3 large egg whites
- ½ cup skim milk
- 10 oz. frozen chopped spinach
- ⅔ cup low-sodium pasta sauce
- ⅓ cup reduced-fat feta

Cook pasta according to package directions, omitting salt and fat.

Meanwhile, melt ½ tsp. butter in an ovenproof nonstick skillet over medium heat. Add onion, and sauté 7 minutes or until lightly browned. Add garlic; sauté 30 seconds. Remove from heat.

Combine eggs, egg whites, and next 2 ingredients in a large bowl; stir well with a whisk. Stir in pasta and onion mixture.

Melt ½ teaspoon butter in same pan; add egg mixture. Cover and cook 12 minutes or until top is almost set.

Preheat broiler.

Spread pasta sauce to within 1½ inches of edges of frittata; sprinkle with cheese.

Broil 5 minutes or until golden. Cut into 4 wedges. Refrigerate remaining servings up to 3 days.

NUTRITION INFO: *Calories 275, Fat (g) 8, Sat fat (g) 4, Protein (g) 19, Carbs (g) 30, Fiber (g) 6, Sodium (mg) 472*

pesto fish

Store-bought pesto turns tilapia into a memorable yet simple supper. We especially like this in summer, paired with a tomato salad.

SERVES 1 PREP TIME 10 minutes COOK TIME 20 minutes

- **4 oz. tilapia**
- **2 tsp. pesto**
- **1 zucchini, sliced**
- **1 cup mushrooms**
- **½ lemon, juiced**
- **½ cup cooked brown rice**

Preheat oven to 350°. Place fish on an oven tray lined with parchment paper, spray with cooking spray, and top with pesto. Place in oven, and bake for 15 minutes or until fish is cooked through.

Meanwhile, steam the vegetables. Stir the vegetables and lemon juice into the rice.

Serve the fish on top of the rice and vegetables.

VEGETARIAN OPTION Sub in 3 oz. tofu for the fish.

NUTRITION INFO: *Calories 311, Fat (g) 8, Sat fat (g) 1, Protein (g) 30, Carbs (g) 32, Fiber (g) 4, Sodium (mg) 148*

DESSERTS

orange & mango ice pops

This two-ingredient treat is easily adaptable and will keep in the freezer for up to 1 month. Swap in any fruit or juice you like.

SERVES 4 PREP TIME 5 minutes FREEZE TIME 4 hours

- **½ cup diced mango**
- **8 oz. orange juice**

Divide mango pieces into 4 ice-block molds, and then pour in the juice.

Adjust an ice-pop stick into each mold.

Freeze at least 4 hours before serving.

NUTRITION INFO: *Calories 40, Fat (g) 0, Sat fat (g) 0, Protein (g) 0, Carbs (g) 10, Fiber (g) 1, Sodium (mg) 2*

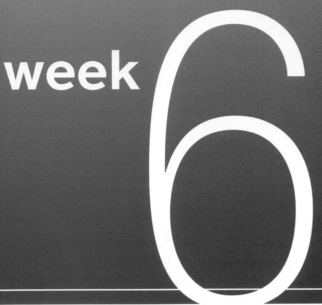

week 6

WOW, it's Week 6 already—what a journey it has been so far! (Can you believe you have just three weeks left?) Give yourself credit for sticking with the Bootcamp. It's intense, and your commitment is an achievement in itself.

The journey you have chosen is a tough one—doable, but definitely tough. Tough as it is, you're doing this! Are you ready to make some more real progress and changes this week? You've already seen the progress you are making, and let us tell you, it's huge! This is more than a push-up; it's more than a squat. This process is changing you and helping change the lives of others. You are taking ownership of your emotions and actions. You now know you can always look for ways to improve instead of ignoring what's wrong with your life. You continue to surround yourself with good things, people, food, and energy, and find balance in your day. You make yourself proud every day.

The aim of your weekly goals is to teach you how to be accountable—to yourself. So what will you do for you this week? Don't forget to write down your goal in your notebook or online.

What are we waiting for? Off we go to Week 6!

WEEKLY WORKOUTS

MONDAY	Seriously?!
TUESDAY	Off the Richter
WEDNESDAY	DYOW
THURSDAY	Mama Got a Makeover
FRIDAY	Pump It Up
SATURDAY	Last-Chance Workout—Sione
SUNDAY	Active Rest Day

WEEK 6 MEALS

MONDAY

B Oatmeal Pancakes

L Quick Quesadilla

D Prosciutto-Wrapped Fish with Smashed Peas

TUESDAY

B Breakfast Bacon & Egg Grilled Cheese

L Stuffed Portobello Pizzas

D Santa Fe Turkey Skillet

WEDNESDAY

B Peanut Butter Toast

L Santa Fe Turkey Skillet Wrap

D Vegetable Lasagna with Ricotta

THURSDAY

B Overnight Oats

L Vegetable Lasagna with Ricotta

D Chicken Gyro Lettuce Wraps

FRIDAY

B Yogurt with Granola & Fruit

L Herbed Chicken & Grapefruit Salad

D Pork with Sautéed Kale with Cranberries, Feta & Walnuts

SATURDAY

B Morning Oatmeal

L Quick Tortilla Pizza

D Goat Cheese & Garlic Mashed Cauliflower with Chicken

SUNDAY

B Cinnamon Roll with Greek Yogurt Frosting

L Tex Mex Stuffed Sweet Potato

D Marinated Beef with Veggies

coaches' corner

WHAT DO YOU WANT TO FOCUS ON? Now that you've been following the Bootcamp for five weeks, you've had a chance to see what types of foods and exercises work well for you and have probably come up with some ideas for other changes you want to make. And you've also learned what doesn't work well or appeal to you. As you begin to tailor your approach, whether it's immediately after the Bootcamp or sometime down the road, you'll want to truly make it your own by focusing on the changes you feel inspired to make and are READY to make. You can continue to see progress with your weight and health by choosing specific behaviors that you want to continue or to put into practice. Now let's bring these ideas into focus.

Create three columns. In the first column, list the healthy behaviors you're currently doing that you can envision continuing even after the Bootcamp is done. These are your "go to" behaviors that you believe are both crucial to your success and manageable for the foreseeable future. In the second column, list healthy behaviors that have not been part of this Bootcamp experience, but that you'd like to begin exploring. For example, perhaps you've not had a chance to work on stress reduction while putting all your effort into Bootcamp, and now you can begin to see a time after the eight weeks is finished when this could be a priority. Finally, in the third column, list those healthy behaviors that you would like to set aside for a while, or permanently, after Bootcamp. These are the behaviors that you think of as tedious, unrewarding, or overly demanding.

Your lists will be an important part of the next week's exercise, so give it some careful thought and consideration!

day 1

nutrition bite:

You Control Your Food.

We know this journey is our choice, but we know that sometimes we don't "hear" that message. Keep reminding yourself that you control everything that goes into your mouth. You can't always control what goes on around you, but your hand is governed by your head—and it controls what goes into your mouth. Eating right is a choice, one you have to make up to six times a day. It's not always easy, and you won't get it right all the time. But it is one thing you can begin to control. Today, stop and think before you eat. Remind yourself who's in control!

WORKOUT
seriously?!

39 MINUTES | WARM UP FOR 5 MINUTES

It's Week 6 and we're kicking it into high gear! We've got longer cardio intervals with back-to-back strength moves—oh yeah! You're getting so much stronger, and your endurance is building every day. You can do this—SERIOUSLY!

Optional weights can be added to the moves marked with an asterisk (*). You do not need any equipment for the remaining moves.

THE WORKOUT

1 Jumping Jacks X 30 seconds
2 Lunge Twists X 30 seconds
3 Skater Jumps X 30 seconds
4 Traveling Squats with Pivot X 30 seconds
5 Squats with Biceps Curls* X 1 minute
— Lunge Twists X 30 seconds
6 Squats with Overhead Presses* X 1 minute
7 Seated Woodchops* X 1 minute
8 Walking X 1 minute
— Jumping Jacks X 30 seconds
9 Curtsies X 30 seconds
10 Forward Lunges X 30 seconds
— Skater Jumps X 30 seconds
11 Burpees X 30 seconds

(CONTINUES)

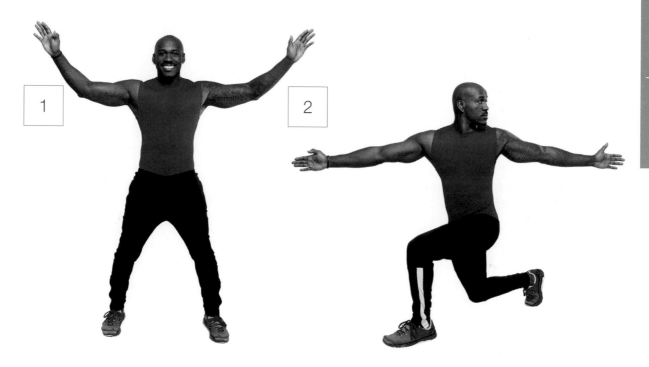

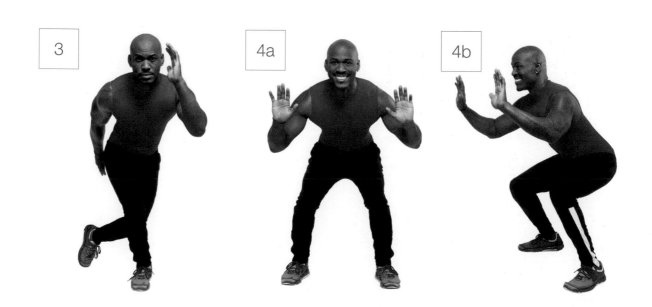

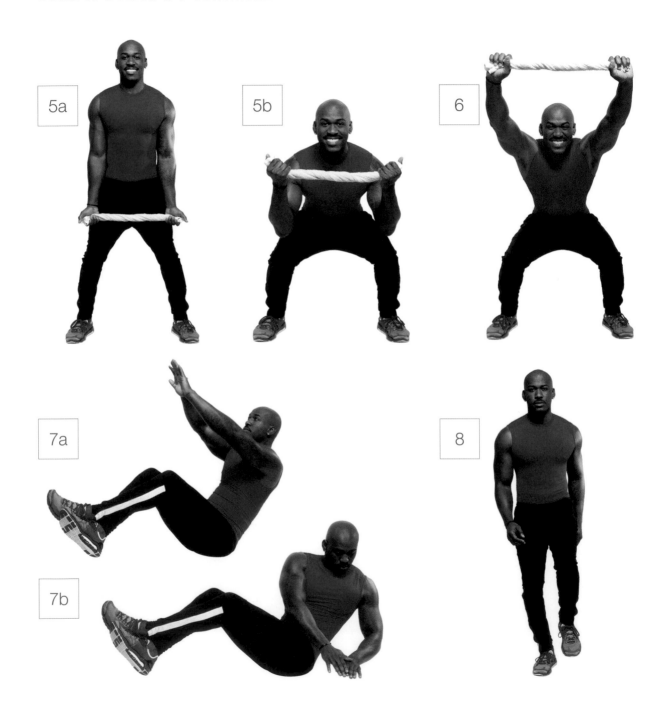

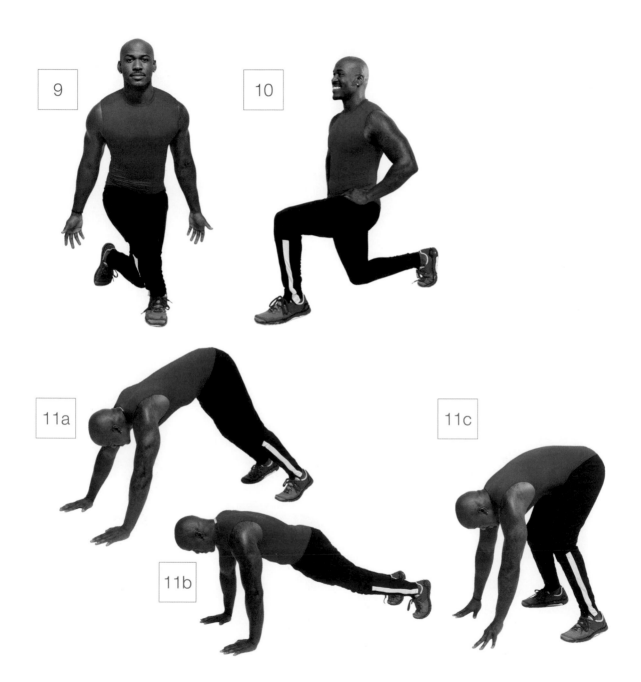

THE WORKOUT
CONTINUED

12 Rear-Stepping Lunges with One-Arm Rows* X 1 minute

13 Woodchops* X 1 minute

14 Bicycle Crunches X 1 minute

— Easy Cardio X 1 minute (Your choice)

— Hard Cardio X 2.5 minutes (Your choice)

— Lunge Twists X 30 seconds

— High Knees X 30 seconds

15 Air Jump Rope X 30 seconds

16 Mountain Climbers X 30 seconds

17 Traveling Squats X 30 seconds

18 Squats with Rear Fly* X 1 minute

19 Side Lunges X 1 minute

20 Plank X 1 minute

— Walking X 1 minute

— Air Jump Rope X 30 seconds

— Lunge Twists X 30 seconds

— Skater Jumps X 30 seconds

(CONTINUES)

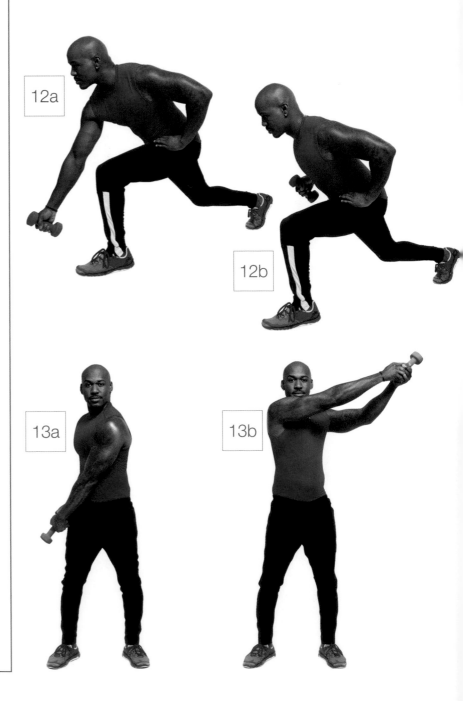

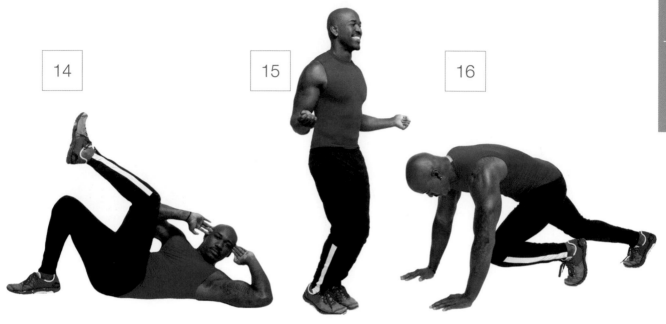

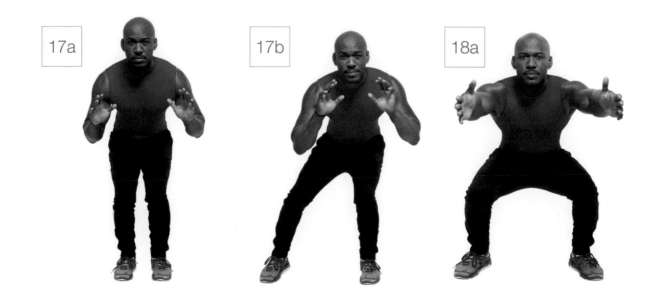

THE WORKOUT
CONTINUED

— Jogging X 30 seconds
— Traveling Squats with Pivot X 30 seconds
21 Jump Squats X 1 minute
22 Walk-Out Push-Ups X 1 minute
23 Crunches X 1 minute
— Walking X 1 minute

COOL DOWN FOR 5 MINUTES

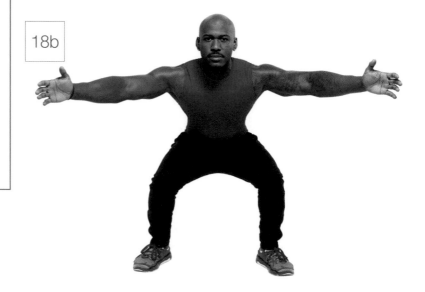

18b

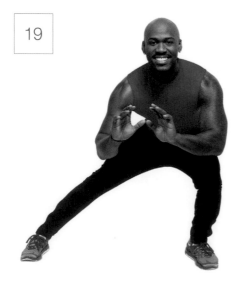

19

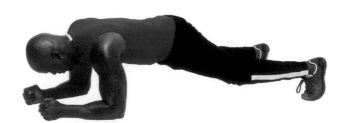

20

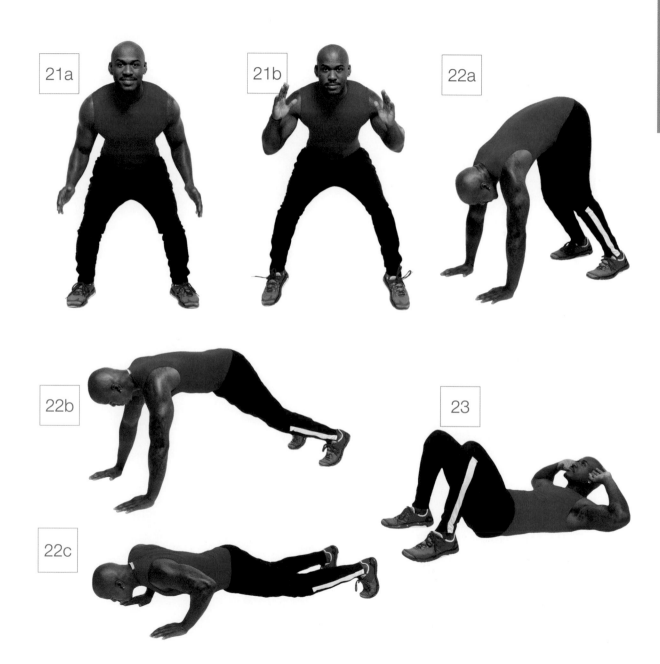

MEALS

BREAKFAST

oatmeal pancakes

Serve with 1 cup strawberries and 1 Tbsp. maple syrup.

Blend 2 egg whites with ½ cup oats and ½ banana, plus a pinch of cinnamon and ¼ tsp. vanilla extract. Pour into a greased skillet, and cook as you would pancakes.

NUTRITION INFO: *Calories 342, Fat (g) 4, Sat fat (g) 0, Protein (g) 14, Carbs (g) 69, Fiber (g) 6, Sodium (mg) 113*

LUNCH

quick quesadilla

Serve with 1 orange.

Mash ½ cup black or pinto beans. Spread onto half of 1 whole-wheat tortilla along with 2 Tbsp. shredded reduced-fat cheddar or pepper Jack cheese. Fold in half, and cook until the tortilla is crispy and the cheese has melted. Serve with low-sodium salsa for dipping and 1 cup bell pepper strips with ¼ avocado, mashed.

NUTRITION INFO: *Calories 362, Fat (g) 11, Sat fat (g) 2, Protein (g) 24, Carbs (g) 43, Fiber (g) 20, Sodium (mg) 488*

DINNER

prosciutto-wrapped fish with smashed peas

See recipe on page 252.

Serve with 1 extra cup of peas or green beans.

SNACKS

Choose up to 300 calories of snacks to reach your calorie goal for the day. See the lists in Chapter 3 for snack ideas.

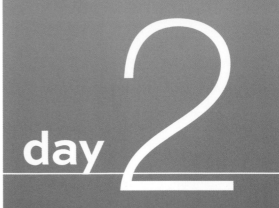

day 2

morning motivation:

Mind *And* Body.

Remember—this journey is about your mind AND your body. To be healthy, you need both aspects of you to be in good health. Choose activities that feed your body AND your soul. Balance exercise with activities that calm you and ground you—consider trying gentle yoga, tai chi, or simply a walk in nature for your Wednesday workout. In addition to grounding physical activities, take time for you: hot baths, pedicures, and other forms of self-care; an evening of "me" time with a call to your BFF or a couple of episodes of your favorite show; or a daily ritual that reminds you of your beliefs and motivations, such as prayer, meditation, or journaling. Don't neglect your mind (and your spirit) along this journey—they're along for the ride, too.

WORKOUT off the richter

33 MINUTES | WARM UP FOR 5 MINUTES

Get ready for an energy-packed workout! We call this Off the Richter to describe your intensity and exertion! Breathe! What's your number on the Richter scale? We predict it's off the charts!

THE WORKOUT

REPEAT A MINIMUM OF 5 TIMES—OR A MAXIMUM OF 10!

1   Jumping Jacks X 30 seconds

2   Lunge Twists X 30 seconds

3   Skater Jumps X 30 seconds

4   Jogging X 30 seconds

5   Traveling Squats with Pivot X 30 seconds

HARD CARDIO X 1 MINUTE—CHOOSE ONE EACH TIME!

—   Jumping Jacks

6   Mountain Climbers

7   High Knees

8   Burpees

9   Air Jump Rope

—   Walking X 1 minute

COOL DOWN FOR 5 MINUTES

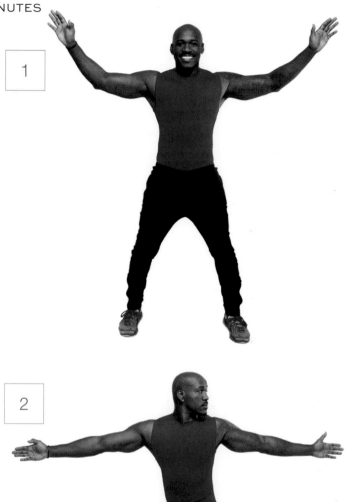

227

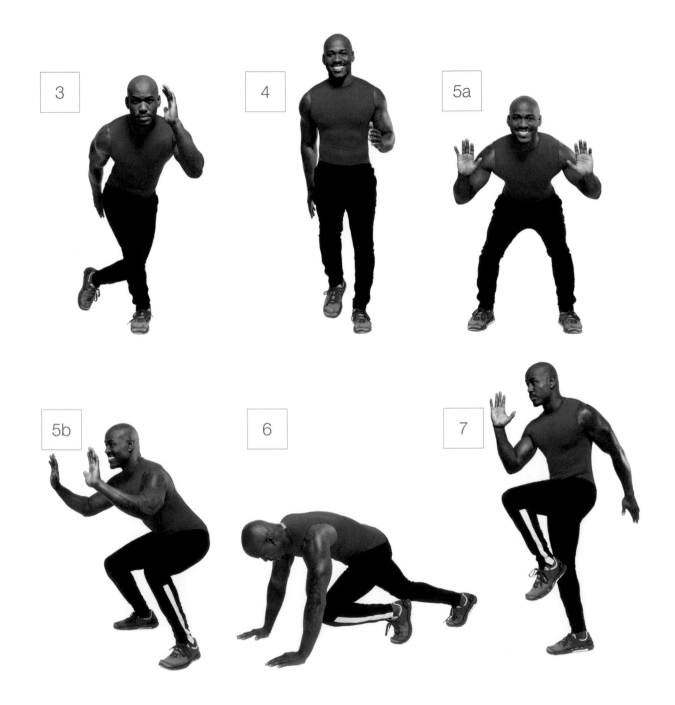

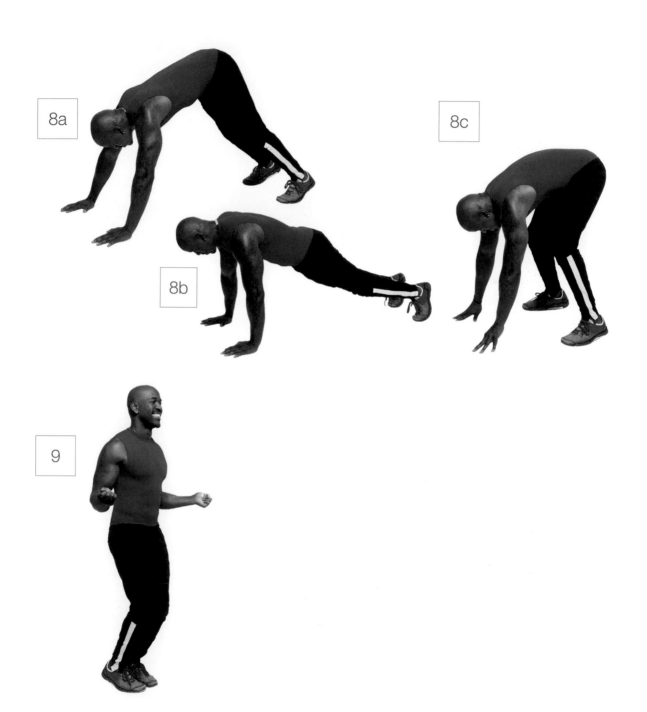

8a

8b

8c

9

MEALS

BREAKFAST

breakfast bacon & egg grilled cheese

Serve with 1 orange and 1 cup skim milk.
Spread 1 tsp. margarine on 1 slice whole-wheat bread. Toast the bread on one side in a skillet, then top with 2 cooked egg whites, 1 slice crumbled turkey bacon, ½ cup chopped fresh spinach, and 2 Tbsp. shredded reduced-fat cheddar cheese. Continue cooking over low heat until the cheese has melted.

NUTRITION INFO: *Calories 221, Fat (g) 11, Sat fat (g) 3, Protein (g) 19, Carbs (g) 14, Fiber (g) 2, Sodium (mg) 460*

LUNCH

stuffed portobello pizzas

Serve with 3 oz. chicken, 2 cups broccoli, and 1 cup skim milk.
Grill or broil 2 portobello mushrooms sprinkled with ¼ tsp. Italian seasonings until juicy and tender. Drain any juices, then top with ¼ cup low-sodium pasta sauce and 2 Tbsp. shredded part-skim mozzarella cheese. Broil until the cheese melts.

NUTRITION INFO: *Calories 91, Fat (g) 5, Sat fat (g) 2, Protein (g) 7, Carbs (g) 11, Fiber (g) 3, Sodium (mg) 166*

DINNER

santa fe turkey skillet

See recipe on page 252.

Serve with ½ cup cooked brown rice. You'll eat a leftover portion for lunch tomorrow.

SNACKS

Choose up to 300 calories of snacks to reach your calorie goal for the day. See the lists in Chapter 3 for snack ideas.

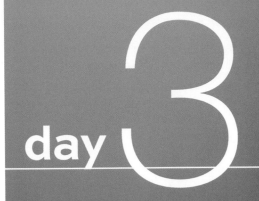

day 3

check-in:

How Are You Doing Today?

You're six weeks in, with less than three weeks left. We want you to take a moment to think about the workouts. How many did you do last week? What about the week before that? How many did you do during Week 1? Are you increasing your reps or the weight of your dumbbells, if you are using them? Doing more each week? Or are you struggling? You don't have to share these answers with anyone, but we DO want you to think about your progress. And beyond the number on the scale, how are you measuring your success? No sugarcoating it. Keep it real!

WORKOUT

do your own workout (dyow)

Wednesday means you get to do your own workout, so what will it be this week? Walking with a friend? Dancing with your daughter? Or biking alone? Choose your sweat today, and we'll see you tomorrow for another Bootcamp workout.

> ❝There's no traffic on the extra mile. Just when you think you've done enough, do more. Challenge yourself. The only traffic that exists is in your mind. The road is wide open for you to make more change in your day. What will you do to go the extra mile?❞ —*The Biggest Loser* trainer Jessie Pavelka

MEALS

BREAKFAST

peanut butter toast

Serve 2 slices whole-wheat bread, 1 Tbsp. peanut butter, and 1 orange with 1 cup skim milk.

NUTRITION INFO: *Calories 395, Fat (g) 10, Sat fat (g) 1, Protein (g) 20, Carbs (g) 59, Fiber (g) 7, Sodium (mg) 390*

LUNCH

santa fe turkey skillet

Serve 1 leftover portion with ½ cup cooked brown rice.

DINNER

vegetable lasagna with ricotta

See recipe on page 253.

Serve with 3 cups mixed salad greens, 1 cup cucumbers, and 2 Tbsp. low-fat vinaigrette. You'll eat this a couple more times this week.

DESSERT

peanut butter chocolate popcorn

Pop 1 single-serve bag low-fat microwave popcorn or 3 cups air-popped popcorn. Shake on 1 tsp. each powdered peanut butter and unsweetened cocoa powder, plus a pinch of salt and sugar.

NUTRITION INFO: *Calories 107, Fat (g) 2, Sat fat (g) 0, Protein (g) 4, Carbs (g) 33, Fiber (g) 5, Sodium (mg) 33*

SNACKS

Choose up to 300 calories of snacks to reach your daily goal. See the lists in Chapter 3 for snack ideas. Don't forget to include your dessert in your food journal (dessert gets included with your snack calories).

day 4

morning motivation:

Your Next Decision Is Your *Best* Decision.

What matters most is your next decision—not the one you made five minutes ago or all the ones that you made before starting Bootcamp. What can you do right now that is a healthy step in the right direction? One of the biggest pitfalls of any effort to lose weight or to get more fit is the potential to feel like quitting or throwing in the towel after making one unhealthy choice or action, or after having a day (or a week) where you didn't meet your goals. Recognize that pitfall and work around it. Don't let it derail you. Make a positive choice—take a positive action after experiencing a setback or negative feeling. Look forward and keep going.

WORKOUT
mama got a makeover

39 MINUTES

WARM UP FOR 5 MINUTES

You started your makeover six weeks ago—and the journey continues! Transformation happens on the outside and the inside. Let's carry on! Dig deep and knock this out of the park. Note that there are two sets of cardio intervals you will repeat at various times during the workout.

Optional weights can be added to the moves marked with an asterisk (*). You do not need any equipment for the remaining moves.

❝Unseen victories. Fitting into "that" pair of jeans. Saying no to that piece of chocolate cake. Clocking 10,000 steps per day. Yes, these are non-scale victories—BUT these are huge! I say include these benchmarks in your weekly goals and you'll find the rhythm you've been looking for.❞ —*The Biggest Loser* trainer Jennifer Widerstrom

THE WORKOUT

INTERVAL A

1 Jumping Jacks X 30 seconds

2 Curtsies X 30 seconds

3 Forward Lunges X 30 seconds

4 Skater Jumps X 30 seconds

5 Burpees X 30 seconds

6 Squats with Biceps Curls* X 1 minute

7 Squats with Rear Fly X 1 minute

8 Russian Twists* X 1 minute

9 Walking X 1 minute

INTERVAL B

10 Lunge Twists X 30 seconds

11 High Knees with Torso Twist X 30 seconds

12 Air Jump Rope X 30 seconds

13 Mountain Climbers X 30 seconds

14 Traveling Squats X 30 seconds

15 Squats with Overhead Presses* X 1 minute

16 Woodchops* X 1 minute

17 Plank with Straight Leg Lifts X 1 minute

— Walking X 1 minute

(CONTINUES)

INTERVAL A

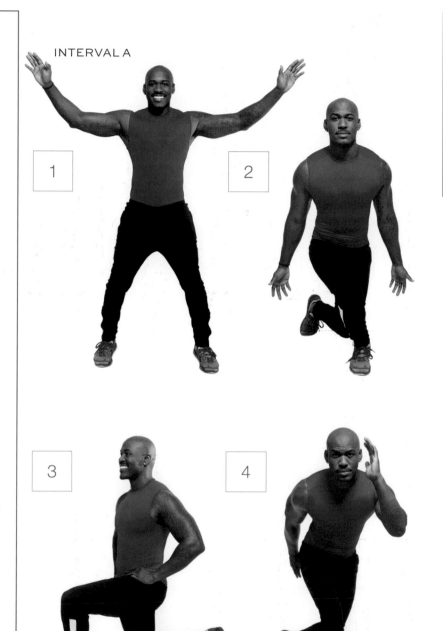

1

2

3

4

233

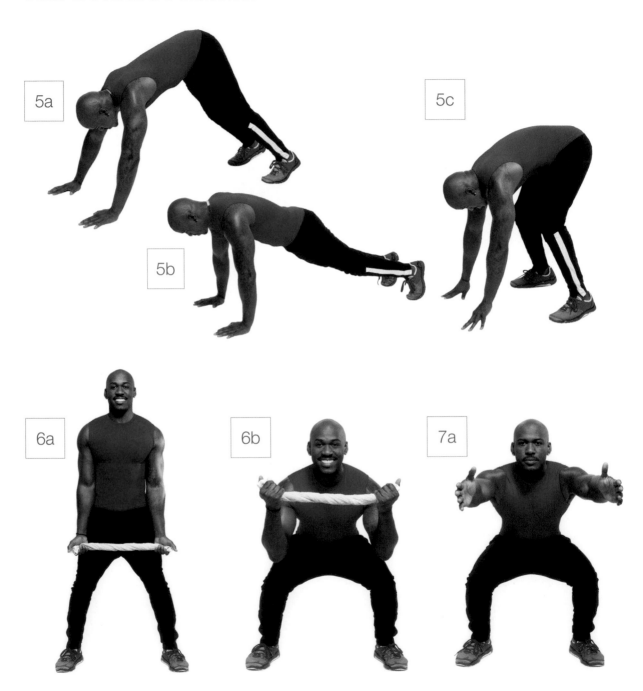

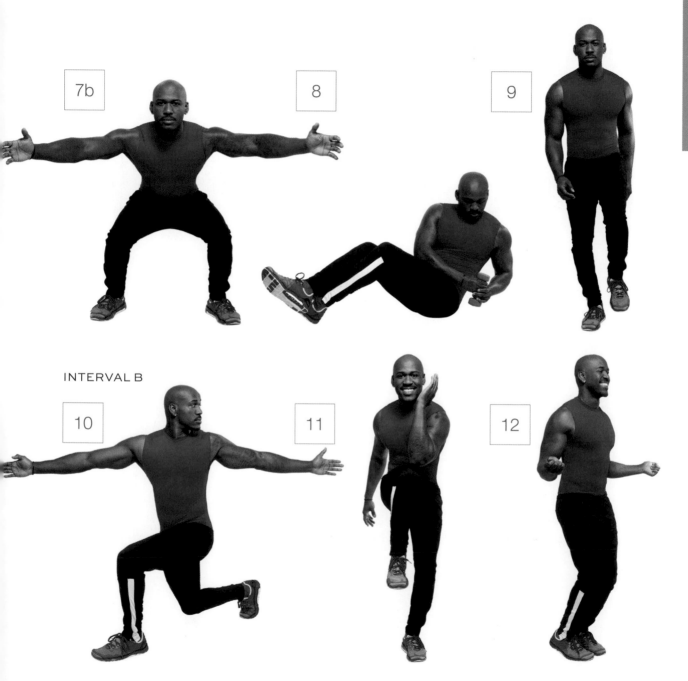

7b

8

9

INTERVAL B

10

11

12

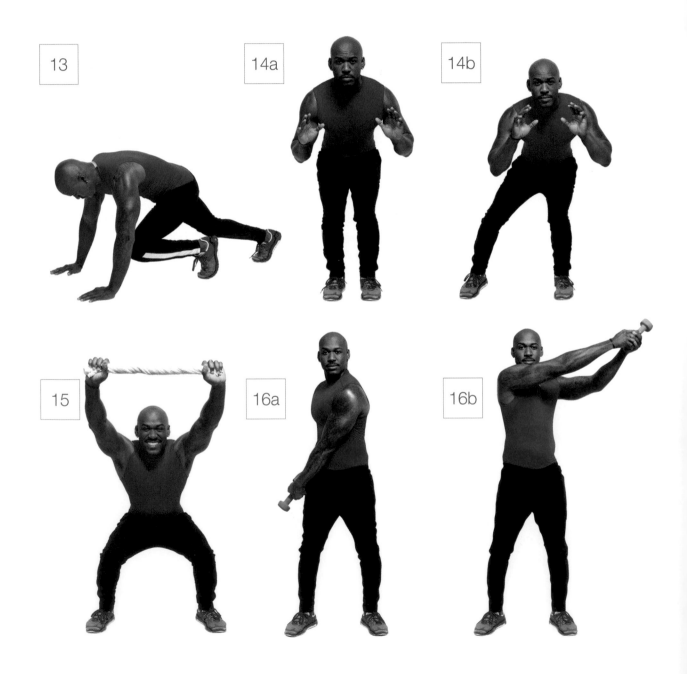

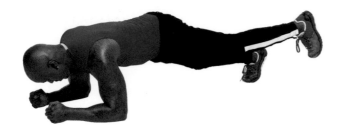

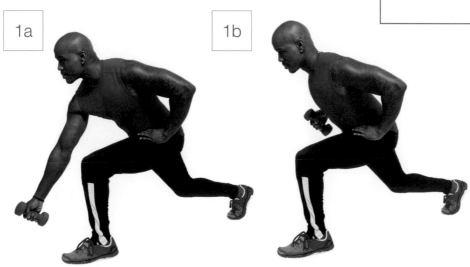

THE WORKOUT
CONTINUED

Repeat Interval A, then do

1 Rear-Stepping Lunges with One-Arm Rows* X 1 minute

2 Walk-Out Push-Ups X 1 minute

3 Crunches X 1 minute

— Walking X 1 minute

Repeat Interval B, then do

4 Jump Squats X 1 minute

5 Side Lunges with Single Arm Lateral Raises* X 1 minute

6 Side Plank with Rear Fly X 1 minute

— Walking X 1 minute

COOL DOWN FOR 5 MINUTES

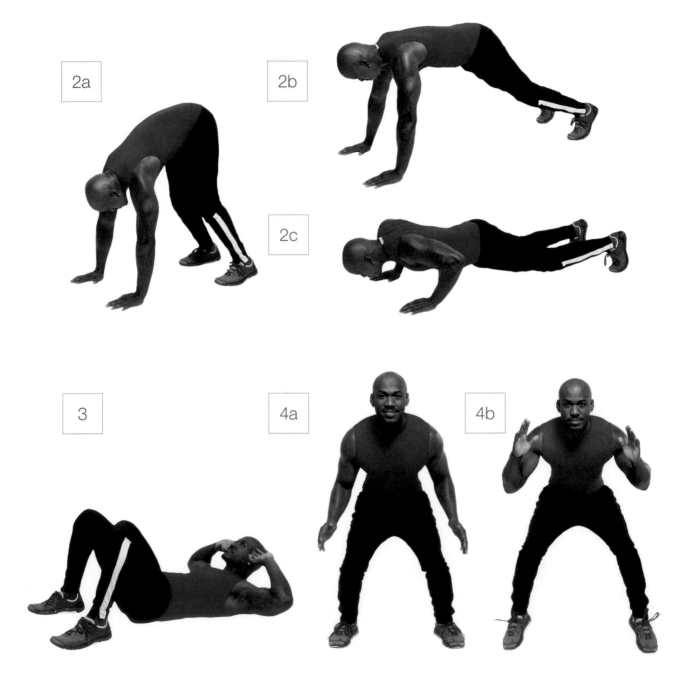

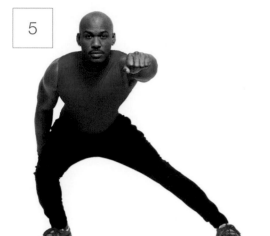

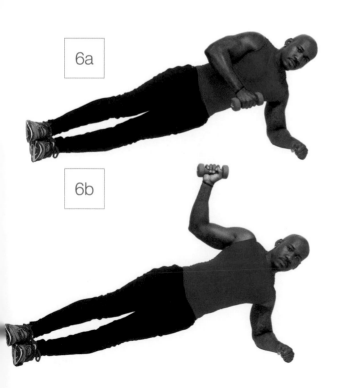

MEALS

BREAKFAST

overnight oats

See recipe on page 250.

Serve with 1 cup berries.

LUNCH

vegetable lasagna with ricotta

See recipe on page 253.

Serve leftovers with 3 cups mixed salad greens, 1 cup cucumbers, and 2 Tbsp. low-fat vinaigrette.

DINNER

chicken gyro lettuce wraps

Serve with 1 portion whole-wheat crackers and 1 medium-size piece of fruit.

Fill 6 large lettuce leaves with 3 oz. cooked chicken and ½ cup each chopped tomatoes, cucumbers, and onions. Combine 2 Tbsp. plain fat-free Greek yogurt with a pinch each of dill and mint, plus a squeeze of lemon juice and plenty of black pepper. Drizzle over the lettuce wraps.

NUTRITION INFO: *Calories 218, Fat (g) 2, Sat fat (g) 1, Protein (g) 34, Carbs (g) 20, Fiber (g) 5, Sodium (mg) 109*

SNACKS

Choose up to 300 calories of snacks to reach your calorie goal for the day. See the lists in Chapter 3 for snack ideas.

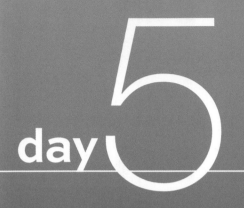

day 5

nutrition bite:

Size Matters.

Choose smaller plates, bowls, and containers whenever you can. This simple strategy has been shown to help people eat less.

Our dinner plates and even our cupboards are larger than our grandparents', so choose today's salad bowls and bread plates instead of giant cereal bowls and dinner plates. Your appropriate portions will look bigger in the smaller context. And use those bowls and plates: Eating from a bag, can, or box will trick you into thinking you're eating less than you are—and soon one serving turns into three!

WORKOUT
pump it up

32 MINUTES | WARM UP FOR 5 MINUTES

Who is ready to get pumped? We are progressing each week and building a solid foundation—congrats on becoming an athlete! Put your game face on; we're going to Pump It Up!

THE WORKOUT
REPEAT A MINIMUM OF 5 TIMES—A MAX OF 10!

1. Forward Lunges X 30 seconds
2. High Knees with Torso Twist X 30 seconds
3. Air Jump Rope X 30 seconds
4. Mountain Climbers X 30 seconds
5. Traveling Squats X 30 seconds
6. Jogging X 1 minute
7. Walking X 1 minute

COOL DOWN FOR 5 MINUTES

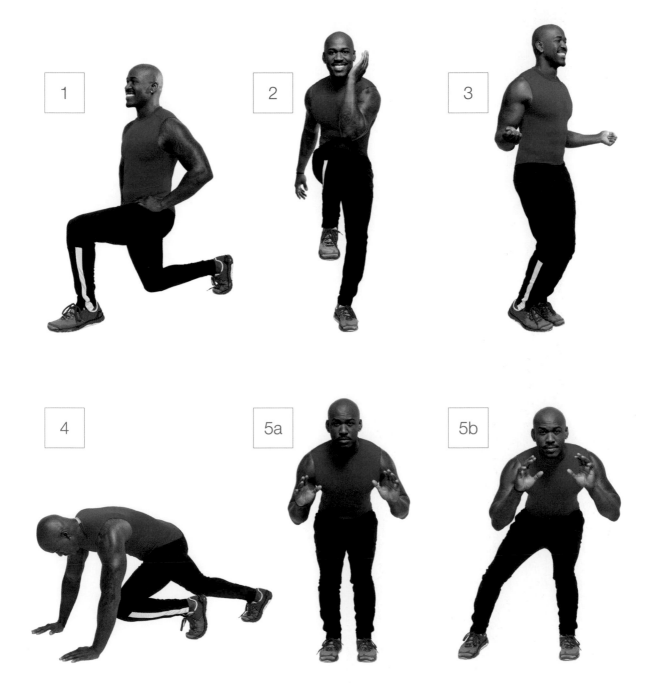

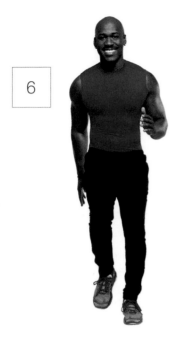

6

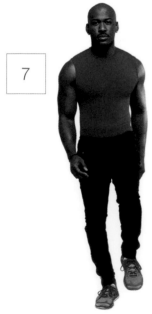

7

MEALS

BREAKFAST

yogurt with granola & fruit

Serve 1 (6-oz.) container plain fat-free Greek yogurt with ¼ cup low-fat granola, 7 chopped walnuts (½ oz.), and 1 cup strawberries.

NUTRITION INFO: *Calories 417, Fat (g) 12, Sat fat 1 (g), Protein (g) 31, Carbs (g) 52, Fiber (g) 9, Sodium (mg) 102*

LUNCH

herbed chicken & grapefruit salad

See recipe on page 250.

DINNER

pork with sautéed kale with cranberries, feta & walnuts

Serve with 1 cup cooked brown rice.
Saute 2 Tbsp. chopped onion, then add 2 cups chopped kale, and cook until tender. Season with black pepper and stir in 1 Tbsp. chopped walnuts, 2 Tbsp. crumbled feta cheese, and 1 tsp. dried cranberries. Serve with 3 oz. cooked lean pork.

VEGETARIAN OPTION Sub in ½ cup cooked lentils or beans for the pork.

NUTRITION INFO: *Calories 269, Fat (g) 11, Sat fat (g) 2, Protein (g) 26, Carbs (g) 18, Fiber (g) 3, Sodium (mg) 313*

SNACKS

Choose up to 300 calories of snacks to reach your calorie goal for the day. See the lists in Chapter 3 for snack ideas.

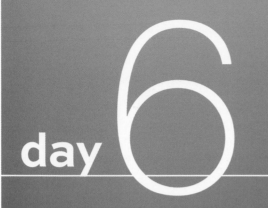

day 6

last chance:

Your Saturday Workout Is
Here Again!

But what if it really *were* your last
chance to work out? How would
you make the most of it?
Please don't tell us you'd skip it.
Would you? Not today!

WORKOUT

last-chance
workout—
sione

61 MINUTES

WARM UP FOR 5 MINUTES

This week, your Last-Chance Workout uses some
of the toughest elements found in your workouts
up to now—back-to-back sets working the same
areas of the body, long cardio sections at high
intensity, holding sustained yoga poses—you
name it, it's in here!

We're dedicating this workout to Sione from
Season 7. Sione inspired us then by losing a whop-
ping 146 pounds, and he continues to inspire
through his work as a personal trainer and motivational speaker. Here's to you, Sione!

Note that there is a set of cardio intervals you
will repeat at various times during the workout.

Optional weights can be added to the moves
marked with an asterisk (*). You do not need any
equipment for the remaining moves.

THE WORKOUT

2 ROUNDS

1 Skater Jumps X 30 seconds

2 High Knees with Torso Twist X 30 seconds

3 Air Jump Rope X 30 seconds

4 Squats with Biceps Curls* X 1 minute

5 Squats with Overhead Presses* X 1 minute

6 Seated Woodchops* X 1 minute

7 Warrior 1 X 1 minute

8 Walking X 30 seconds

9 Lat Pulldowns X 1 minute

10 Push-Ups X 1 minute

— Seated Woodchops* X 1 minute

11 Warrior 2 X 1 minute

— Walking X 30 seconds

12 Squats with Rear Fly X 1 minute

13 Side Lunges X 1 minute

14 Plank X 1 minute

— Warrior 1 X 1 minute

— Walking X 30 seconds

Repeat for Round 2

COOL DOWN FOR 5 MINUTES

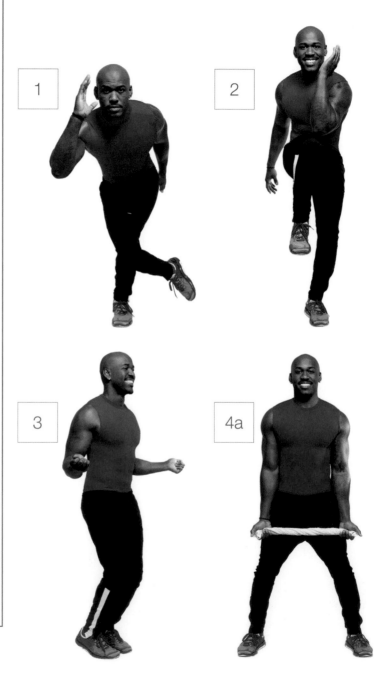

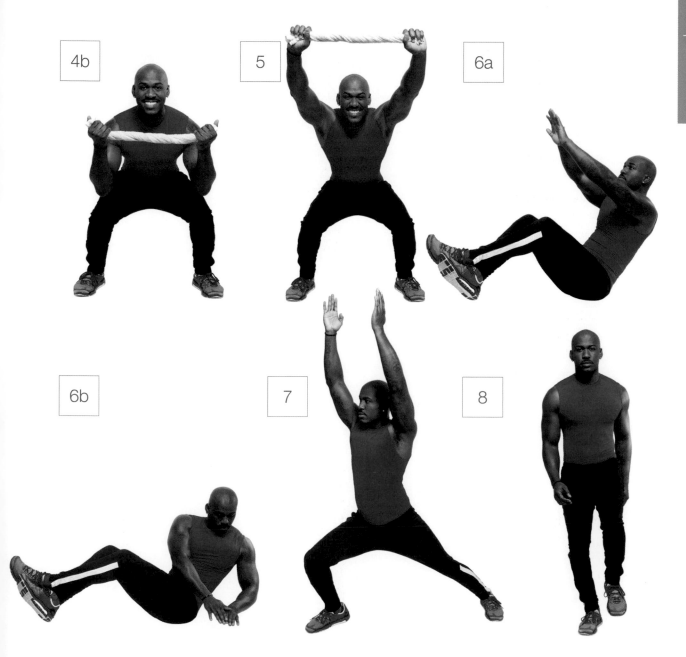

4b

5

6a

6b

7

8

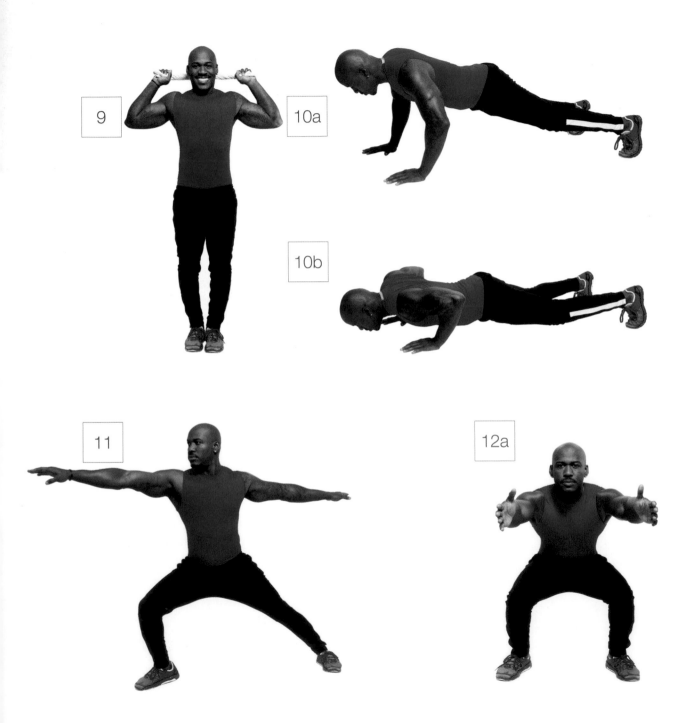

9   10a   10b   11   12a

12b

13

14

MEALS

BREAKFAST

morning oatmeal

Prepare ½ cup oats with ½ to ¾ cup water. Top with 1 sliced peach and 7 chopped walnuts (½ oz.). Serve with 1 cup skim milk.

NUTRITION INFO: *Calories 387, Fat (g) 12, Sat fat (g) 1, Protein (g) 17, Carbs (g) 58, Fiber (g) 7, Sodium (mg) 121*

LUNCH

quick tortilla pizza

See recipe on page 251.

DINNER

goat cheese & garlic mashed cauliflower with chicken

Steam 2 cups cauliflower with 2 cloves garlic, then mash with 2 Tbsp. crumbled goat cheese, plenty of black pepper, and enough fat-free chicken broth to achieve the desired consistency. Serve with 3 oz. cooked chicken.

VEGETARIAN OPTION Sub 3 oz. tofu or beans for the chicken.

NUTRITION INFO: *Calories 239, Fat (g) 5, Sat fat (g) 3, Protein (g) 26, Carbs (g) 10, Fiber (g) 2, Sodium (mg) 283*

SNACKS

Choose up to 300 calories of snacks to reach your calorie goal for the day. See the lists in Chapter 3 for snack ideas.

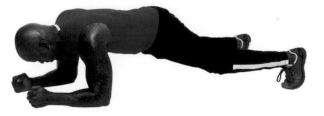

day 7

morning motivation:

Think Positive.

Just as you have to make an effort to eat the right foods, you also have to make an effort to keep your thoughts healthy and positive. We so often hear self-defeating talk in our own minds. Today, practice positive and affirming thoughts. Each time a negative thought arises, immediately catch yourself and turn it around. Instead of thinking "I will never be able to do all those burpees," think "I am going to do as many burpees as I can today." Think back to the exercise earlier in Bootcamp where you wrote yourself a letter and started it "Dear Friend." Today, take that same approach with your thoughts about yourself.

WORKOUT
active rest day

Enjoy this rest day. You've completed six weeks of workouts, with just two more left. That's something to make you feel proud! As usual, we'll remind you that you don't have to rest entirely. You can get up and go for a walk, do some tai chi, or clean your closets! As you progress with your workouts, you might find yourself doing more active things even beyond exercise! That's a sign you're really changing your life. You'll get there, even if you aren't there already.

MEALS

BREAKFAST

cinnamon roll with greek yogurt frosting

Serve with 1 cup skim milk and 1 medium-size apple.
Combine ¼ cup plain fat-free Greek yogurt with ¼
tsp. vanilla extract and ¼ tsp. ground cinnamon, plus
1 tsp. powdered sugar. Dip 2 slices cinnamon-raisin
toast into the "frosting."

NUTRITION INFO: *Calories 230, Fat (g) 1, Sat fat (g) 1, Protein (g)
14, Carbs (g) 40, Fiber (g) 2, Sodium (mg) 263*

LUNCH

tex mex stuffed sweet potato

Serve with 1 cup bell pepper strips.
Microwave or bake 1 small potato. Split open and fill
with 3 oz. ground turkey cooked with taco seasonings, ¼ cup low-sodium salsa, and 2 Tbsp. reduced-fat
shredded cheese of your choice, and heat until the
cheese melts. Top with 1 Tbsp. plain fat-free Greek
yogurt, hot sauce, and chopped cilantro.

VEGETARIAN OPTION Sub in ½ cup cooked black beans
for the turkey.

NUTRITION INFO: *Calories 359, Fat (g) 4, Sat fat (g) 1, Protein (g)
30, Carbs (g) 47, Fiber (g) 7, Sodium (mg) 428*

DINNER

marinated beef with veggies

See recipe on page 251.

DESSERT

fruit salad with orange honey syrup

See recipe on page 253.

SNACKS

Choose up to 300 calories of snacks to reach your
daily goal. See the lists in Chapter 3 for snack ideas.
Don't forget to include your dessert in your food journal (dessert gets included with your snack calories).

BREAKFASTS

overnight oats

This updated twist on Bircher muesli is a fast and tasty morning meal.

SERVES 1   PREP TIME 5 minutes

- ¼ cup oats
- ½ apple, grated
- ¼ cup plain fat-free Greek yogurt
- 1 Tbsp. chopped walnuts
- ¼ tsp. ground cinnamon
- 1 cup blueberries

Soak the oats in ¼ cup of water overnight. This will soften the oats without cooking. In the morning, add apple, yogurt, walnuts, and cinnamon, and mix well. Serve topped with blueberries.

NUTRITION INFO: *Calories 322, Fat (g) 11, Sat fat (g) 1, Protein (g) 12, Carbs (g) 48, Fiber (g) 8, Sodium (mg) 23*

LUNCHES

herbed chicken & grapefruit salad

This healthy protein-filled salad with fresh herbs is a delicious treat for lunch!

SERVES 1   PREP TIME 10 minutes   COOK TIME 6 minutes

- ¼ tsp. olive oil
- 4 oz. chicken breast
- 1 tsp. fresh thyme
- 1 tsp. lemon zest
- 1½ tsp. parsley
- 1 Tbsp. fresh basil
- ½ Tbsp. lemon juice
- ½ tsp. honey
- 1 tsp. Dijon mustard
- 1½ cups spinach
- 1 cup arugula
- ½ cup sliced fennel
- ½ cucumber, sliced
- ½ medium-size grapefruit, segmented

Heat the oil in a nonstick pan over medium heat.

Using a knife, butterfly the chicken breast or pound with a meat mallet so it is around ½ inch thick. Season the chicken with a dash of salt and pepper, and sprinkle with thyme, lemon zest, parsley, and basil. Cook for 2 to 3 minutes on each side, or until cooked through. Remove from heat, and let rest in a warm area.

For the dressing, mix together the lemon juice, honey, and mustard.

Meanwhile, place the spinach, arugula, fennel, cucumber, and grapefruit onto a serving plate. Slice the chicken into bite-size pieces, and place on the salad. Drizzle with dressing and serve warm.

VEGETARIAN OPTION Sub in cooked white beans for the chicken in this dish. Sauté ½ cup with the seasonings intended for the chicken.

NUTRITION INFO: *Calories 347, Fat (g) 2, Sat fat (g) 1, Protein (g) 30, Carbs (g) 40, Fiber (g) 5, Sodium (mg) 355*

quick tortilla pizza

Turn a healthy staple, the whole-wheat tortilla, into a lunch you'll look forward to all morning long. You might not consider chicken to be a pizza topping, but it adds a boost of lean protein to give this meal staying power!

SERVES 1 PREP TIME 5 minutes COOK TIME 10 minutes

- 1 (8-inch) whole-wheat tortilla
- 2 Tbsp. tomato-basil sauce
- 2 oz. shredded chicken breast
- 2 Tbsp. chopped bell peppers and/or red onions
- ¼ tsp. oregano
- 1 Tbsp. shredded reduced-fat cheese of your choice

Preheat oven to 400°.

Place tortilla on a baking sheet. Top with the pasta sauce, chicken, peppers, oregano, and cheese.

Bake for 10 minutes or until the pizza base is crisp and the cheese has melted.

NUTRITION INFO: *Calories 226, Fat (g) 6, Sat fat (g) 3, Protein (g) 21, Carbs (g) 23, Fiber (g) 3, Sodium (mg) 364*

DINNERS

marinated beef with veggies

This beef dish tastes like a Sunday supper, but this filling meal is ready in under an hour.

SERVES 1 PREP TIME 15 minutes COOK TIME 22 minutes

- ½ lemon, juiced
- ½ Tbsp. honey
- 1 Tbsp. Dijon mustard
- 1 tsp. red wine vinegar
- 3 oz. lean beef
- ½ small sweet potato
- 2 cups broccoli or cauliflower

In a small bowl, combine the lemon juice, honey, mustard, and vinegar. Coat the beef evenly on both sides.

Spray a nonstick skillet with cooking spray, and heat over medium high-heat. Cook beef for approximately 3 to 4 minutes on each side, or to desired degree of doneness.

Meanwhile, cut the potato into slices, and steam or boil for 8 to 10 minutes.

Add the vegetables, and continue to cook for another 3 to 4 minutes, then serve with the beef.

VEGETARIAN OPTION Sub in 1 cup mushrooms or ½ cup lentils for the beef (add up to ¾ cup water).

NUTRITION INFO: *Calories 356, Fat (g) 6, Sat fat (g) 2, Protein (g) 26, Carbs (g) 42, Fiber (g) 9, Sodium (mg) 298*

prosciutto-wrapped fish with smashed peas

The trick to integrating higher-fat and higher-sodium foods such as prosciutto is to use them as flavorings, as we did in this dish.

SERVES 1   PREP TIME 10 minutes   COOK TIME 20 minutes

1 tsp. olive oil
1 tsp. lemon zest
1 tsp. dried rosemary
4 oz. tilapia
1 slice prosciutto
1 tomato, sliced
½ cup low-sodium chicken broth
½ cup frozen peas
1 wedge lemon

Heat oil in a small nonstick pan.

Place the lemon and rosemary on the fish, and wrap with prosciutto.

Place the fish in the pan with the tomato, and cook for 2 to 3 minutes on each side.

Meanwhile, in a small pan, bring the broth to a boil, and add the peas. Cook for 5 to 6 minutes, until nearly all the broth has evaporated and the peas are tender. Using a fork, slightly smash the peas and set aside.

Serve the fish with the peas, tomato, and a lemon wedge.

NUTRITION INFO: *Calories 264, Fat (g) 9, Sat fat (g) 2, Protein (g) 34, Carbs (g) 24, Fiber (g) 8, Sodium (mg) 443*

santa fe turkey skillet

This spicy supper requires only one pan—gotta love that!

SERVES 2   PREP TIME 5 minutes   COOK TIME 20 minutes

½ (15-oz.) can no-salt-added black beans, drained
½ (10-oz.) can no-salt-added diced tomatoes and green chiles, undrained
½ (8¾-oz.) can no-salt-added whole-kernel corn, drained
1 Tbsp. chopped fresh cilantro or parsley
½ tsp. ground cumin
¼ tsp. hot sauce
½ lb. turkey breast tenderloin, cut into 1-inch pieces
¼ cup plus 2 Tbsp. chopped onion
¼ tsp. bottled minced garlic or 1 small garlic clove, minced

Combine first 6 ingredients in a bowl; set aside.

Coat a large nonstick skillet with cooking spray; place over medium-high heat until hot. Add turkey, onion, and garlic; cook, stirring constantly, until turkey is browned. Stir in bean mixture; bring to a boil. Reduce heat, and simmer, uncovered, 5 to 7 minutes or until turkey is done and most of liquid is evaporated, stirring occasionally.

Refrigerate leftovers for up to 2 days. You'll eat the second serving for lunch the next day.

VEGETARIAN OPTION   Double up on the beans.

NUTRITION INFO: *Calories 288, Fat (g) 2, Sat fat (g) 1, Protein (g) 35, Carbs (g) 28, Fiber (g) 8, Sodium (mg) 327*

vegetable lasagna with ricotta

A comfort food gets lightened up without sacrificing flavor.

SERVES 6   PREP TIME 15 minutes   COOK TIME 60 minutes

- 1 tsp. olive oil
- 1 medium-size onion, diced
- 1 clove garlic, chopped
- 1 (14.5-oz.) can no-salt-added crushed tomatoes
- ¼ tsp. black pepper
- Pinch of salt
- 1 Tbsp. dried oregano
- 2 tsp. sugar (optional)
- ½ cup skim milk
- 1 large egg
- 1 cup part-skim ricotta
- ½ tsp. ground nutmeg
- 6 sheets whole-wheat lasagna
- 8 cups sliced mixed vegetables (butternut squash, zucchini, bell peppers, mushrooms)

Preheat oven to 400°.

Heat oil in a large nonstick skillet over medium heat. Add onion and garlic, and cook for 2 minutes. Stir in crushed tomatoes, pepper, salt, oregano, and sugar (if using), and simmer for 6 to 8 minutes.

Whisk together milk, egg, ricotta, and nutmeg in a bowl until smooth. Season with salt and pepper, and set aside.

Place ½ cup of tomato sauce in the bottom of a baking dish, followed by a layer of 2 pasta sheets, and then a layer of vegetables. Repeat this layering process, alternating the sauce, pasta sheets, and vegetables. Finish with a top layer of pasta sheets, and pour ricotta mixture over the top.

Bake for 30 minutes, remove from oven and cover with foil, then bake for another 15 minutes.

Cut into squares, and refrigerate single-serving portions for up to 3 days or freeze for up to 1 month. You'll eat 1 serving for lunch the next day.

NUTRITION INFO: *Calories 260, Fat (g) 6, Sat fat (g) 3, Protein (g) 13, Carbs (g) 40, Fiber (g) 4, Sodium (mg) 228*

DESSERTS

fruit salad with orange honey syrup

Serve up the flavors of summer with this tasty little number—perfect for breakfast or brunch. For added indulgence, enjoy it with a spoonful of low-fat vanilla yogurt.

SERVES 1   PREP TIME 15 minutes   COOK TIME 5 minutes

- ½ orange, zested and juiced
- ½ tsp. honey
- 2 cups mixed fruit (berries, melon, and citrus)

Combine the orange juice, zest, and honey in a small bowl. Microwave for 30 seconds at HIGH, stirring occasionally, then allow to cool.

Combine all of the fruits in a bowl. Pour the orange honey syrup over the fruit, toss gently, and serve.

NUTRITION INFO: *Calories 136, Fat (g) 1, Sat fat (g) 0, Protein (g) 2, Carbs (g) 34, Fiber (g) 4, Sodium (mg) 18*

week 7

there are only two weeks left of Bootcamp! You should be thrilled with yourself that you have made it this far; we knew you had it in you. You are reaching highs that you haven't experienced before, and we know that they will keep you moving in this new, positive direction.

you made the decision to be a better you

Changing your life is difficult; in fact, it can be downright hard. It's even more challenging when you don't see results in the time you had expected. Here is the truth: Even making an effort to change is a step in the right direction! Changing is a process—a process that doesn't happen overnight. You will see the most success when your decision to change comes from you—you know that if we want something, the only way to make it happen is through focus, determination, and the willingness to take action.

There is no time like the present to truly commit to a program or to your health. We know that you have been seeing results over the past six weeks ... but could you be doing more? Yes, you've been tracking your food and doing the workouts, but could you, or rather, would you be open to turning up the intensity in your fitness? Could you follow the program any better? Re-evaluate your drive and see what more you can bring to the table! For you returning campers, you should be seeing an even more dramatic difference in your strength, endurance, and ability to conquer the workouts. We will say the same thing to you first-timers. You didn't think you could feel this good. Guess what? You can and you do. Keep it up.

Time to set your weekly goal. It's the same every week: setting, accomplishing, completing, and meeting your goal! What will your second-to-last Bootcamp goal be? Remember that your goals do not have to be dramatic or intimidating. How about walking an extra 5,000 steps a day? You've been thinking of signing up for Pilates classes—do it. That garage needs organizing—consider it done. Your goal should be easy, attainable, and designed to be conquered by you.

You know the drill: Write it down. What will it be this week?

WEEKLY WORKOUTS

MONDAY	Homestretch
TUESDAY	Pay It Forward
WEDNESDAY	DYOW
THURSDAY	Power 2U
FRIDAY	Burn It, Baby
SATURDAY	Last-Chance Workout—Happy Campers
SUNDAY	Active Rest Day

" Participate today. Use your day. You have the power to choose how you want to be in your life, in every moment. Remember that moments make minutes and minutes make days. **"**
—*The Biggest Loser* trainer Jennifer Widerstrom

WEEK 7 MEALS

MONDAY

B Carrot, Raisin & Walnut Muffin
L Asian Tuna Salad
D Minestrone Soup

TUESDAY

B Carrot, Raisin & Walnut Muffin
L Chicken Caesar Collard Wraps
D Beef & Vegetable Rigatoni

WEDNESDAY

B Greek Breakfast Pita
L Roasted Vegetable & Couscous Salad
D Minestrone Soup

THURSDAY

B Carrot, Raisin & Walnut Muffin
L Beef & Vegetable Rigatoni
D Cheesy Bean Casserole

FRIDAY

B Fruit & Yogurt Parfait
L Cheesy Bean Casserole
D Zucchini Noodles with Turkey & Pesto

SATURDAY

B Spinach Feta Cups
L Zucchini Noodles with Turkey & Pesto
D BBQ Spiced Chicken with Parsley Salad

SUNDAY

B Blueberry Lemon Stuffed French Toast
L Chicken Salad with Mango Vinaigrette
D Cilantro-Lime Chicken with Cauliflower "Spanish" Rice

coaches' corner

WHAT IS YOUR WELLNESS VISION? To make real, lasting changes in your life, you need a compelling reason to change. A personal, powerful wellness vision puts your reasons for changing into the words or pictures that bring those reasons to life. It helps you find the motivation to make a change because you choose to make the change, not because you feel like you have to.

Answering the following questions will help you put your wellness vision into words.

WHAT HEALTH-RELATED OUTCOMES DO YOU WANT TO ACHIEVE?

EXAMPLES

- Be stronger
- Have more stamina
- Have the energy to do my work without fatigue
- Feel good about how I look
- Decrease or eliminate medications (under the supervision of your doctor)
- Live a more balanced life
- Cope better with stress
- Improve performance at work
- Improve performance in a specific sport/activity
- Be able to travel more easily

WHAT BEHAVIORS WILL YOU ADOPT IN ORDER TO IMPROVE YOUR HEALTH?

(You can draw upon the ideas you listed in columns 1 and 2 in the Week 6 exercise.)

EXAMPLES

- Consistently eat fruits and vegetables
- Exercise (including cardio exercise, strength training, yoga, etc.) consistently
- Go to bed by a specific time
- Be assertive in protecting personal time
- Keep kitchen stocked with healthy foods
- Keep a gratitude journal

WHAT PERSONAL VALUES AND PRIORITIES MAKE THESE OUTCOMES IMPORTANT TO YOU?

EXAMPLES

- Feeling balanced mentally, physically, and spiritually
- Honoring my physical body and what it allows me to do
- Being fit and strong
- Eating more local whole foods
- Being a role model for my children
- Being able to take better care of my family members
- Looking professional and being confident in my work clothes
- Having loving relationships
- Being physically capable and independent

WHAT ARE YOUR STRENGTHS THAT WILL HELP YOU ACHIEVE THESE OUTCOMES?

EXAMPLES

- Determination
- Organizational skills
- Attention to detail
- Adaptability
- Courage
- Willingness to try new things
- Ability to keep perspective

- Sense of humor
- Creativity
- Zest for life
- Reliability

WHAT CHALLENGES WILL YOU OVERCOME IN THE PROCESS OF REACHING YOUR OUTCOMES?

EXAMPLES

- Lack of time
- Lack of support
- Peer pressure
- "All-or-nothing" thinking
- The need to see quick changes on the scale
- Being a "picky" eater
- Financial challenges

WHAT SUPPORT (strategies, systems, people, and environments) DO YOU NEED IN PLACE TO OVERCOME YOUR CHALLENGES?

EXAMPLES

- A tracking system for my weekly goals
- Consistent support from like-minded peers
- Support from my spouse/partner
- The availability of healthier foods at home
- A gym membership
- Support from a therapist, personal trainer, and/or nutritionist
- Kitchen tools for healthy food preparation
- A healthy foods shopping list

Using the important outcomes, essential strengths, personal values, priorities, challenges that you will overcome, and support you will call upon, write your Wellness Vision.

EXAMPLE OF A WELLNESS VISION

"I am energized all day long for work and play. I am disciplined and respect the meaningful boundaries that will allow a balanced life to flourish. I continue to eat a clean, whole-foods diet; I sleep well and exercise consistently during the week. Exercise is a seamless part of my life. I read for pleasure and participate in outdoor activities with my family. I embrace this time being active with my family as it supports my physical, mental, and emotional self. I am open to change and willingly make adjustments as needed to preserve time for myself. My job satisfaction remains incredibly high, and my overall health is good. I continue to draw on the success of past lifestyle experiences to make this so. I am strong and capable in my body as I age and am an eager, full participant in my life, drawing energy from a balanced approach to my work, exercise, and play time with family as I move into the next phase of my life."

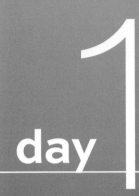

day 1

nutrition bite:

Plan Ahead.

Going to a meeting at work, a book club gathering, or a neighborhood potluck? Volunteer to bring nutritious foods, or ask the person in charge of the meeting to provide healthy fare like fresh fruit, yogurt, and whole-grain foods. Or bring your healthy snack with you, along with your water bottle, and focus on the people instead of the food! (What a shift in perspective that is!)

WORKOUT
homestretch

38 MINUTES | WARM UP FOR 5 MINUTES

It's Week 7, and yes, as this workout says, we are in the Homestretch. Buckle up and give your all these next two weeks.

THE WORKOUT

COMPLETE 2 ROUNDS AND CALL IT A DAY, OR GO FOR ROUND 3

1 Lat Pulldowns X 1 minute
2 Jumping Jacks X 1 minute
3 Push-Ups X 1 minute
4 Jogging X 1 minute
5 Bicycle Crunches X 1 minute
6 Skater Jumps X 1 minute
7 Bent-Over One-Arm Rows X 1 minute
8 Burpees X 1 minute
9 Chest Presses X 1 minute
10 Quick Feet X 1 minute
11 Crunches X 1 minute
— Jumping Jacks X 1 minute
— Lat Pulldowns X 1 minute

Repeat for Round 2

COOL DOWN FOR 5 MINUTES

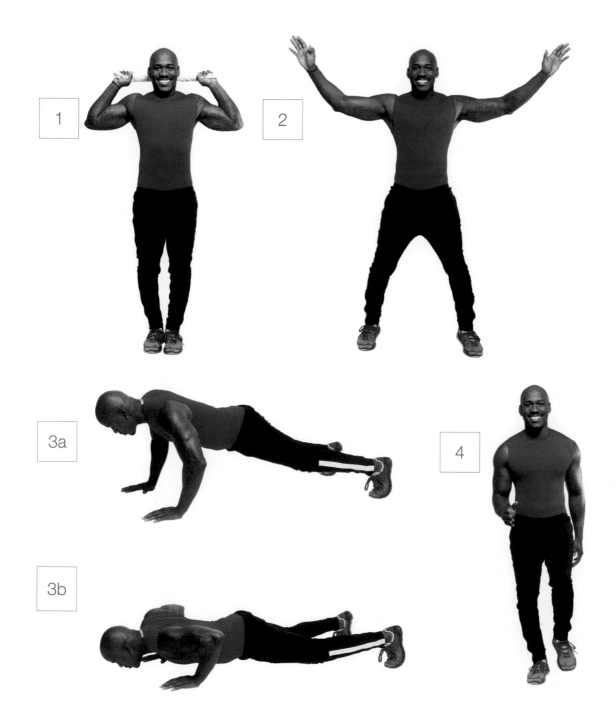

1

2

3a

3b

4

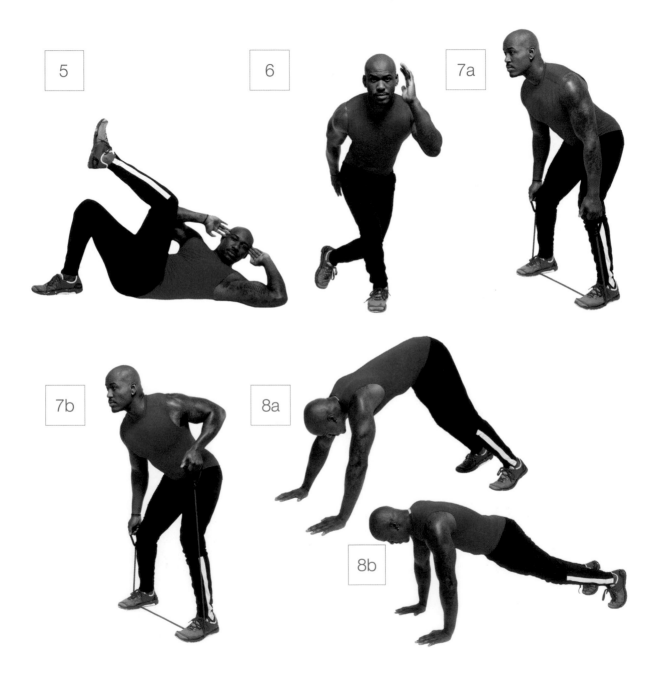

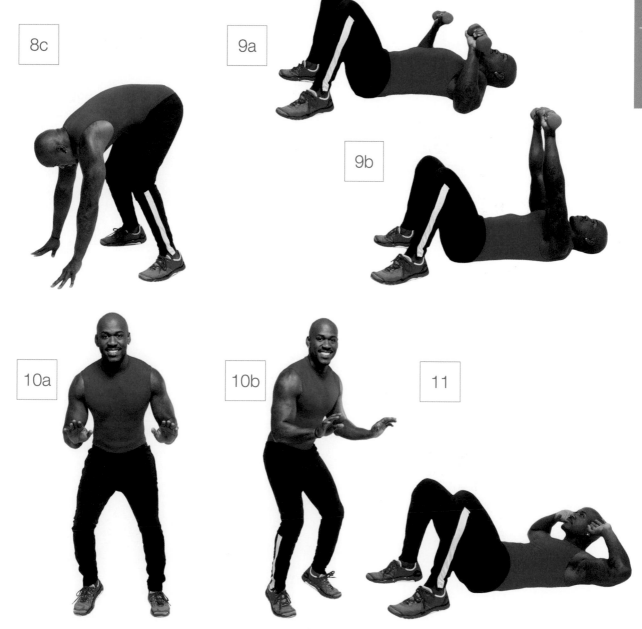

8c

9a

9b

10a

10b

11

MEALS

BREAKFAST

carrot, raisin & walnut muffin

See recipe on page 288.

Serve 1 muffin with 1 Tbsp. natural peanut butter and 1 cup plain fat-free Greek yogurt with 1 Tbsp. all-fruit preserves.

LUNCH

asian tuna salad

Serve with ½ cup cooked brown rice and 1 mandarin orange.
Combine 1 (2.6-oz.) pouch tuna in water with 2 Tbsp. sesame-ginger dressing, 1 cup broccoli slaw, ½ cup chopped red bell pepper, 1 chopped green onion, and 2 Tbsp. chopped cilantro.

VEGETARIAN OPTION Sub in ½ cup shelled edamame for the tuna.

NUTRITION INFO: *Calories 268, Fat (g) 14, Sat fat (g) 0, Protein (g) 2, Carbs (g) 14, Fiber (g) 7, Sodium (mg) 383*

DINNER

minestrone soup

See recipe on page 291.

Serve with 3 oz. extra-lean turkey or ½ cup cooked beans, plus 1 slice whole-wheat bread.

SNACKS

Choose up to 300 calories of snacks to reach your calorie goal for the day. See the lists in Chapter 3 for snack ideas.

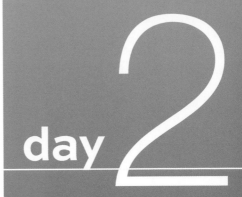

day 2

morning motivation:

Respect Yourself.

Repeat this mantra: I love and respect myself, no matter what.

The more you honor and accept yourself now, the easier it will be for you to stick with your goals—especially after Bootcamp ends. Accepting yourself today doesn't mean you're satisfied with how things are right now. It just puts you in a place where good things can happen. Beating yourself up doesn't make you stronger. And that's what this journey is all about. Right now, stop and think of three reasons why you love and respect yourself. Here are three we can think of: 1. You made it this far. 2. You work hard every day. 3. You're changing your life and the lives of those around you.

WORKOUT pay it forward

41 MINUTES | WARM UP FOR 5 MINUTES

You are about to Pay It Forward. We've got two weeks left to make history. Are you ready to sweat?

THE WORKOUT

COMPLETE 2 ROUNDS AND CALL IT A DAY, OR GO FOR ROUND 3

1 Squats X 1 minute

2 Jumping Jacks X 1 minute

3 Forward Lunges X 1 minute

4 Jogging X 1 minute

5 Plank with Straight Leg Lifts X 1 minute

6 Skater Jumps X 1 minute

7 Rear Lunges X 1 minute

8 Walking X 1 minute

9 Burpees X 1 minute

10 Side Lunges X 1 minute

11 Quick Feet X 1 minute

12 Bicycle Crunches X 1 minute

— Jumping Jacks X 1 minute

— Walking X 1 minute

Repeat for Round 2

COOL DOWN FOR 5 MINUTES

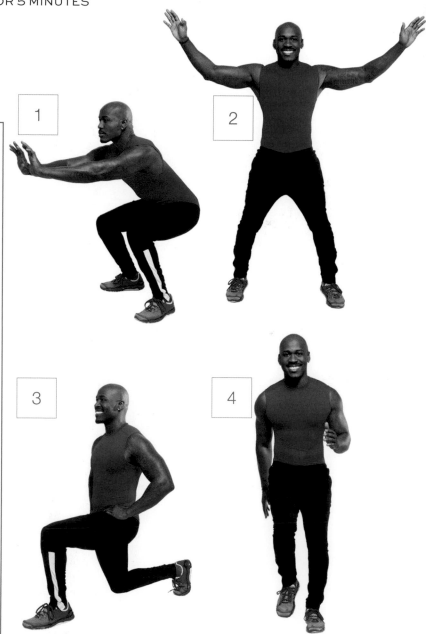

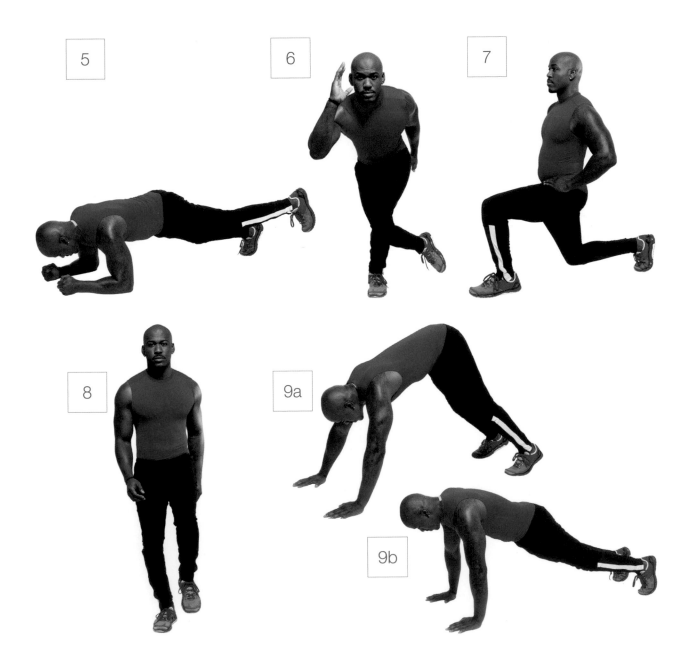

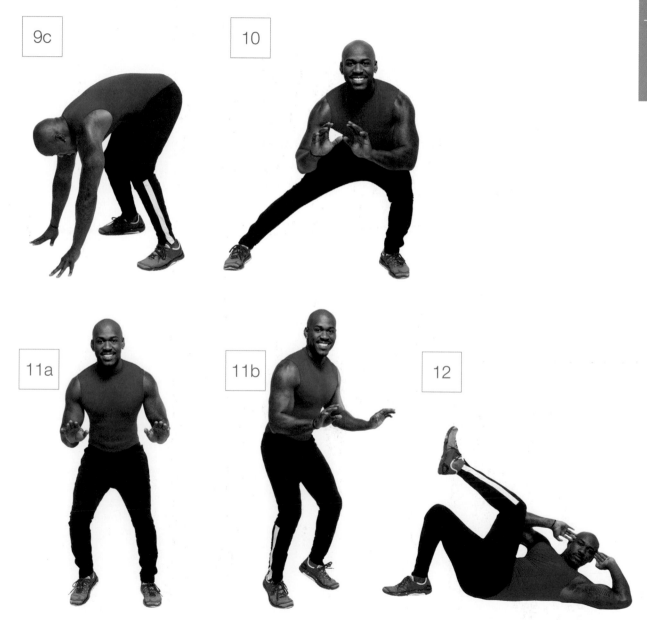

9c

10

11a

11b

12

MEALS

BREAKFAST

carrot, raisin & walnut muffin

Serve 1 leftover muffin with 1 Tbsp. natural peanut butter and 1 cup plain fat-free Greek yogurt with 1 Tbsp. all-fruit preserves.

LUNCH

chicken caesar collard wraps

Serve with 1 apple, sliced, sprinkled with cinnamon. Remove the stems from 2 large collard leaves. Microwave for 30 seconds to soften, if desired. Combine 6 oz. cooked chicken with 2 Tbsp. low-fat Caesar dressing, 1 cup chopped tomatoes, and 2 tsp. grated Parmesan cheese. Season with plenty of black pepper. Place half the mixture in the center of each leaf, and roll like a burrito.

VEGETARIAN OPTION Sub in ½ cup chopped chickpeas or 3 oz. tofu for the chicken.

NUTRITION INFO: *Calories 328, Fat (g) 6, Sat fat (g) 2, Protein (g) 49, Carbs (g) 18, Fiber (g) 3, Sodium (mg) 203*

DINNER

beef & vegetable rigatoni

See recipe on page 290.

DESSERT

creamy pineapple soft serve

Blend 1 cup frozen pineapple chunks with ½ cup skim milk and 1 tsp. sugar or 1 packet stevia.

NUTRITION INFO: *Calories 130, Fat (g) 0, Sat fat (g) 0, Protein (g) 5, Carbs (g) 26, Fiber (g) 3, Sodium (mg) 65*

SNACKS

Choose up to 300 calories of snacks to reach your daily goal. See the lists in Chapter 3 for snack ideas. Don't forget to include your dessert in your food journal (dessert gets included with your snack calories).

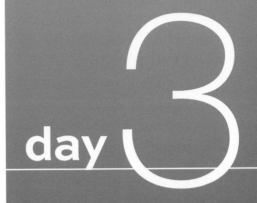

day 3

weekly check-in:

With the End in Sight, You're Probably Thinking About How Far You've Come.

In addition to weight loss and fitness gains, what about food? Have you tried something new and like it? Kale? Quinoa? Avocado? Salmon? Is there a healthy food you always avoided (or never tried) that you now love? That's quite an accomplishment. What would you like to try that you haven't? Many people are surprised to find that when they start to ditch the junk food from their diets, they actually find more variety and more choices. What have you always wanted to eat but have been hesitant to try? If it is a whole food, go for it!

WORKOUT

do your own workout (dyow)

Everybody loves Wednesdays! It's DYOW Day! So what's it going to be today? Hiking? Dancing? Biking? Whatever you choose, give it your all. We'll see you tomorrow for another Bootcamp workout.

"My favorite treat: I make healthy popcorn using walnut oil and Himalayan salt. When the popcorn is still hot, I sprinkle it with nutritional yeast. The final product mimics popcorn sprinkled with cheddar cheese. I said it was a treat, right?**"**
—*The Biggest Loser* trainer Jessie Pavelka

MEALS

BREAKFAST

greek breakfast pita

Serve with 1 apple and 1 cup skim milk.
Sauté ½ cup red bell peppers and onions with a pinch of oregano, then add 1 egg and 1 egg white, scrambled. Stir in 2 Tbsp. reduced-fat feta. Toast half of a whole-wheat pita and fill with 1 cup arugula or spinach, 2 slices tomato, and the egg mixture.

NUTRITION INFO: *Calories 270, Fat (g) 7, Sat fat (g) 2, Protein (g) 19, Carbs (g) 36, Fiber (g) 6, Sodium (mg) 461*

LUNCH

roasted vegetable & couscous salad

See recipe on page 289.

DINNER

minestrone soup

See recipe on page 291.

Serve with 3 oz. extra-lean turkey or ½ cup cooked beans, plus 1 slice whole-wheat bread. This soup tastes even better the next day, which is good because you'll have it again later this week.

SNACKS

Choose up to 300 calories of snacks to reach your calorie goal for the day. See the lists in Chapter 3 for snack ideas.

day 4

morning motivation:

Choices Change Your Life.

The choices you make today are changing your life. In the same way that a journey of 1,000 miles is a series of single steps, you are building a healthier you every day with every choice that you make. A journey takes patience and is measured not only by its outcome but also by the many small moments and experiences you have along the way. Congratulate yourself for each and every positive choice you make and positive action you take. What choices have you made so far in your journey that have made the biggest impact on your life? What choices have you made today to reach your goal?

power 2u

35 MINUTES
WARM UP FOR 5 MINUTES

This is all about strength and determination. This workout is designed to build your power. That's right: Power 2U!

THE WORKOUT

COMPLETE 1 ROUND OR GO FOR A TOTAL OF 2 ROUNDS

1   Bent-Over One-Arm Rows* X 1 minute
2   Jumping Jacks X 1 minute
3   Push-Ups X 1 minute
4   Jogging X 1 minute
5   Bicycle Crunches X 1 minute
6   Skater Jumps X 1 minute
7   Biceps Curls to Overhead Presses X 1 minute
8   Burpees X 1 minute
9   Side Plank with Rear Fly X 1 minute
10 Quick Feet X 1 minute
11 Seated Woodchops X 1 minute
—   Jumping Jacks X 1 minute

(CONTINUES)

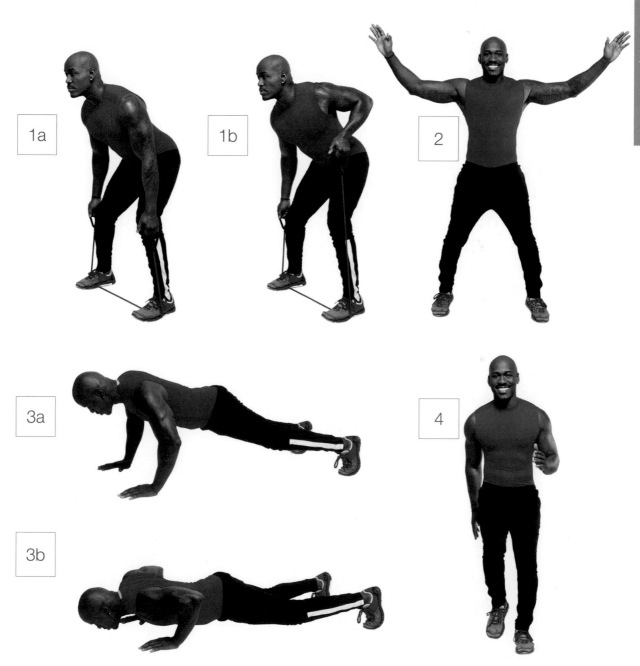

1a

1b

2

3a

3b

4

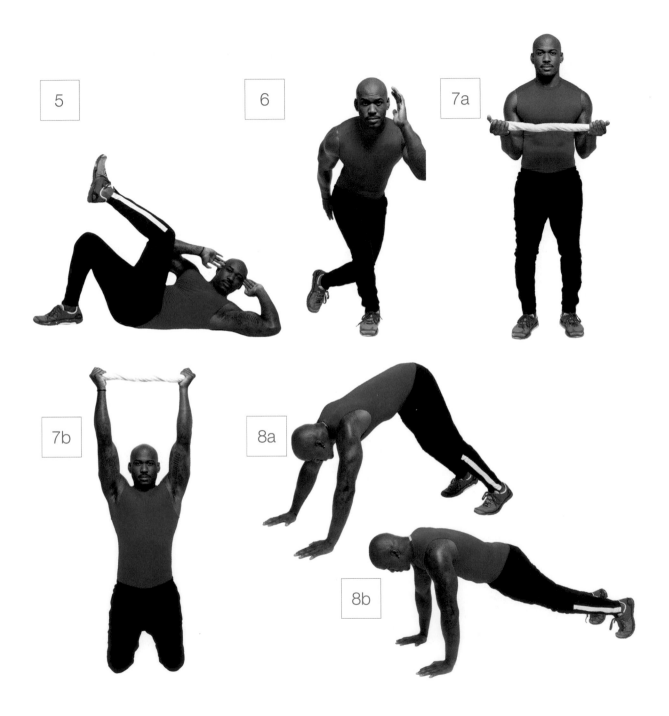

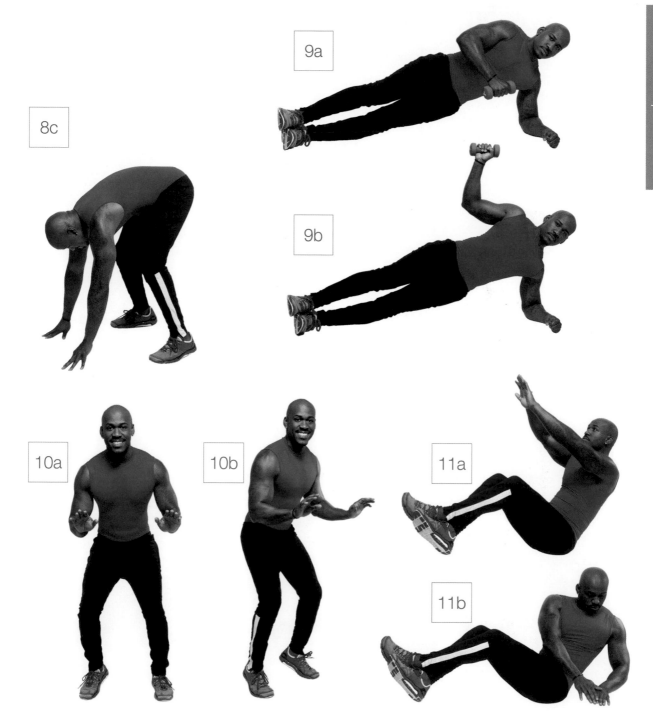

8c

9a

9b

10a

10b

11a

11b

THE WORKOUT
CONTINUED

12 Lat Pulldowns X 1 minute

— Jogging X 1 minute

13 Overhead Presses X 1 minute

14 Mountain Climbers X 1 minute

15 Hip Bridge X 1 minute

16 Air Jump Rope X 1 minute

17 Renegade Rows X 1 minute

18 High Knees with Torso Twist X 1 minute

19 Chest Presses X 1 minute

— Skater Jumps X 1 minute

Repeat for Round 2

COOL DOWN FOR 5 MINUTES

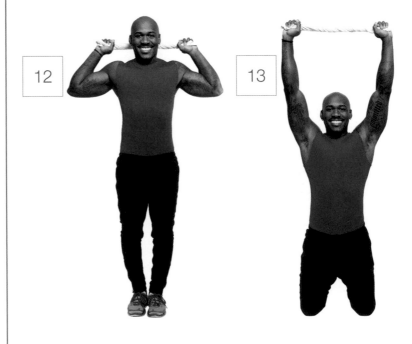

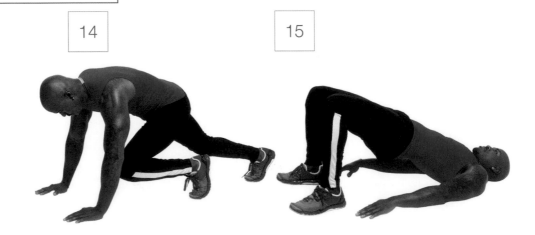

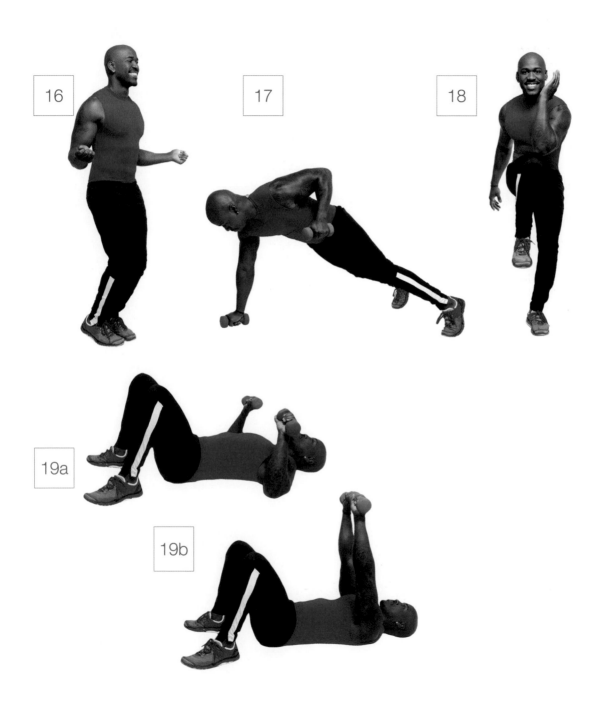

MEALS

BREAKFAST

carrot, raisin & walnut muffin

Serve 1 leftover muffin with 1 Tbsp. natural peanut butter and 1 cup plain fat-free Greek yogurt with 1 Tbsp. all-fruit preserves.

LUNCH

beef & vegetable rigatoni

Serve leftovers from Tuesday.

DINNER

cheesy bean casserole

See recipe on page 290.

Serve with 3 cups spinach and ½ cup cooked brown rice. You'll save 1 portion for tomorrow's lunch.

SNACKS

Choose up to 300 calories of snacks to reach your calorie goal for the day. See the lists in Chapter 3 for snack ideas.

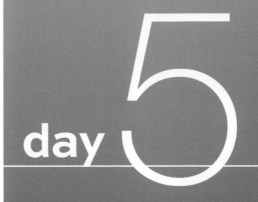

day 5

nutrition bite:

What's Plan B?

When you're visiting friends or invited to a social gathering, how are you going to have fun AND take care of yourself in the process? What is your Plan A? Don't stop there. Create a Plan B in the event that things take an unexpected turn. Having a solid Plan B can help you navigate the most difficult situations. For example, if you plan to order a healthy dish at a family dinner, but the restaurant no longer offers it, what's your back-up choice? Will you give in and eat something deep-fried and heavy, or will you ask your server to help you create a lighter meal that's heavy on the veggies?

WORKOUT burn it, baby

34 MINUTES | WARM UP FOR 5 MINUTES

Intervals are one of the most effective ways to build muscle and endurance. You are going to feel this one, so let's not wait any longer—Burn It, Baby!

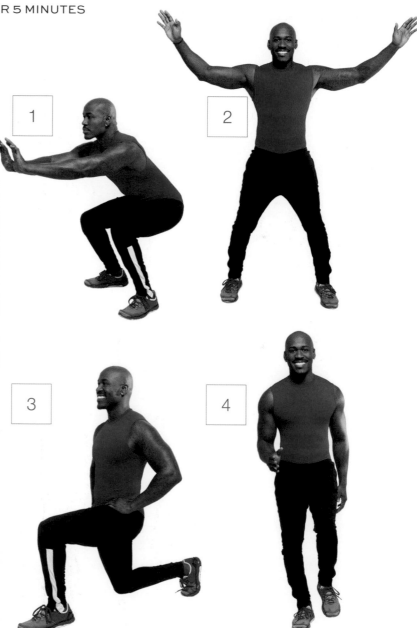

THE WORKOUT

COMPLETE 1 ROUND OR GO FOR A TOTAL OF 2 ROUNDS

1   Squats X 1 minute
2   Jumping Jacks X 1 minute
3   Forward Lunges X 1 minute
4   Jogging X 1 minute
5   Plank with Straight Leg Lifts X 1 minute
6   Skater Jumps X 1 minute
—   Forward Lunges X 1 minute
7   Walking X 1 minute
8   Burpees X 1 minute
9   Rear Lunges X 1 minute
10 Quick Feet X 1 minute
11 Jump Squats X 1 minute

(CONTINUES)

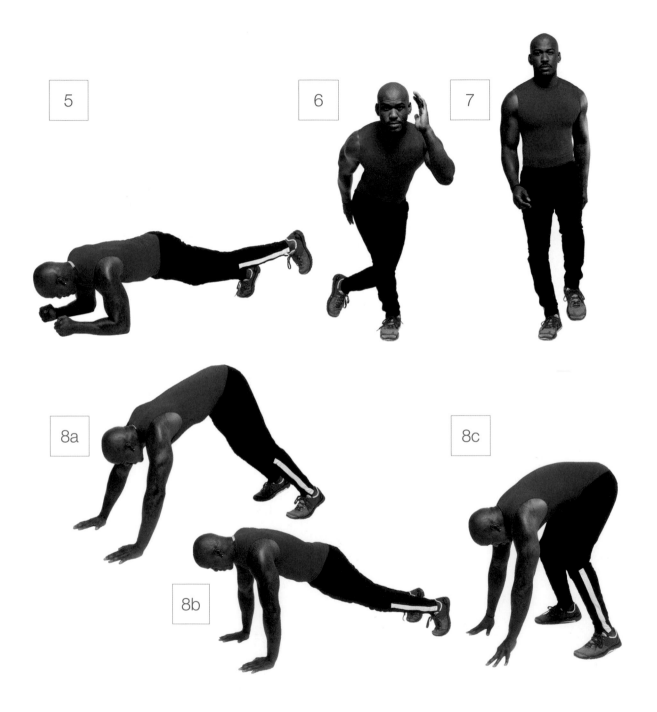

5

6

7

8a

8b

8c

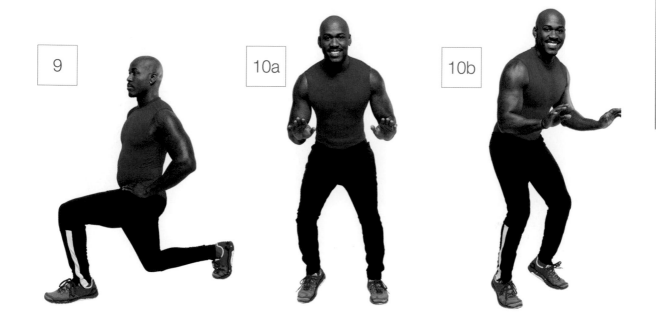

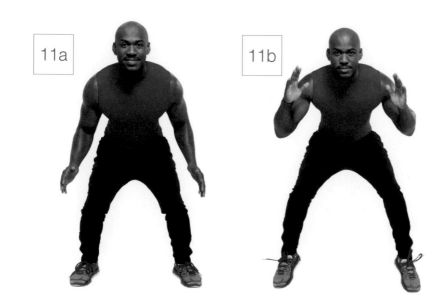

THE WORKOUT

CONTINUED

— Jumping Jacks X 1 minute

12 Bicycle Crunches X 1 minute

— Jogging X 1 minute

— Walking X 1 minute

13 Side Lunges X 1 minute

14 Mountain Climbers X 1 minute

15 Curtsies X 1 minute

16 Air Jump Rope X 1 minute

17 Lunge Twists X 1 minute

18 High Knees with Torso Twist X 1 minute

Repeat for Round 2

COOL DOWN FOR 5 MINUTES

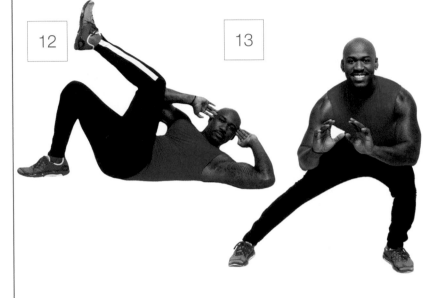

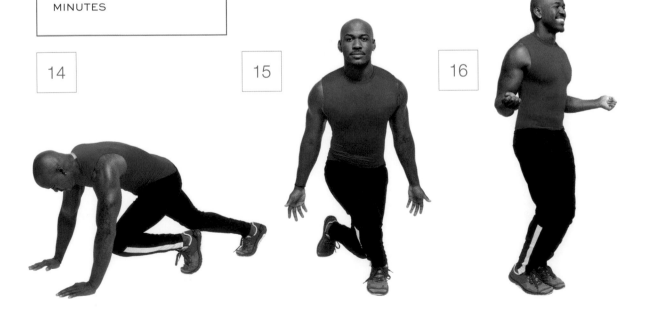

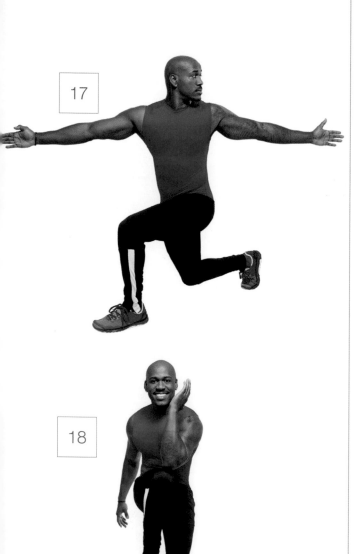

17

18

MEALS

BREAKFAST

fruit & yogurt parfait

See recipe on page 288.

LUNCH

cheesy bean casserole

Serve last night's leftovers in a whole-grain wrap with 1 cup vegetables (tomatoes, onions, and peppers).

DINNER

zucchini noodles with turkey & pesto

Serve with 1 slice whole-grain bread.
Use a spiralizer, food processor, or vegetable peeler to create zucchini "noodles" using 4 medium-size zucchini. Microwave or sauté until hot. Top with 6 oz. cooked extra-lean turkey and ¼ cup prepared pesto. Save half for tomorrow's lunch.

NUTRITION INFO: *Calories 295, Fat (g) 16, Sat fat (g) 2, Protein (g) 27, Carbs (g) 15, Fiber (g) 4, Sodium (mg) 281*

SNACKS

Choose up to 300 calories of snacks to reach your calorie goal for the day. See the lists in Chapter 3 for snack ideas.

day 6

last chance:

We Want Everything You've Got In Today's Last-Chance Workout.

And if your mind is saying you can't, tell it to be quiet. Go to the cliff in this workout. Not over the cliff— just to the edge, where the view is beautiful. Have a great workout!

last-chance workout— happy campers

55 MINUTES

WARM UP FOR 5 MINUTES

It's time for another Last-Chance Workout! Once you've completed this doozy of a workout, you will all be Happy Campers. We think you'll really enjoy your active rest day tomorrow after this one!

Optional weights can be added to the moves marked with an asterisk (*). You do not need any equipment for the remaining moves.

> **If you're hungry you should eat! You're working out and your body needs fuel. Make your focus healthy foods and you will fuel the fire. Choose lean protein, a piece of fruit, or a handful of almonds. Waiting too long to eat almost always leads to bad eating behaviors.**
> —*The Biggest Loser* trainer Jennifer Widerstrom

THE WORKOUT

COMPLETE 2 ROUNDS,
AND IF YOU FEEL LIKE
REALLY KICKING BUTT
TODAY, GO FOR A THIRD
ROUND.

1 Squats* X 1 minute

2 Jumping Jacks X 1
minute

3 Bent-Over One-Arm
Rows* X 1 minute

4 Air Jump Rope X 1
minute

(CONTINUES)

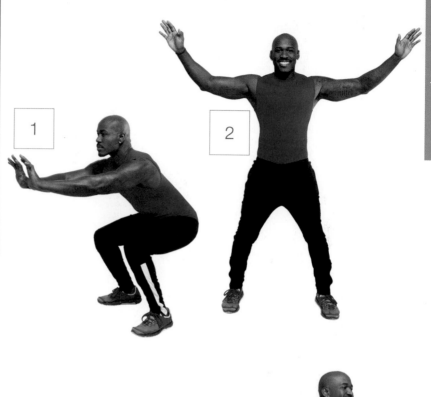

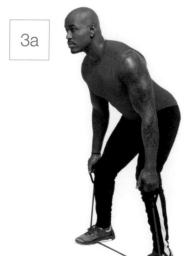

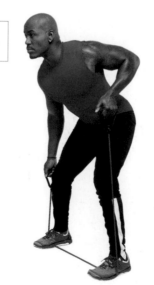

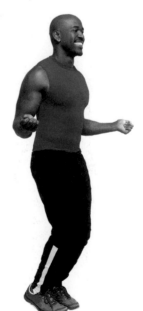

THE WORKOUT

CONTINUED

5 Forward Lunges X 1 minute

6 Jogging X 1 minute

7 Plank with Straight Leg Lifts X 1 minute

8 Skater Jumps X 1 minute

9 Push-Ups X 1 minute

10 Walking X 1 minute

11 Burpees X 1 minute

12 Rear Lunges X 1 minute

13 Quick Feet X 1 minute

14 Biceps Curls to Overhead Presses* X 1 minute

15 Mountain Climbers X 1 minute

16 Jump Squats X 1 minute

— Jumping Jacks X 1 minute

17 Bicycle Crunches X 1 minute

— Air Jump Rope X 1 minute

— Walking X 1 minute

Repeat for Round 2

COOL DOWN FOR 5 MINUTES

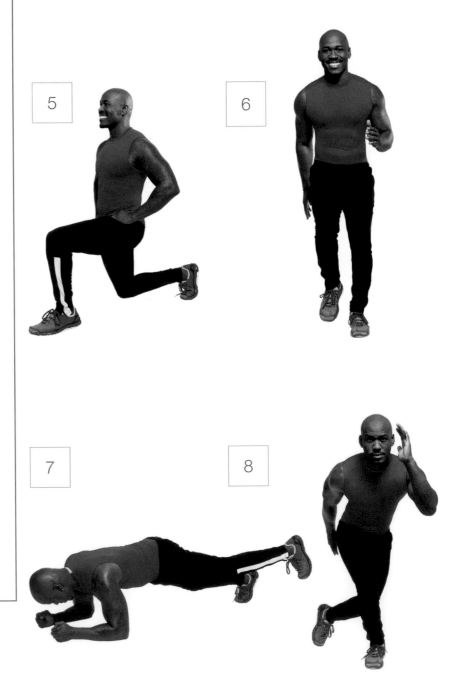

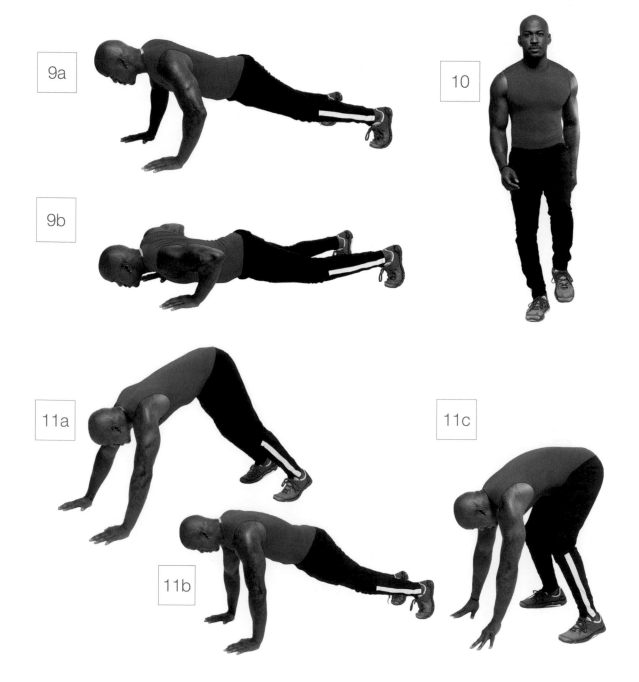

9a

9b

10

11a

11b

11c

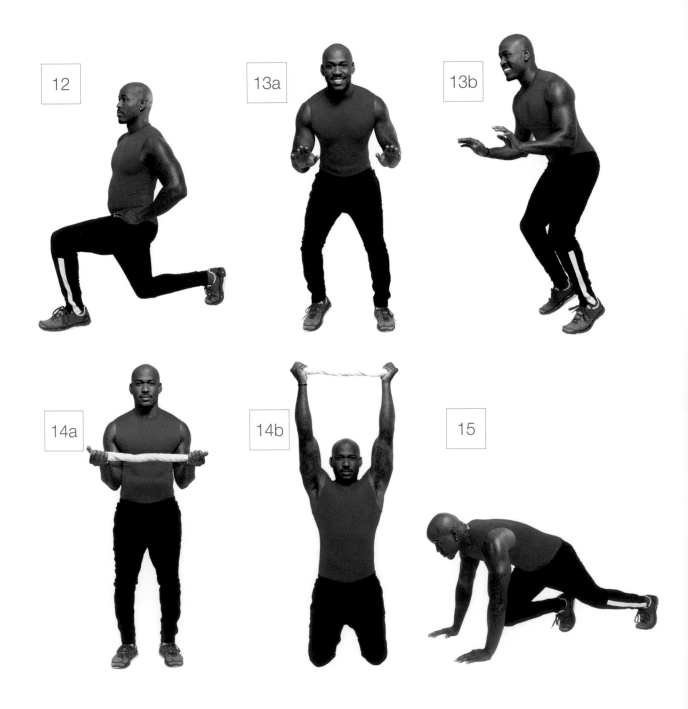

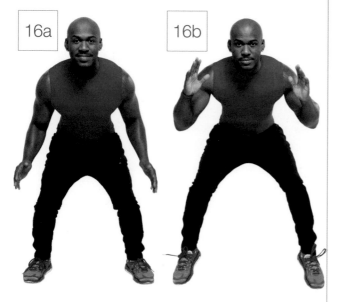

16a 16b

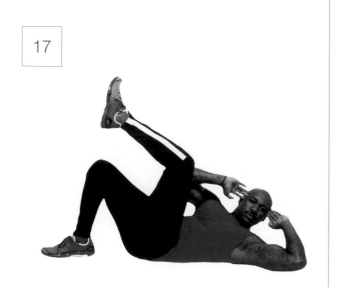

17

MEALS

BREAKFAST

spinach feta cups

Serve with 1 slice whole-wheat toast, 1 cup skim milk, and 1 cup grape tomatoes.

Combine 1 cup chopped spinach, ½ tsp. minced garlic, 2 Tbsp. reduced-fat feta cheese, and 1 egg plus 1 egg white. Season with a pinch of nutmeg and black pepper. Pour into 3 wells of a greased muffin tin. Bake at 350° for about 15 minutes, until the eggs have set. Serve with 1 slice whole-wheat toast.

NUTRITION INFO: *Calories 191, Fat (g) 8, Sat fat (g) 3, Protein (g) 17, Carbs (g) 16, Fiber (g) 3, Sodium (mg) 460*

LUNCH

zucchini noodles with turkey & pesto

Serve last night's leftovers for lunch.

DINNER

bbq spiced chicken with parsley salad

See recipe on page 289.

SNACKS

Choose up to 300 calories of snacks to reach your calorie goal for the day. See the lists in Chapter 3 for snack ideas.

day 7

morning motivation:

Trust Yourself And You'll Get There.

I trust myself to make enough healthy decisions to get me where I want to go.

Trust yourself, not that you'll be perfect, but that you have the tools to become healthier and to stick with your program. When you trust yourself more, and forgive yourself for the slips that you make, you'll begin to make better choices more often.

active rest day

What will you do today with your day off from exercise? Will you do something active? Prep meals for next week? Catch up on your chores? Whatever you do, give it your all! See you tomorrow for the start of Week 8!

MEALS

BREAKFAST

blueberry lemon stuffed french toast

Serve with 1 link lower-sodium turkey breakfast sausage and 1 cup skim milk.

Combine 1 egg white, 2 Tbsp. skim milk, and a dash of vanilla extract. Dredge 2 slices whole-wheat bread in the mixture, then cook on both sides until firm. Sprinkle with ½ tsp. powdered sugar. Spread 2 Tbsp. fat-free lemon Greek yogurt and ½ cup blueberries on 1 slice, then top with the other.

NUTRITION INFO: *Calories 242, Fat (g) 3, Sat fat (g) 0, Protein (g) 16, Carbs (g) 45, Fiber (g) 6, Sodium (mg) 365*

LUNCH

chicken salad with mango vinaigrette

See recipe on page 212 for the dressing.

Combine 1 serving dressing with 3 cups kale (leaves only, chopped), 1 chopped cooked chicken breast (3 oz.), and 2 Tbsp. unsalted peanuts.

NOTE You can toss the kale and dressing up to 1 day in advance; this will tenderize the kale.

VEGETARIAN OPTION Sub in ½ cup cooked chickpeas for the chicken.

NUTRITION INFO: *Calories 347, Fat (g) 10, Sat fat (g) 2, Protein (g) 37, Carbs (g) 31, Fiber (g) 6, Sodium (mg) 170*

DINNER

cilantro-lime chicken with cauliflower "spanish" rice

Serve with 1 Tbsp. low-sodium salsa and a corn tortilla. Marinate 4 oz. chicken breast in 1 tsp. each lime juice and cilantro, ½ tsp. each olive oil and ground cumin, and a pinch of salt and pepper. Grill or bake as desired until cooked through. Finely mince 2 cups cauliflower, and steam. Stir in ½ cup cooked peas and ¼ cup low-sodium salsa of your choice. Serve chicken over "rice" with additional low-sodium salsa.

VEGETARIAN OPTION Sub in 3 oz. tofu for the chicken.

NUTRITION INFO: *Calories 291, Fat (g) 3, Sat fat (g) 0, Protein (g) 33, Carbs (g) 24, Fiber (g) 6, Sodium (mg) 281*

DESSERT

chocolate banana split

See recipe on page 291.

SNACKS

Choose up to 300 calories of snacks to reach your daily goal. See the lists in Chapter 3 for snack ideas. Don't forget to include your dessert in your food journal (dessert gets included with your snack calories).

BREAKFASTS

carrot, raisin & walnut muffins

Satisfy your sweet cravings with these delicious muffins. They're perfect for breakfast or a snack.

SERVES 10   PREP TIME 10 minutes   COOK TIME 20 minutes

½ cup self-rising flour
1¼ cups whole-wheat flour
⅓ cup light brown sugar
1½ tsp. ground cinnamon
6 oz. orange juice
2 Tbsp. plain fat-free Greek yogurt
1 large egg
1 carrot, grated
⅓ cup raisins
1 Tbsp. chopped walnuts

Preheat oven to 350°.

Mix the flours, sugar, and cinnamon in a large bowl. In a separate bowl combine orange juice, Greek yogurt, and egg.

Fold the egg mixture into the flour mixture; add carrot, raisins, and walnuts and stir until well combined. Spoon into a greased muffin tin and bake for 20 minutes until golden and firm to the touch. Cool on a wire rack before freezing.

Freeze muffins in a resealable plastic bag for up to 1 month. You'll eat three muffins for breakfasts this week, and you can eat them as snacks, too.

NUTRITION INFO: *Calories 140, Fat (g) 1, Sat fat (g) 0, Protein (g) 4, Carbs (g) 30, Fiber (g) 3, Sodium (mg) 89*

fruit & yogurt parfait

This tasty breakfast is delicious year-round. Change it up by using different fruit each season. This recipe is courtesy of The Biggest Loser Resorts Niagara.

SERVES 1   PREP TIME 5 minutes

1 (6-oz.) container plain fat-free Greek yogurt
1 tsp. coconut palm sugar (optional)
1 tsp. fresh lime juice (or to taste)
½ cup seasonal fresh fruit
1 tsp. honey
2 Tbsp. sliced almonds
1 Tbsp. hemp seeds

Combine yogurt, coconut palm sugar (if using), and lime juice. Make the parfait by layering the yogurt mixture, fruit, honey, almonds, and seeds.

NUTRITION INFO: *Calories 332, Fat (g) 7, Sat fat (g) 1, Protein (g) 25, Carbs (g) 39, Fiber (g) 5, Sodium (mg) 105*

LUNCHES

roasted vegetable & couscous salad

Couscous is a great alternative to brown rice—it's super-healthy and delicious.

SERVES 1   PREP TIME 15 minutes   COOK TIME 30 minutes

- ½ cup chopped butternut squash
- ½ cup chopped eggplant
- ½ cup chopped zucchini
- ½ cup whole-wheat couscous
- 1 clove garlic, minced
- 1 tsp. balsamic vinegar
- 1 tsp. extra-virgin olive oil
- ¼ tsp. honey
- ¼ cup diced onion
- ¼ cup diced red bell pepper
- 2 cups arugula

Preheat oven to 450°.

Place butternut squash in a deep baking tray and spray lightly with cooking spray. Bake for 10 minutes, then add the eggplant and zucchini (also sprayed lightly with cooking spray). Roast for another 20 minutes or until cooked. Remove from oven and set aside.

Place couscous in a heatproof bowl and cover with boiling water. Stir to coat the grains, and then set aside for 5 minutes to absorb. Using a fork, fluff the grains to separate.

To make the dressing, place the garlic, balsamic vinegar, oil, and honey in an airtight jar, and shake until combined.

Loosen the couscous with a fork until light and fluffy. Add the roasted vegetables, onion, bell pepper, and arugula. Mix the dressing through the salad until coated.

NUTRITION INFO: *Calories 462, Fat (g) 5, Sat fat (g) 1, Protein (g) 18, Carbs (g) 66, Fiber (g) 5, Sodium (mg) 248*

DINNERS

bbq spiced chicken with parsley salad

This Middle Eastern-inspired meal is impressive yet simple to prepare, and it's a fun twist on your favorite grilled chicken.

SERVES 1   PREP TIME 15 minutes   COOK TIME 10 minutes

- 1 whole-wheat tortilla
- 4 oz. chicken breast
- 1 tsp. ground cumin
- 1 tsp. ground cinnamon
- ½ Tbsp. honey
- ½ lemon, juiced
- 1 cup parsley
- 1 tsp. fresh mint (optional)
- ½ cucumber, sliced
- 1 tomato, chopped
- ½ cup chopped green or red bell pepper
- 2 Tbsp. hummus (try the Roasted Red Pepper Hummus—see recipe on page 68)

Preheat oven to 350°. Place tortilla on a baking sheet, and cook for 3 to 4 minutes, or until toasted and crisp. Remove from oven and set aside to cool.

Heat a nonstick skillet over medium-high heat. Coat the chicken with cumin, cinnamon, and a pinch of salt and pepper, and add to pan. Spray a little olive oil spray onto the chicken, and cook for 3 minutes on each side, or until golden and cooked through. Remove from pan, and keep warm.

Mix together honey and lemon juice in a large bowl. Chop parsley, mint (if using), cucumber, tomato, and bell pepper, and add to the bowl, tossing to coat.

Spread hummus onto a serving plate. Top with the salad, and break the tortilla into small pieces on top. Top with cooked chicken and serve with extra black pepper and a lemon wedge.

NUTRITION INFO: *Calories 431, Fat (g) 6, Sat fat (g) 1, Protein (g) 37, Carbs (g) 55, Fiber (g) 11, Sodium (mg) 384*

beef & vegetable rigatoni

This hearty, homemade sauce is packed with vegetables. It tastes even better the next day!

SERVES 2   PREP TIME 15 minutes   COOK TIME 30 minutes

- 4 oz. whole-wheat rigatoni
- 1 small onion, chopped
- 2 cloves garlic, chopped
- 8 oz. extra-lean ground beef
- 1 cup eggplant, cubed
- 1 large red bell pepper, chopped
- 2 small zucchini, chopped
- 2 tomatoes, chopped
- 1 Tbsp. no-salt-added tomato paste
- ⅔ cup low-sodium beef broth
- 2 tsp. raw sugar (optional)
- ¼ cup fresh basil, chopped

Place the pasta in a pot of boiling water and cook just until softened. Drain and set aside.

Meanwhile, spray a large nonstick skillet with cooking spray, and heat over medium heat. Add onion and garlic and cook, stirring, for 2 to 3 minutes. Add the beef and cook, stirring with a wooden spoon to break up any lumps, for 6 to 8 minutes or until beef has browned. Season with a dash of salt and pepper.

Add eggplant, bell pepper, zucchini, tomato, tomato paste, and broth, and cook for another 12 to 14 minutes, stirring occasionally. Add a dash of water if needed to thin the sauce.

Add the pasta, sugar (if using), and basil to the sauce, and stir for 3 minutes or until pasta is warmed through.

Transfer half to a serving bowl and top with extra basil to serve. Refrigerate the remaining portion for lunch later in the week.

VEGETARIAN OPTION Sub ½ cup cooked lentils for the beef.

NOTE Adjust the quantities and types of vegetables as desired.

NUTRITION INFO: *Calories 418, Fat (g) 6, Sat fat (g) 2, Protein (g) 34, Carbs (g) 53, Fiber (g) 9, Sodium (mg) 160*

cheesy bean casserole

This comforting casserole is quick and easy yet filling.

SERVES 2   PREP TIME 15 minutes   COOK TIME 15 minutes

- ½ large white onion, chopped
- 1 (14.5-oz.) can dark red kidney beans, drained and rinsed
- ½ (14.5-oz.) can no-salt-added diced tomatoes
- Pinch of garlic powder
- Pinch of black pepper
- ¼ cup reduced-fat cheddar cheese, shredded

Preheat oven to 400°.

Coat a nonstick skillet with cooking spray; place over medium-high heat until hot. Add onion; sauté until tender. Stir in beans and next 3 ingredients. Cook 3 minutes or until thoroughly heated, stirring well.

Spoon mixture into 1 (8-inch) square baking dish; sprinkle with cheese. Bake, uncovered, for 5 minutes or until cheese melts. Let stand 5 minutes.

Refrigerate the second portion for tomorrow's lunch.

NUTRITION INFO: *Calories 183, Fat (g) 3, Sat fat (g) 1, Protein (g) 11, Carbs (g) 35, Fiber (g) 9, Sodium (mg) 169*

minestrone soup

This veggie-packed soup is the perfect way to warm up on a cold day. We love it as the basis for a light meal or as a starter. Thanks to The Biggest Loser Resorts Niagara, you've just found your new favorite soup.

SERVES 6   PREP TIME 15 minutes   COOK TIME 75 minutes

- ½ cup Spanish onion, diced
- 1 clove garlic, minced
- 1½ tsp. extra-virgin olive oil
- 1 qt. low-sodium vegetable broth
- 1 cup tomatoes, diced
- ¾ cup yellow squash, diced
- 1 cup zucchini, diced
- 1 cup cannellini beans
- 1½ cups escarole, washed and chopped
- ½ cup green beans, chopped
- 1½ tsp. fresh basil, chopped
- 2 tsp. Italian parsley, chopped
- ¼ tsp. salt
- 4 tsp. Parmesan cheese

Sauté onion and garlic in oil. Add broth and bring to a boil; reduce heat and bring to a simmer. Add the tomatoes, squash, zucchini, cannellini beans, escarole, and green beans. After simmering for 1 hour, add basil and parsley. Add salt. Garnish with cheese before serving.

Refrigerate one portion for dinner later this week, and freeze the remaining servings individually for up to 1 month.

NUTRITION INFO: *Calories 86, Fat (g) 1, Sat fat (g) 0, Protein (g) 4, Carbs (g) 12, Fiber (g) 3, Sodium (mg) 124*

DESSERTS

chocolate banana split

Treat yourself to an irresistible dessert made with reduced-fat vanilla frozen yogurt and chocolate, topped with nuts.

SERVES 1   PREP TIME 5 minutes

- 1 cup strawberries, sliced
- 1 banana, sliced
- ½ cup slow-churned low-fat vanilla frozen yogurt
- ½ Tbsp. chopped walnuts
- 1 tsp. mini chocolate chips

Place strawberries in a dessert dish. Top with the banana slices and a scoop of frozen yogurt.

Sprinkle with walnuts and chocolate chips, then serve.

NUTRITION INFO: *Calories 235, Fat (g) 7, Sat fat (g) 3, Protein (g) 4, Carbs (g) 40, Fiber (g) 3, Sodium (mg) 47*

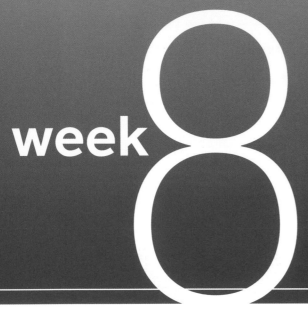

week 8

you're here:

Week 8 of Bootcamp. The finish line is in sight. You've begun your transformation into the newer, healthier version of you. Congratulations! We don't consider Week 8 to be the "end" of Bootcamp or your journey.

It marks the end of the first phase of the rest of your life. What comes next is up to you. This week you'll spend some time visualizing your future, and you'll start to set goals for the next month, the next three months, and even the next year.

Right now, as you head into Day 50 (oh, yeah, that's right!) of Bootcamp, we want you to consider where you were when you started. What couldn't you do then that's easy for you now? What was a struggle and no longer is? Think back to that first workout, on Day 1 of Week 1. "Ready to Rock" was your first taste of Bootcamp, and after a quick warm-up, you started doing push-ups, air jump rope, planks, and even skater jumps! We bet you were pretty wiped out after that 33-minute workout. Now think about your last workout of Week 7: The "Last Chance Workout" called "Happy Campers." Not only were you doing some of the same moves you did during your

inaugural Bootcamp workout, but you were doing more of them, plus optional weights and more complicated movements. And the workout was almost twice as long!

It doesn't matter whether the scale budged 1 pound or 20, whether you used no weights or 8-pound dumbbells for every move, or whether you struggled with your eating or followed the plan closely. In Week 1, we told you: "You have to keep coming back to the program, doing your workouts, and setting your goals."

Did you do those three things? If you did, then great job! If you struggled a bit more than expected, that's OK. Start where you are, do the Bootcamp again starting next week, and see how far you get the second time around. We were looking for progress, not perfection, remember? And we know you made progress—after all, you're still here!

You're so much stronger now, inside and out, and there's still time to push yourself or even turn it around! We want you to give this final week everything you've got. Don't hold back. Don't be afraid to push yourself. In fact, that's the goal we'd like you to focus on this week.

We want you to push yourself in the workouts by trying at least one of the more advanced moves. For example, if you've been doing push-ups on your knees, try it on your toes. Even if it's just for a rep or two. You'll surprise yourself at what you can do.

Enjoy this last week!

WEEKLY WORKOUTS

MONDAY	Stronger
TUESDAY	Faster
WEDNESDAY	DYOW
THURSDAY	Survivor
FRIDAY	My Time to Shine
SATURDAY	Last-Chance Workout— Thank You, All
SUNDAY	Active Rest Day

WEEK 8 MEALS

MONDAY

B Breakfast Tostada
L Grown-Up PBJ
D Garlic Shrimp

TUESDAY

B Protein Mocha Shake
L Roast Beef Lettuce Pockets with Horseradish Mayo
D Lisa Rambo's Chicken Pizza

WEDNESDAY

B Overnight Oats
L Salmon Wrap
D Salsa Verde Smothered Turkey Burger

THURSDAY

B Sweet Waffle Sandwich
L Salsa Verde Smothered Turkey Burger
D Three-Bean Vegetarian Chili

FRIDAY

B Peanut Butter Toast
L Zucchini "Pasta" Salad
D Peanut Noodles with Tofu & Broccoli

SATURDAY

B Fernanda's Sweet & Savory Breakfast
L Three-Bean Vegetarian Chili Stuffed Sweet Potato
D Spaghetti Squash Chicken Alfredo

SUNDAY

B Banana Yogurt Smoothie
L Simple Spaghetti Squash
D Grass-Fed Beef Kabobs with Goat Cheese Stuffed Tomatoes & Roasted Vegetables

coaches' corner

WHAT DOES THE FUTURE HOLD FOR YOU? Now that you have identified some outcomes that are important to you (your wellness vision), it's time to create the steps that will help you get there.

THREE-MONTH AND WEEKLY GOALS

Your three-month goals are the long-term goals designed to lead you to your wellness vision. They are set far enough in the future to allow time for a meaningful change, yet not so far that you find them daunting or lose interest before you can reach them.

You want to be confident that you can achieve your three-month goals, but that doesn't mean that you need to play it totally safe. Because these goals do allow time for significant changes to take place, step outside your comfort zone and challenge yourself.

Write these with as much detail and specificity as you can. However, it is worth noting that three-month goals are, by nature, going to be less detailed than weekly goals. For example, when setting three-month goals it is enough detail to include how many days per week you anticipate doing a particular behavior ("I will do 45 minutes of cardio exercise four days per week"). But, when setting weekly goals, you have more control over your schedule and know what you are motivated to do. You are able to see exactly which days will work best for achieving a particular goal and, perhaps, even what time of day you will work on that goal ("I will do 45 minutes of cardio on the treadmill before breakfast on Monday, Wednesday, Thursday, and Saturday this week").

TIPS FOR THREE-MONTH GOALS

Focus on just one behavior per goal. For instance, the goal "I will eat five servings of vegetables and do 30 minutes of cardiovascular exercise on five days per week" is actually two separate goals.

Remember, if you set a three-month goal that is an outcome ("I will lose 10 pounds" or "I will finish a 5K"), be sure to come up with at least one behavior that leads to that outcome.

Set a total of two to three three-month goals.

EXAMPLES OF THREE-MONTH GOALS

- I will complete 30 minutes of strength-training exercise two days each week.
- I will practice meditation for 10 minutes prior to breakfast four mornings each week.
- Three evenings each week I will journal three positive things that happened to me or that I accomplished that day.
- I will use a stress-reduction technique for five minutes before my daily staff meetings.
- I will eat four servings of vegetables five days each week.

TIPS FOR WEEKLY GOALS

Your weekly goals are steps toward your three-month goals (just as three-month goals are steps toward your wellness vision). Because of the short time frame, your weekly goals are smaller in scope than your three-month goals.

Focus on just one behavior per goal. For instance, the goal "I will eat five servings of vegetables and do 30 minutes of cardiovascular exercise five days per week" is actually two separate goals.

Focus on specific behaviors rather than outcomes.

Set a total of two to three weekly goals.

EXAMPLES OF WEEKLY GOALS

- I will complete 15 minutes of strength-training exercise on Tuesday afternoon at 5 p.m. this week.
- I will practice meditation for one minute before breakfast on Monday and Thursday mornings this week.
- On Tuesday and Thursday evenings at 9 p.m., I will journal three positive things that happened to me or that I accomplished that day.
- I will use deep breathing to relax for five minutes before my 2 p.m. staff meetings on Monday, Wednesday, and Friday this week.
- I will eat two servings of vegetables on Monday, Wednesday, and Friday this week.

day 1

nutrition bite:

Stick With It.

Something we hear time and again from Bootcamp Success Stories and our former *The Biggest Loser* contestants is that their daily eating habits haven't changed much since they reached their goal weight. That's because this isn't a diet, and there is no expiration date. If you go back to eating the way you did, you will undo all your hard work. This whole-foods-based plan is meant to carry you through the rest of your journey. Don't be afraid to experiment with new recipes and foods, but you also don't need to change much. Swapping different proteins and vegetables into the recipes and quick meals you've been eating these past two months is a great way to fend off boredom while still eating foods that fuel your body.

WORKOUT stronger

54 MINUTES | WARM UP FOR 5 MINUTES

This is it! Our final week of Biggest Loser Bootcamp! You
are much stronger than you were seven short weeks ago. We
are kicking up the intensity right now! Three rounds of only
strength moves—let's get started!

Optional weights can be added to the moves marked with
an asterisk (*). You do not need any equipment for the remaining moves.

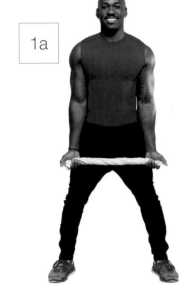

THE WORKOUT
3 ROUNDS

1 Squats with Biceps
Curls* X 1 minute

2 Squats with Overhead
Presses* X 1 minute

3 Side Lunges with Single
Arm Lateral Raises* X 1
minute

4 Lat Pulldowns X 1
minute

5 Bent-Over One-Arm
Rows* X 1 minute

6 Bicycle Crunches X 1
minute

(CONTINUES)

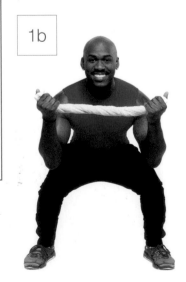

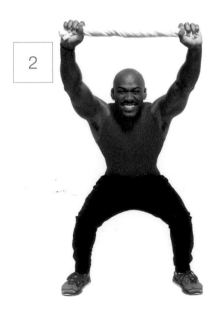

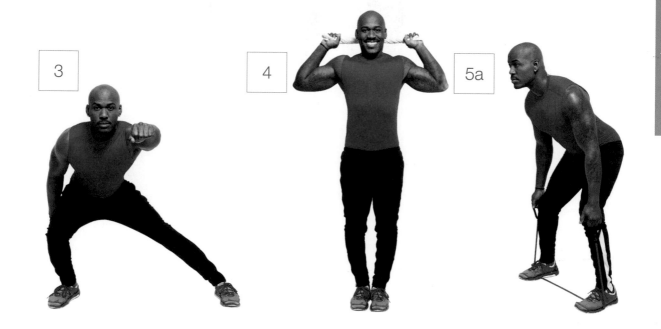

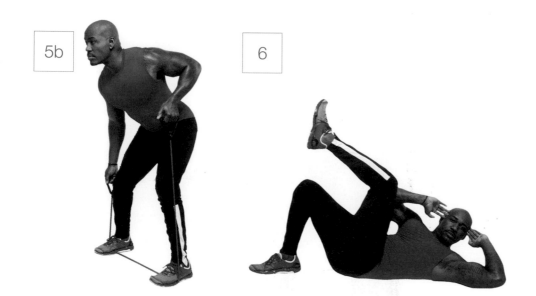

THE WORKOUT
CONTINUED

7 Woodchops* X 1 minute

8 Rear-Stepping Lunges with One-Arm Rows X 1 minute

9 Squats with Rear Fly* X 1 minute

10 Chest Presses* X 1 minute

11 Overhead Presses* X 1 minute

12 Plank with Straight Leg Lifts X 1 minute or 30 seconds per side

13 Squats with Biceps Curls* X 1 minute

Repeat for Rounds 2 and 3

COOL DOWN FOR 5 MINUTES

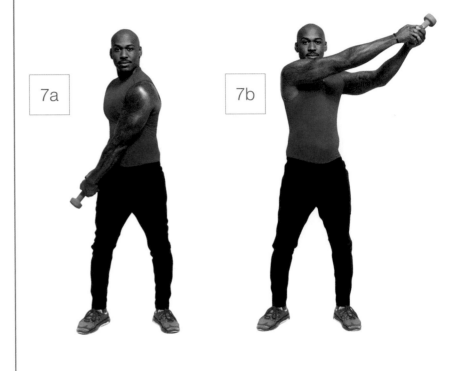

7a 7b

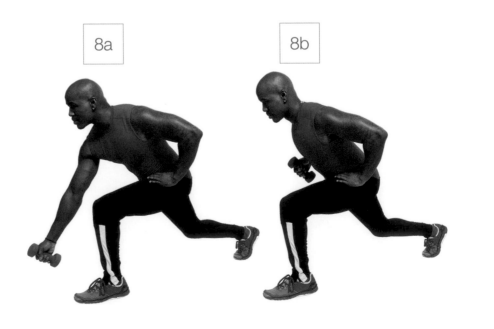

8a 8b

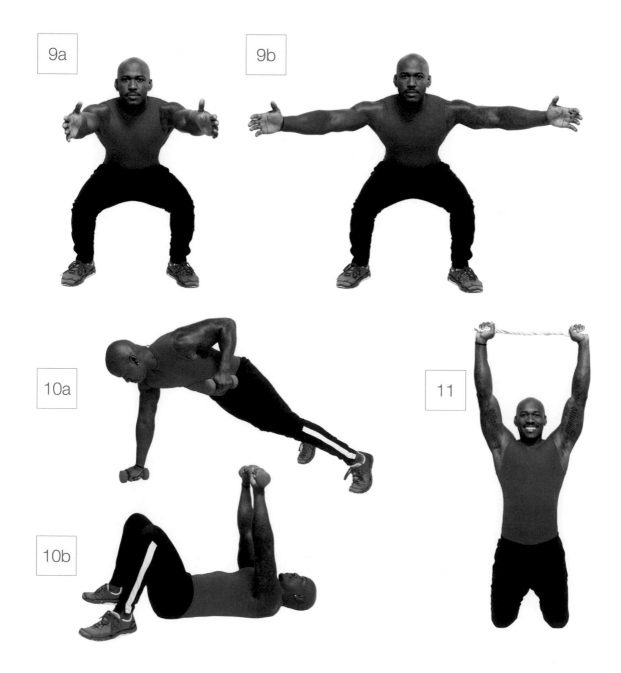

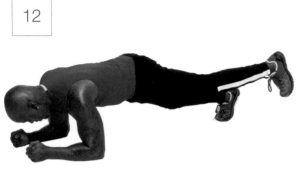

12

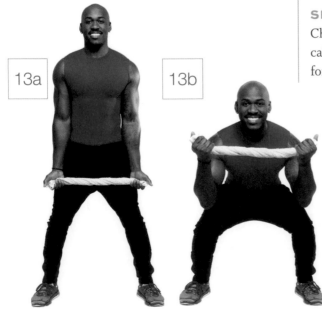

13a 13b

MEALS

BREAKFAST

breakfast tostada

See recipe on page 324.

Serve with 1 cup strawberries and 1 (6-oz.) container plain fat-free Greek yogurt.

LUNCH

grown-up pbj

Serve with 1 cup skim milk.
Mix 2 Tbsp. nut butter (cashew, sunflower seed, or almond) with a pinch of sea salt and dried ground ginger. Spread onto 2 slices whole-wheat bread. Top with ½ cup sliced strawberries.

NUTRITION INFO: *Calories 336, Fat (g) 18, Sat fat (g) 1, Protein (g) 13, Carbs (g) 39, Fiber (g) 9, Sodium (mg) 231*

DINNER

garlic shrimp

See recipe on page 326.

SNACKS

Choose up to 300 calories of snacks to reach your calorie goal for the day. See the lists in Chapter 3 for snack ideas.

day 2

morning motivation:

Healthier Every Day.

Remind yourself: "Every day, in every way, I am becoming healthier." Regular exercise and healthier eating mean whole-body health. You might not always be able to see it or feel it immediately, but you're getting stronger and improving your health. You're moving more easily and are able to do more, and by having more nourishing foods in your body, you're more likely to be feeling great! With each day that goes by, your healthy actions will continue to make you stronger, inside and out. What you put in, you get out. The food, the exercise, and the motivation—they're changing you!

WORKOUT
faster

28 MINUTES | WARM UP FOR 5 MINUTES

Let's get your heart pumping! We're doing easy and hard cardio intervals—this will knock your socks off! You're in the home stretch now—you are getting stronger, and you're moving faster—you can do this! Enjoy this cardio crusher.

THE WORKOUT

COMPLETE 2 ROUNDS OF THE FOLLOWING SEQUENCE. YOU HAVE THE OPTION TO ADD A ROUND 3 IF YOU FEEL UP TO IT!

1 Skater Jumps X 1 minute
2 High Knees with Torso Twist X 1 minute
3 Air Jump Rope X 1 minute
4 Jogging X 30 seconds
5 Walking X 15 seconds
6 Quick Feet X 30 seconds
— Walking X 1 minute
7 Forward Lunges X 1 minute
— Jogging X 1 minute
8 High Knees X 1 minute
9 Jumping Jacks X 30 seconds
— Walking X 15 seconds
— Air Jump Rope X 30 seconds
— Walking X 1 minute

(CONTINUES)

COOL DOWN FOR 5 MINUTES

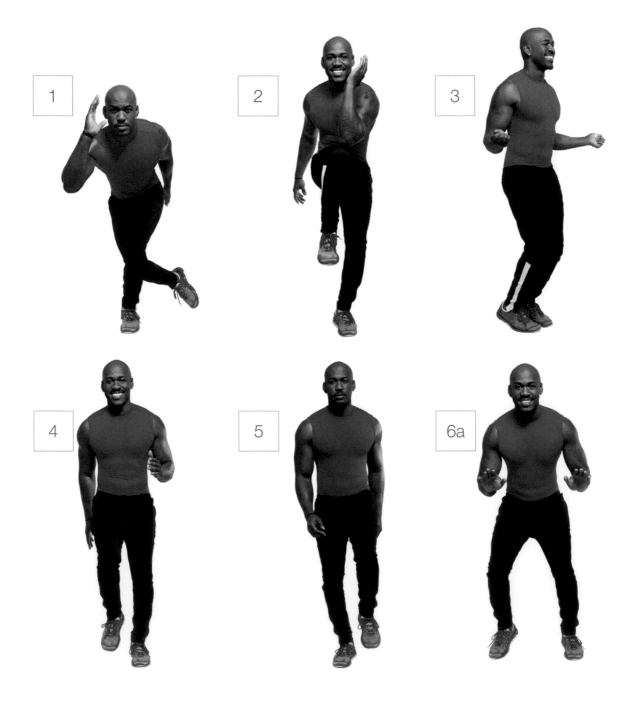

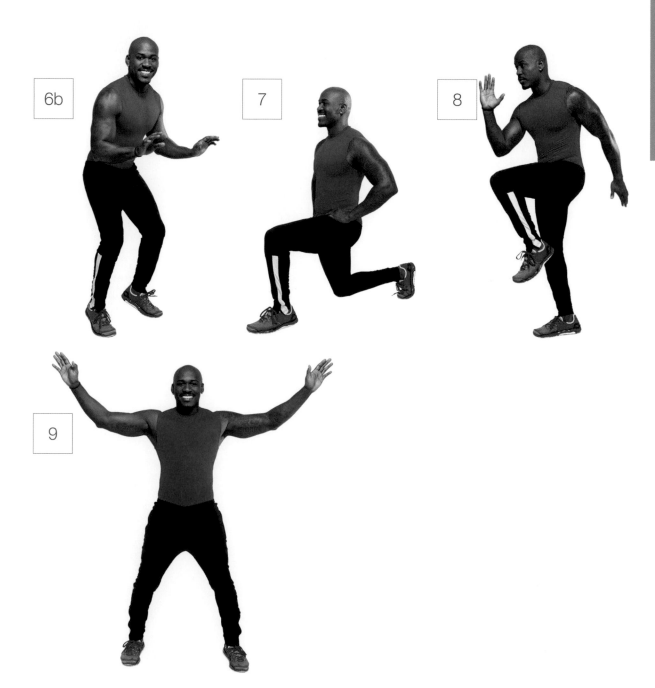

6b

7

8

9

MEALS

BREAKFAST

protein mocha shake

Serve with 8 almonds (½ oz.).
In a blender, combine 1 cup skim milk, ½ cup ice, 1 scoop chocolate protein powder, 1 banana, and 1 tsp. instant coffee.

NUTRITION INFO: *Calories 296, Fat (g) 2, Sat fat (g) 0, Protein (g) 28, Carbs (g) 44, Fiber (g) 6, Sodium (mg) 170*

LUNCH

roast beef lettuce pockets with horseradish mayo

Serve with 2 medium-size carrots and 2 Tbsp. hummus. Mix ¼ tsp. horseradish (or to taste) with 1 Tbsp. reduced-fat mayonnaise, and spread inside half of a whole-wheat pita. Add 3 oz. lean deli roast beef, 1 cup salad greens, and 3 slices of tomato.

NUTRITION INFO: *Calories 259, Fat (g) 8, Sat fat (g) 2, Protein (g) 22, Carbs (g) 29, Fiber (g) 4, Sodium (mg) 458*

DINNER

lisa rambo's chicken pizza

See recipe on page 325.

Serve with 1 cup skim milk and 2 cups green beans.

DESSERT

berry delight ice pops

See recipe on page 327.

SNACKS

Choose up to 300 calories of snacks to reach your daily goal. See the lists in Chapter 3 for snack ideas. Don't forget to include your dessert in your food journal (dessert gets included with your snack calories).

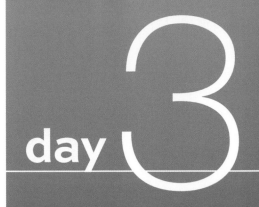

day 3

weekly check-in:

In Our Final Week Of Bootcamp, We Want To Know What YOU Are Most Proud Of!

What have you achieved over the past eight weeks? We don't mean the weight loss. We want to know about the small victories. This is a week for reflection and recognition. Write it down, and share it with those you love the most.

WORKOUT

do your own workout (dyow)

It's the most wonderful time of the week: DYOW! Wednesday means you get to do what you want, whether that's yoga, cycling, walking, or anything else that gets you up and gets you moving. How will you get your sweat on today?

"Fall in love with the feeling of exercise. There are apps and fitness devices that provide you with a ton of information. That's well and good, but remember to check in and become aware of how you feel versus what information you are reading."
—*The Biggest Loser* trainer Jessie Pavelka

MEALS

BREAKFAST

overnight oats

See recipe on page 250.

Serve with 1 cup raspberries and ½ oz. chopped almonds.

LUNCH

salmon wrap

See recipe on page 324.

Serve with 1 cup cucumber slices and 1 medium-size banana.

DINNER

salsa verde smothered turkey burger

Top 2 (3-oz.) cooked turkey burgers with 2 oz. reduced-fat Monterey Jack cheese, 4 slices red onion, and ¼ cup salsa verde. Place in an ovenproof dish, and broil until cheese melts. Serve with ½ cup brown rice, 1 cup bell pepper strips, and ¼ avocado.

VEGETARIAN OPTION Sub in 2 low-sodium veggie burgers for the turkey burgers.

NOTE Save 1 burger for tomorrow's lunch.

NUTRITION INFO: *Calories 416, Fat (g) 12, Sat fat (g) 3, Protein (g) 36, Carbs (g) 44, Fiber (g) 11, Sodium (mg) 334*

SNACKS

Choose up to 300 calories of snacks to reach your calorie goal for the day. See the lists in Chapter 3 for snack ideas.

day 4

morning motivation:

Be Grateful For Today.

Tell yourself: I am grateful for this new day.

Noticing why you're grateful and then speaking or journaling about those things has been shown to help people make big changes and stick with them. It also increases your happiness level and helps you to not sweat the small stuff. Consider making gratitude a practice, even for a little while, to get in the habit of thinking this way. Grab a notebook or journal and write down what you're grateful for as you go through your day, or before bed as you review your day. Today, we know we're grateful for you being part of this Bootcamp experience with us. What are you grateful for?

WORKOUT
survivor

61 MINUTES | WARM UP FOR 5 MINUTES

Strong, determined and focused! That's who you are. This workout will fly by—you know the moves. Give it more than your all; you won't just survive, you will dominate this workout!

Optional weights can be added to the moves marked with an asterisk (*). You do not need any equipment for the remaining moves.

THE WORKOUT
2 ROUNDS

1 Squats with Biceps Curls* X 1 minute
2 Squats with Rear Fly X 1 minute
3 Rear-Stepping Lunges with One-Arm Rows* X 1 minute
4 Lat Pulldowns X 1 minute
5 Bent-Over One-Arm Rows* X 1 minute
6 Seated Woodchops* X 1 minute
7 Bicycle Crunches X 1 minute
8 Squats with Overhead Presses* X 1 minute
9 Side Lunges with Single Arm Lateral Raises* X 1 minute
10 Woodchops* X 1 minute
11 Chest Presses* X 1 minute

(CONTINUES)

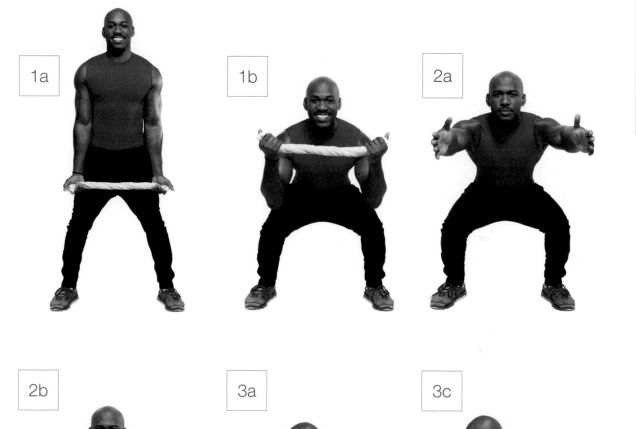

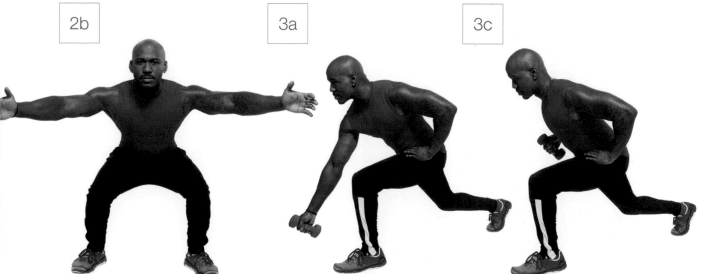

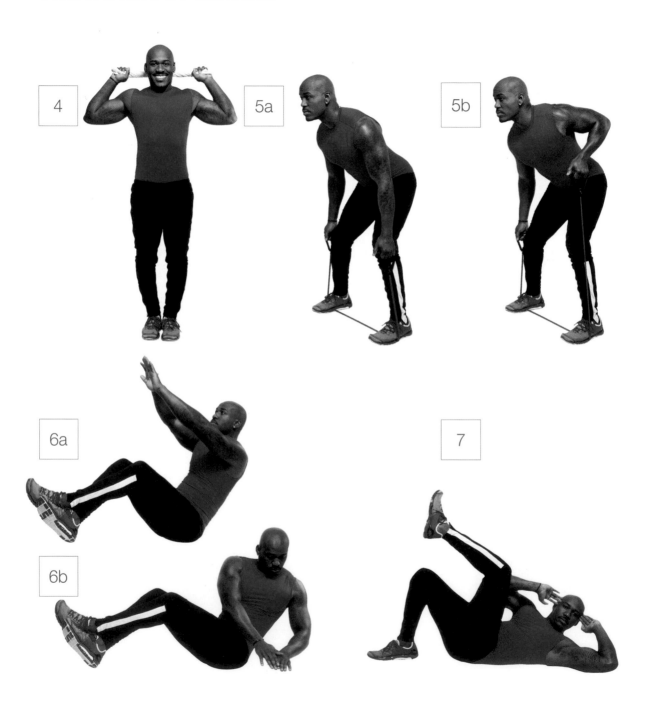

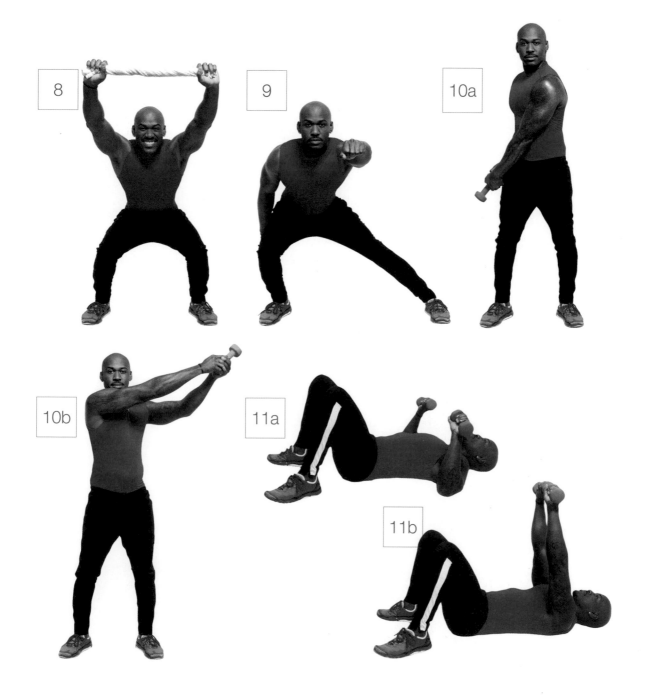

THE WORKOUT

CONTINUED

12 Overhead Presses* X 1 minute

13 Plank X 1 minute

14 Russian Twists* X 1 minute

— Squats with Biceps Curls* X 1 minute

— Squats with Overhead Presses* X 1 minute

15 Renegade Rows* X 1 minute

16 Walk-Out Push-Ups X 1 minute

17 Two-Arm Rows X 1 minute

18 Plank with Straight Leg Lifts X 1 minute or 30 seconds per side

19 Crunches X 1 minute

Repeat for Round 2

COOL DOWN FOR 5 MINUTES

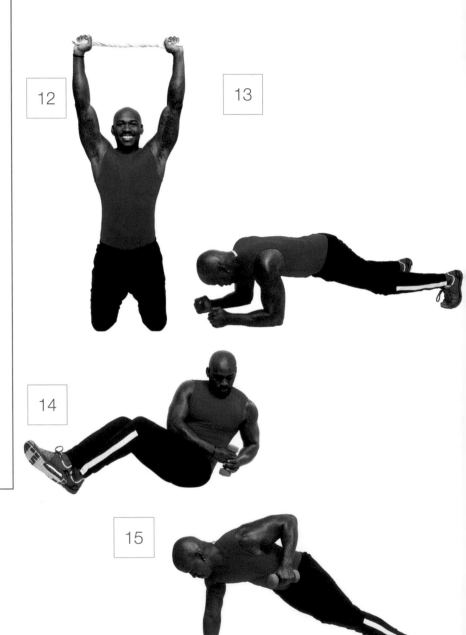

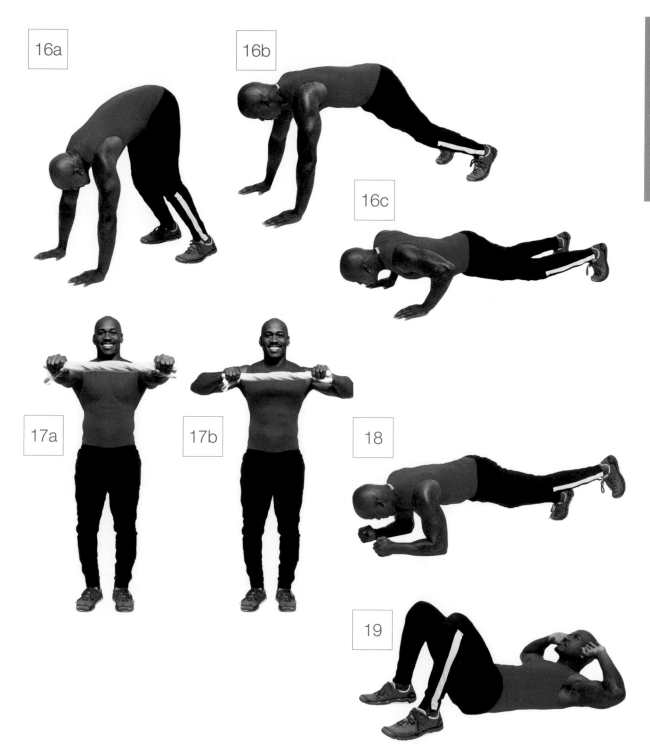

MEALS

BREAKFAST

sweet waffle sandwich

Toast 2 whole-grain waffles. Spread with 2 Tbsp. peanut butter, 1 Tbsp. all-fruit preserves, and ¼ cup sliced strawberries. Sprinkle on 1 tsp. ground flaxseed.

NUTRITION INFO: *Calories 424, Fat (g) 18, Sat fat (g) 3, Protein (g) 13, Carbs (g) 48, Fiber (g) 13, Sodium (mg) 352*

LUNCH

salsa verde smothered turkey burger

Serve last night's leftovers.

DINNER

three-bean vegetarian chili

See recipe on page 327.

Serve with 1 Tbsp. shredded reduced-fat cheddar cheese and ½ cup cooked brown rice.

SNACKS

Choose up to 300 calories of snacks to reach your calorie goal for the day. See the lists in Chapter 3 for snack ideas.

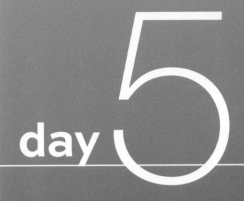

day 5

nutrition bite:

Commit To Eat Right Today.

Next week, you're going to be doing this without a daily meal plan. So when you wake up on Week 9, Day 1, tell yourself: "I will stick to my eating plan today."

Make this commitment to yourself even though Bootcamp is "over." Commit to sticking to your eating plan for just that one day. Don't think about tomorrow yet. Commit to that one day. Then, the next day, focus on today again. And so on. You'll stick with the healthy habits you worked so hard to build these past two months. Focusing on one small goal and meeting it will build confidence and momentum for the weeks and even months ahead.

WORKOUT my time to shine

33 MINUTES | WARM UP FOR 5 MINUTES

As you reach the end of Bootcamp, we think you're probably feeling like it's your time to shine. And shine you will with this workout (of course, by shine, we also mean sweat). We challenge you to do three rounds of this workout. We know you have it in you.

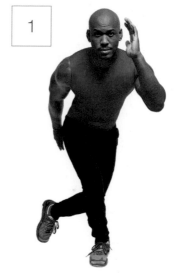

THE WORKOUT

2 ROUNDS. ADD A ROUND 3 IF YOU FEEL UP TO IT!

1 Skater Jumps X 1 minute
2 High Knees with Torso Twist X 1 minute
3 Air Jump Rope X 1 minute
4 Jumping Jacks X 30 seconds
5 Walking X 15 seconds
6 Burpees X 30 seconds
— Walking X 1 minute
7 Rear-Stepping Lunges with Woodchops X 1 minute
8 Jogging X 1 minute
9 Mountain Climbers X 1 minute
— Jumping Jacks X 30 seconds
— Walking X 15 seconds
— Mountain Climbers X 30 seconds
— Walking X 1 minute

Repeat for Round 2

COOL DOWN FOR 5 MINUTES

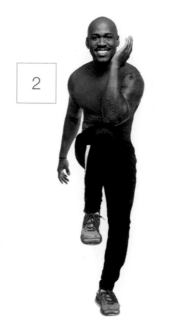

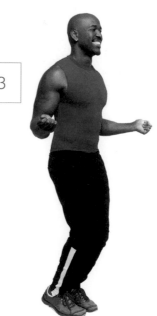

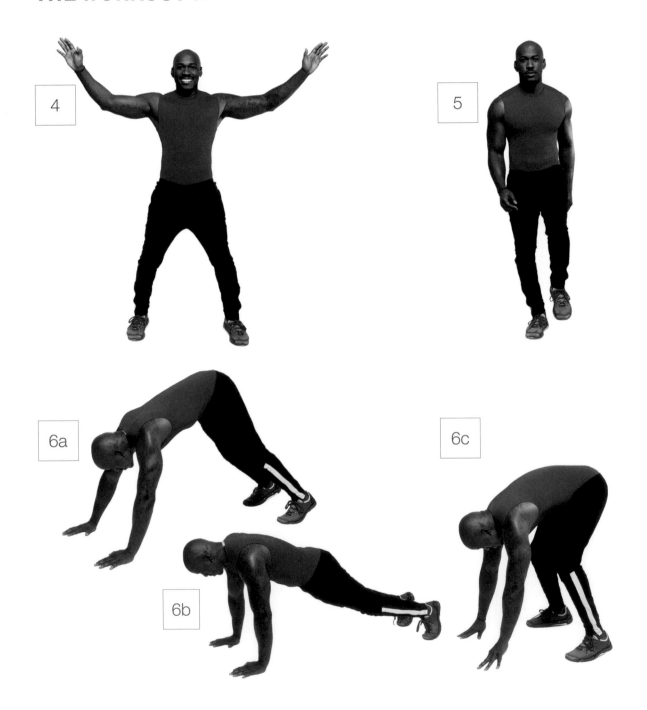

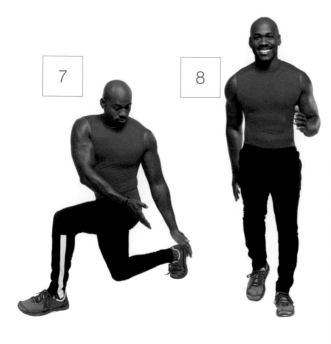

7

8

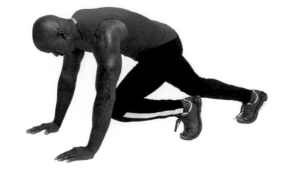

9

MEALS

BREAKFAST

peanut butter toast

Serve 2 slices whole-wheat bread, 1 Tbsp. peanut butter, and 1 small banana with 1 cup skim milk.

NUTRITION INFO: *Calories 395, Fat (g) 10, Sat fat (g) 1, Protein (g) 20, Carbs (g) 59, Fiber (g) 7, Sodium (mg) 390*

LUNCH

zucchini "pasta" salad

See recipe on page 325.

Serve with 1 stalk celery and 1 Tbsp. hummus, plus 1 cup skim milk.

DINNER

peanut noodles with tofu & broccoli

Cook 1 cup whole-wheat noodles. Combine 2 Tbsp. peanut sauce with 3 oz. cooked tofu, 1 cup cooked broccoli, and 1 cup additional vegetables (peppers, onions, carrots, snow peas, etc.), and toss with the noodles.

NUTRITION INFO: *Calories 501, Fat (g) 13, Sat fat (g) 1, Protein (g) 20, Carbs (g) 72, Fiber (g) 7, Sodium (mg) 415*

SNACKS

Choose up to 300 calories of snacks to reach your calorie goal for the day. See the lists in Chapter 3 for snack ideas.

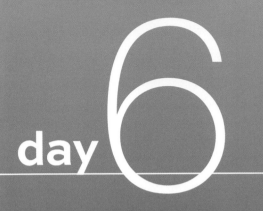

day 6

last chance:

Thank You, All!

This is it. This is the last "Last-Chance Workout" of *The Biggest Loser Bootcamp*, and it's somewhat of a grand finale. While you're giving this workout your all, think about the person you were eight weeks ago and how far you've come. By committing to this, you've been focusing on yourself. Make yourself proud today!

last-chance workout— thank you, all

78 MINUTES | WARM UP FOR 5 MINUTES

This is one of our longest workouts of the program. In this workout, you'll use many of the cardio and strength moves you've come to know and love during Bootcamp. Thank you, all!

THE WORKOUT

REPEAT THIS 2 TIMES!

1 Skater Jumps X 30 seconds
2 High Knees with Torso Twist X 30 seconds
3 Air Jump Rope X 30 seconds
4 Jumping Jacks X 30 seconds
5 Walking X 15 seconds
6 Squats with Biceps Curls X 1 minute
7 Squats with Rear Fly X 1 minute
— Walking X 15 seconds
8 Mountain Climbers X 30 seconds
— Walking X 15 seconds
9 Renegade Rows X 1 minute
10 Push-Ups X 1 minute
— Walking X 15 seconds
11 Jogging X 30 seconds
— Walking X 15 seconds
12 Seated Woodchops X 1 minute
13 Bicycle Crunches X 1 minute
— Walking X 15 seconds

(CONTINUES)

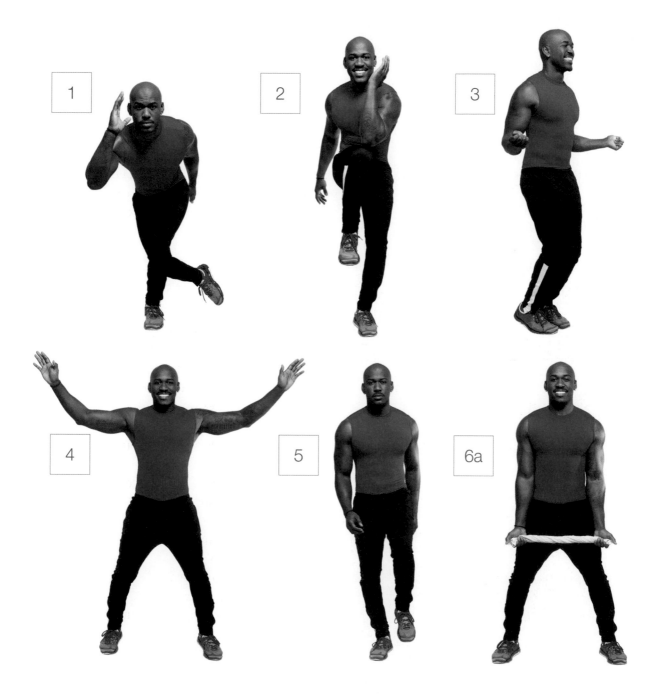

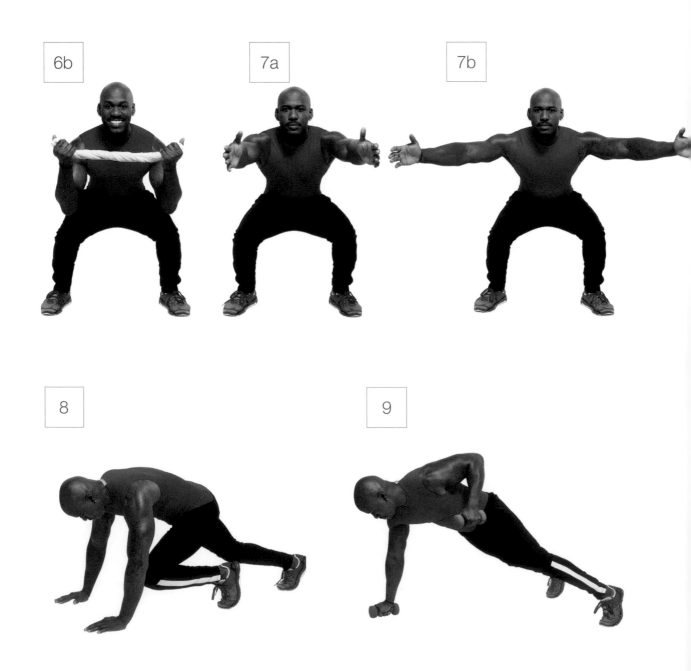

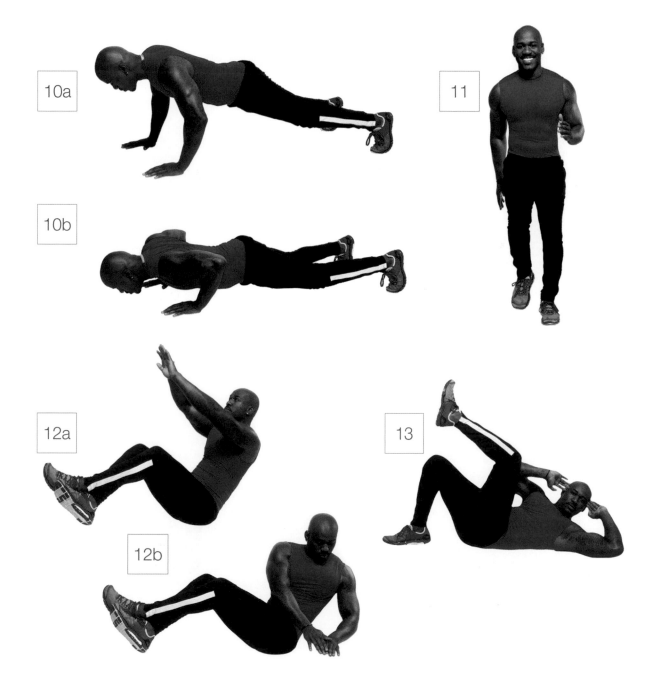

10a

10b

11

12a

12b

13

THE WORKOUT
CONTINUED

14 Burpees X 30 seconds

— Walking X 15 seconds

15 Squats with Overhead Presses X 1 minute

16 Side Lunges with Single Arm Lateral Raises* X 1 minute

— Walking X 15 seconds

— Jumping Jacks X 30 seconds

— Walking X 15 seconds

17 Bent-Over One-Arm Rows* X 1 minute

18 Overhead Presses X 1 minute

— Walking X 15 seconds

Repeat for Round 2

COOL DOWN FOR 5 MINUTES

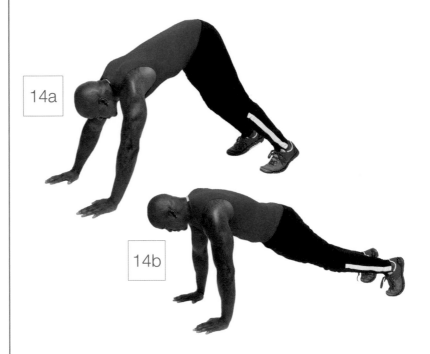

14a

14b

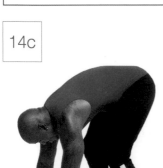

14c

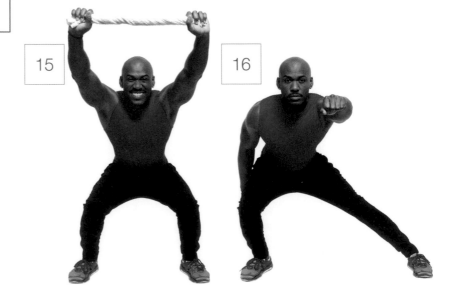

15

16

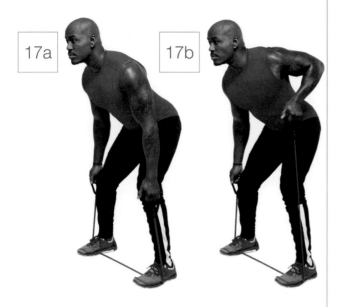

17a

17b

18

MEALS

BREAKFAST

fernanda's sweet & savory breakfast

See recipe on page 324.

Serve with 1 cup skim milk and 1 orange.

LUNCH

three-bean vegetarian chili stuffed sweet potato

Serve leftovers over 1 small baked sweet potato with 1 Tbsp. shredded reduced-fat cheddar cheese.

DINNER

spaghetti squash chicken alfredo

Serve with 2 cups green beans sautéed with ½ oz. chopped almonds.

Combine 2 Tbsp. plain fat-free Greek yogurt, 2 Tbsp. Parmesan cheese, ½ tsp. minced garlic, and plenty of black pepper. Toss with 1 cup cooked spaghetti squash and 3 oz. cooked chicken breast, and heat through.

VEGETARIAN OPTION Sub in ½ cup cooked white beans or 3 oz. tofu for the chicken.

NUTRITION INFO: *Calories 327, Fat (g) 5, Sat fat (g) 2, Protein (g) 48, Carbs (g) 14, Fiber (g) 3, Sodium (mg) 330*

SNACKS

Choose up to 300 calories of snacks to reach your calorie goal for the day. See the lists in Chapter 3 for snack ideas.

day 7

morning motivation:

You Did It!

Congratulations! You did it. You completed all eight weeks of *The Biggest Loser Bootcamp* and built strength, inside and out. Two months ago, you set out on the journey of a lifetime. You decided the time was right to change your life, and you started taking steps toward losing weight and getting healthier. For 56 days, you kept your eye on the prize, and you kept working toward your goal—and setting and crushing smaller goals along the way. It wasn't always easy. The road was long, and you encountered detours, setbacks, and rough terrain. But you kept going—and now you're here.

The journey isn't over, as we said at the start of this week. In fact, it's just beginning, in a way. As Bootcamp ends, we want you to remember that if something doesn't challenge you, it doesn't change you. Boy, have you changed! And that's because you've challenged yourself and not given up. There were days when you were tired and needed a break. And there will be more just like that. There were days when you felt like you could conquer the world. And those days aren't behind you, either! When the going gets tough, we want you to look back at these eight weeks and remember how much strength you've built and how far you've come. Maybe the scale budged and maybe it didn't. Maybe you lost inches. Maybe you learned to love exercise or found passion in healthy cooking. If you didn't, that's OK. What matters is that you set goals, and you stuck with them. You gave it your all!

We knew you could do this—and now you have. What comes next is entirely up to you. Whether you hit your goal weight or have a ways to go, know this: Whatever you set out to do in life, you can.

So what about tomorrow? Though you don't have a day-by-day plan to follow, we're guessing you already have a workout in mind. If not, put one on the calendar. The healthy habits you've built over the past two months will give you the momentum you need to keep going. You can start to weave in your own workouts or continue to use ours. The same goes for your meals and snacks. The way you eat now is the way you'll continue to eat to fuel your body for this new life you've created.

Any time you feel yourself getting off track, remember that you have this Bootcamp to help you and you have the power to get back on track with one workout, one meal, and one healthy decision. You can start the Bootcamp again at any time and for any reason, and you can also lean on your favorite meals and workouts whenever you want.

So go out there and show the world the new you. You did this. Stand tall, hold your head up high, and know that whatever comes next, you're going to succeed!

WORKOUT
active rest day

Enjoy it! Remember that "rest day" does not mean "sit on the couch all afternoon day." It means take it easy from regular exercise, but get up and do something: yoga, a short walk, or cleaning the house.

❝Don't let the scale weigh you down. Your scale is simply a tool that provides you with information on where you are on your weight-loss journey. It's just a number. A scale doesn't tell you how beautiful or generous you are, or how much your family and friends love you. Weigh yourself in awesomeness, how great your smile is, and how kind you are!❞ —*The Biggest Loser* trainer Jennifer Widerstrom

MEALS

BREAKFAST
banana yogurt smoothie
See recipe on page 134.

Serve with 16 almonds (1 oz.) or walnuts.

LUNCH
simple spaghetti squash
Serve with 1 cup skim milk.
Sauté ½ cup each onions and peppers with 3 oz. extra-lean ground turkey. Toss with ½ cup low-sodium pasta sauce and 2 cups spaghetti squash. Top with 2 tsp. Parmesan.

VEGETARIAN OPTION Sub in ½ cup cooked beans or 3 oz. vegetarian "meat" crumbles for the turkey.

NUTRITION INFO: *Calories 296, Fat (g) 5, Sat fat (g) 2, Protein (g) 24, Carbs (g) 35, Fiber (g) 8, Sodium (mg) 296*

DINNER
grass-fed beef kabobs with goat cheese stuffed tomatoes & roasted vegetables
See recipe on page 326.

DESSERT
chocolate peanut butter fudge
See recipe on page 71.

SNACKS
Choose up to 300 calories of snacks to reach your daily goal. See the lists in Chapter 3 for snack ideas. Don't forget to include your dessert in your food journal (dessert gets included with your snack calories).

BREAKFASTS

breakfast tostada

This savory Tex Mex breakfast is a quick and easy take on huevos rancheros.

SERVES 1 **PREP TIME** 5 minutes **COOK TIME** 10 minutes

- 1 (8-inch) whole-wheat tortilla
- 2 Tbsp. refried black beans
- 2 Tbsp. low-sodium salsa
- 1 Tbsp. reduced-fat cheddar cheese, shredded
- 1 large egg
- 1 Tbsp. cilantro, chopped
- 1 green onion, sliced

Preheat oven to 400°.

Place the tortilla on a foil-lined baking sheet. Spread with beans, salsa, and cheese, and bake for 10 minutes, until the tortilla is crunchy and the cheese has melted.

Top with an egg cooked to your liking, plus cilantro and green onions.

NUTRITION INFO: *Calories 255, Fat (g) 11, Sat fat (g) 3, Protein (g) 14, Carbs (g) 25, Fiber (g) 6, Sodium (mg) 468*

fernanda's sweet & savory breakfast

Why choose sweet or savory when you can kick off your morning with both? Fernanda, a fan favorite from Season 15, shares her go-to breakfast.

SERVES 1 **PREP TIME** 5 minutes **COOK TIME** 5 minutes

- 3 cups cooked spinach
- 3 egg whites
- 2 slices cinnamon-raisin bread, toasted
- 1 slice turkey bacon

Sauté the spinach in a small skillet coated with olive oil spray. Add the egg whites, and cook until set.

Serve with the toast and bacon.

VEGETARIAN OPTION Skip the turkey bacon.

NUTRITION INFO: *Calories 256, Fat (g) 4, Sat fat (g) 1, Protein (g) 21, Carbs (g) 40, Fiber (g) 6, Sodium (mg) 450*

LUNCHES

salmon wrap

Omega-3s are a super-healthy fat, and they are packed into this yummy salmon wrap! Use canned salmon to make this an even faster meal.

SERVES 1 **PREP TIME** 5 minutes

- 1 Tbsp. low-fat cream cheese
- 1 (8-inch) whole-wheat tortilla
- 3 oz. cooked salmon
- 1 cup spinach

Spread cream cheese over the tortilla. Fill with salmon and spinach, and roll tortilla over the ingredients. Cut into 2 pieces.

VEGETARIAN OPTION Sub in 1 hard-boiled egg and 1 additional hard-boiled egg white for the salmon.

NUTRITION INFO: *Calories 295, Fat (g) 12, Sat fat (g) 4, Protein (g) 23, Carbs (g) 24, Fiber (g) 4, Sodium (mg) 457*

zucchini "pasta" salad

Super-quick and a fun alternative to pasta, this zucchini noodle salad is going to be a new favorite.

SERVES 1   PREP TIME 15 minutes

---

1 medium zucchini
3 oz. cooked chicken breast
½ carrot, shredded
½ cup chopped red bell peppers
1 Tbsp. fat-free ranch dressing

Use a spiralizer or food processor to shred the zucchini into noodle shapes.

Place in a colander with a pinch of salt for 10 minutes and let any excess water drain away.

Toss with the cooked chicken, shredded carrots, bell peppers, and ranch dressing. Season liberally with fresh cracked black pepper.

VEGETARIAN OPTION Sub in ½ cup white beans for the chicken.

NUTRITION INFO: *Calories 213, Fat (g) 1, Sat fat (g) 0, Protein (g) 24, Carbs (g) 25, Fiber (g) 5, Sodium (mg) 423*

DINNERS

lisa rambo's chicken pizza

Season 14 contestant Lisa Rambo's family loves this quick and simple dish. A cross between pizza and chicken Parmesan, it's high in protein and a huge hit with kids. You can even let every family member top their "pizza" themselves.

SERVES 1   PREP TIME 5 minutes   COOK TIME 20 minutes

---

4 oz. chicken breast
1 tsp. olive oil (optional)
¼ tsp. salt-free Italian seasoning
¼ tsp. garlic powder
2 Tbsp. tomato-basil pizza sauce
4 slices turkey pepperoni
2 medium-size fresh mushrooms, sliced
2 Tbsp. green bell pepper, diced
2 Tbsp. part-skim mozzarella, shredded

Preheat oven to 400°. Flatten the chicken breast between 2 pieces of plastic wrap to make it an even thickness all over. Brush with olive oil (if using), and season with salt, pepper, Italian seasoning, and garlic powder. Place on a foil-lined baking sheet. Spread the pizza sauce over the chicken, then top with pepperoni, raw mushrooms, and green pepper. Bake at 400° for 15 minutes, then top with mozzarella. Bake another 5 minutes or until the cheese is melted and the chicken is done.

VEGETARIAN OPTION Sub hollowed-out zucchini for the chicken.

NUTRITION INFO: *Calories 245, Fat (g) 9, Sat fat (g) 2, Protein (g) 32, Carbs (g) 3, Fiber (g) 1, Sodium (mg) 353*

garlic shrimp

This light and spicy dinner will liven up your week.

SERVES 1 PREP TIME 15 minutes COOK TIME 15 minutes

- ½ lemon, juiced
- 1 clove garlic, minced
- ⅛ tsp. chili flakes (optional)
- 4 oz. shrimp, peeled and deveined
- 2 cups asparagus spears
- ½ cup chopped red bell pepper
- ½ cup cooked brown rice

Mix together lemon juice, garlic, and chili flakes (if using) in a medium-size bowl. Add shrimp, and toss through.

Spray a nonstick pan with cooking spray. Add shrimp and cook for 5 to 10 minutes, or until shrimp are just pink and cooked through.

Meanwhile, steam the vegetables, and serve alongside the shrimp and rice.

NUTRITION INFO: *Calories 364, Fat (g) 2, Sat fat (g) 0, Protein (g) 43, Carbs (g) 47, Fiber (g) 19, Sodium (mg) 164*

grass-fed beef kabobs with goat cheese stuffed tomatoes & roasted vegetables

This is a festive recipe from The Biggest Loser Resorts Niagara. We made this dinner on the last night of Bootcamp, so you can share this healthy recipe with your loved ones. Go ahead—celebrate the healthy way!

SERVES 6 PREP TIME 15 minutes COOK TIME 18 minutes

- 30 oz. grass-fed filet or sirloin steak
- 1 Tbsp. extra-virgin olive oil, plus more for rubbing the grill
- ¾ cup zucchini, sliced 1 inch thick
- ¾ cup yellow squash, sliced 1 inch thick
- ¾ cup red bell pepper, sliced 1 inch thick
- 6 Goat Cheese Stuffed Tomatoes (see recipe, below)
- 6 oz. Golden Tomato Dressing (see recipe, page 174)

Preheat oven to 350°. Prepare grill. Cube steak into 1" x 1" pieces. Skewer 5 oz. of beef on each of 6 metal skewers. Rub grill with a small amount of oil. Grill skewers until medium rare. Toss zucchini, squash, and bell pepper in 1 Tbsp. oil and spread out on baking sheet. Bake for 10 minutes until softened. Bake stuffed tomatoes for 7 minutes. Place 1 stuffed tomato on each plate, and fan out the vegetables, 1 of each color. Lay skewered meat alongside vegetables, and drizzle with dressing.

NUTRITION INFO: *Calories 373, Fat (g) 15, Sat fat (g) 2, Carbs (g) 13, Protein (g) 46, Fiber (g) 3, Sodium (mg) 239*

goat cheese stuffed tomatoes

SERVES 6 PREP TIME 7 minutes COOK TIME 12 minutes

- 6 tomatoes, cored and seeded
- ¼ tsp. sea salt
- ¼ tsp. coarsely ground black pepper
- 2 tsp. minced garlic
- ½ cup minced Spanish onion
- 3 cups cremini mushrooms, chopped
- ¼ cup crumbled goat cheese
- 1 Tbsp. chopped Italian parsley

Sprinkle the cored and seeded tomatoes with salt and pepper, and place upside down to drain. In a ceramic nonstick pan, add garlic and onion. Cook until translucent. Add mushrooms and cook for about 5 minutes or until most of mushroom liquid is absorbed. Season the mushroom mixture with salt and pepper, and remove from heat. Preheat oven to 350°. Mix together room-temperature goat cheese and parsley. Stuff each tomato with the mushroom stuffing and top with a thin layer of goat cheese mixture. Place the tomatoes on a baking sheet and bake for 7 minutes or until cheese is slightly melted and golden.

NOTE The nutrition info for the tomatoes is included in the beef kabob recipe. If you want to serve them separately, see below.

NUTRITION INFO: *Calories 90, Fat (g) 3, Sat fat (g) 1, Protein (g) 6, Carbs (g) 9, Fiber (g) 2, Sodium (mg) 60*

three-bean vegetarian chili

Slow cookers make quick work of dinner. This recipe freezes well, so you can have a healthy dinner in mere minutes.

SERVES 8 PREP TIME 15 minutes COOK TIME 8 hours

- 1¾ cups low-sodium vegetable broth
- 1 onion, chopped
- 2 jalapeño peppers, chopped
- 1 Tbsp. chili powder
- 2 tsp. ground cumin
- 2 cloves garlic, chopped
- 1 (14.5-oz.) can no-salt-added diced tomatoes
- 1 (14.5-oz.) can black beans, drained and rinsed
- 1 (14.5-oz.) can pinto beans, drained and rinsed
- 1 (14.5-oz.) can dark red kidney beans, drained and rinsed
- ½ cup plain fat-free Greek yogurt
- 2 oz. reduced-fat cheddar or pepper Jack cheese, shredded
- 2 Tbsp. chopped cilantro

Combine first 10 ingredients in a 6-qt. slow cooker. Cover and cook on LOW for 8 hours.

Ladle chili into bowls; top with yogurt, cheese, and cilantro.

Refrigerate single-serving portions for up to 3 days or freeze for up to 1 month. Reserve one portion for lunch later in the week.

NUTRITION INFO: *Calories 205, Fat (g) 3, Sat fat (g) 1, Protein (g) 12, Carbs (g) 35, Fiber (g) 11, Sodium (mg) 207*

DESSERTS

berry delight ice pops

These are a low-calorie treat that will satisfy your sweet tooth. A serving size is just one, but the remainder keeps for up to 1 month in the freezer.

SERVES 4 PREP TIME 5 minutes FREEZE TIME 4 hours

- 1 cup 100% fruit juice
- ½ cup berries, any variety

Place juice and berries in a blender, and mix for 30 seconds. Divide mixture into 4 ice-block molds. Insert an ice-pop stick into each mold.

Freeze at least 4 hours before serving.

NUTRITION INFO: *Calories 34, Fat (g) 0, Sat fat (g) 0, Protein (g) 0, Carbs (g) 9, Fiber (g)1, Sodium (mg) 3*

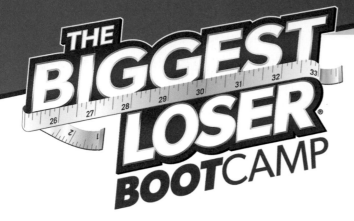
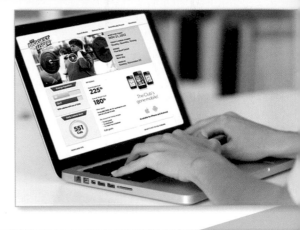
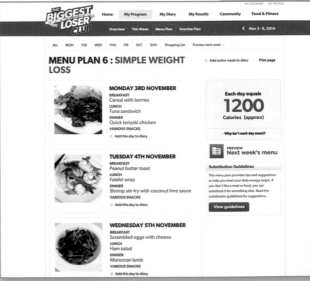
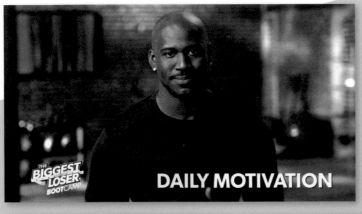
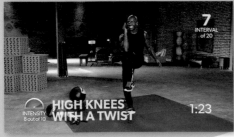
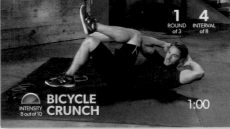
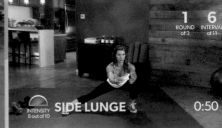